A Pocket Guide to Epidemiology

D1054131

David G. Kleinbaum
Kevin M. Sullivan
Nancy D. Barker

A Pocket Guide to Epidemiology

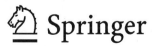 Springer

David G. Kleinbaum
Department of Epidemiology
Rollins School of Public Health
Emory University
1518 Clifton Road, NE
Atlanta, GA 30322
USA
dkleinb@sph.emory.edu

Kevin M. Sullivan
Department of Epidemiology
Rollins School of Public Health
Emory University
1518 Clifton Road, NE
Atlanta, GA 30322
USA
cdckms@sph.emory.edu

Nancy D. Barker
2465 Traywick Chase
Alpharetta, GA 30004
USA
ndbarker@eathlink.net

Library of Congress Control Number: 2006933294

ISBN-10: 0-387-45964-2   e-ISBN-10: 0-387-45966-9
ISBN-13: 978-0-387-45964-6   e-ISBN-13: 978-0-387-45966-0

Printed on acid-free paper.

© 2007 Springer Science+Business Media, LLC
All rights reserved. This work may not be translated or copied in whole or in part without the written
permission of the publisher (Springer Science+Business Media, LLC, 233 Spring Street, New York,
NY 10013, USA), except for brief excerpts in connection with reviews or scholarly analysis. Use
in connection with any form of information storage and retrieval, electronic adaptation, computer
software, or by similar or dissimilar methodology now known or hereafter developed is forbidden.
The use in this publication of trade names, trademarks, service marks, and similar terms, even if they
are not identified as such, is not to be taken as an expression of opinion as to whether or not they are
subject to proprietary rights.

9 8 7 6 5 4 3 2 1

springer.com

Preface

Four years ago (2002), I (DGK) authored a unique educational program, *ActivEpi* (Springer Publishers), developed in CD-ROM format to provide a multimedia interactive "electronic textbook" on basic principles and methods of epidemiology. In 2003, the *ActivEpi* **Companion Text,** authored by myself (DGK), KM Sullivan and ND Barker and also published by Springer, was developed to provide a hard-copy of the material contained in the *ActivEpi* CD-ROM. The CD-ROM contains 15 chapters, with each consisting of a collection of "activities" including narrated expositions, interactive study questions, quizzes, homework questions, and web links to relevant references on the Internet.

In the nearly three years since the publication of the *ActivEpi* CD-ROM, we have received several suggestions from instructors of introductory epidemiology courses as well as health and medical professionals to produce an abbreviated version that narrows the discussion to the most "essential" principles and methods. Instructors expressed to us their concern that the material covered by the CD-ROM (and likewise, the Companion Text) was too comprehensive to conveniently fit the amount of time available in an introductory course. Professionals expressed their desire for a more economically time-consuming version that would conveniently fit their "after hours" availability.

To address these suggestions, we have herewith produced **A Pocket Guide to Epidemiology** which provides a much shorter, more "essential" version of the material covered by the *ActivEpi* CD-ROM and Companion Text. We realize that determining what is "essential" is not a simple task, especially since, from our point of view, the original CD-ROM was already restricted to "essential" topics. Nevertheless, to produce this text, we decided to remove from the original material a great many fine points of explanation and complicated topics/issues about epidemiologic principles and methods, with our primary goal a "quicker read".

A Pocket Guide to Epidemiology contains less than half as many pages as the *ActivEpi* Companion Text. We have continued to include in **A Pocket Guide to Epidemiology** many of the study questions and quizzes that are provided in each Lesson of the CD ROM, but we have eliminated homework exercises, computer exercises, and Internet linkages from the original CD-ROM. Nevertheless, we indicate throughout **A Pocket Guide to Epidemiology** how and where the interested reader can turn to the *ActivEpi* CD ROM (or the Companion Text) to pursue more detailed information.

We authors view **A Pocket Guide to Epidemiology** as a stand-alone introductory text on the basic principles and concepts of epidemiology. Our primary audience for this text is the public health student or professional, clinician, health journalist, and anyone else at any age or life experience that is interested in learning what epidemiology is all about in a convenient, easy to understand format with timely, real-world health examples. We believe that the reader of this text will also benefit from using the multi-media learner-interactive features of the *ActivEpi* CD ROM electronic textbook to further clarify and enhance what is covered in this more abbreviated (non-electronic) text. Nevertheless, we suggest that, on its own, **A Pocket Guide to Epidemiology** will provide the interested reader with a comfortable, time-efficient and enjoyable introduction to epidemiology.

About the Authors
David G. Kleinbaum, Kevin M. Sullivan, and Nancy Barker

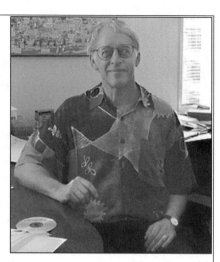

David G. Kleinbaum is a Professor of Epidemiology at Emory University's Rollins School of Public Health in Atlanta, GA, and an internationally recognized expert in teaching biostatistical and epidemiological concepts and methods at all levels. He is the author of several widely acclaimed textbooks including, *Applied Regression Analysis and Other Multivariable Methods*, *Epidemiologic Research: Principles and Quantitative Methods*, *Logistic Regression-A Self-Learning Text*, and *Survival Analysis-A Self-Learning Text*.

Dr. Kleinbaum has more than 25 years of experience teaching over 100 short courses on statistical and epidemiologic methods to a variety of international audiences, and has published widely in both the methodological and applied public health literature. He is also an experienced and sought-after consultant, and is presently an ad-hoc consultant to all research staff at the Centers for Disease Control and Prevention.

On a personal note, Dr. Kleinbaum is an accomplished jazz flutist, and plays weekly in Atlanta with his jazz combo, The Moonlighters Jazz Band.

Dr. Kevin M. Sullivan is an Associate Professor of Epidemiology at Emory University's Rollins School of Public Health. He has worked in the area of epidemiology and public health for over 30 years and has over 80 publications in peer-reviewed journals and has published chapters in several books. Dr. Sullivan has used the *ActivEpi* Companion Textbook and CD-ROM in a number of courses he teaches, both in traditional classroom-based courses and distance learning courses. He is one of the developers of Epi Info, a freely downloadable web-based software package for the analysis of epidemiologic data published by the Centers for Disease Control and Prevention. He is also the co-author of OpenEpi, a freely downloadable web-based calculator for epidemiologic data (www.OpenEpi.com).

Ms. Nancy Barker is a statistical consultant who formerly worked at the Centers for Disease Control and Prevention. She is an Instructor in the Career MPH at the Rollins School of Public Health at Emory University where she teaches a distance learning course on Basic Epidemiology that uses *ActivEpi* CD and *ActivEpi* Companion Text as the course textbooks. She also has been co-instructor in several short courses on beginning and intermediate epidemiologic methods in the Epi in Action Program sponsored by the Rollins School of Public Health.

Contents

CHAPTER 1

A POCKET-SIZE INTRODUCTION

Epidemiology is the study of health and illness in human populations. For example, a randomized clinical trial conducted by Epidemiologists at the Harvard School of Public Health showed that taking aspirin reduces heart attack risk by 20 to 30 percent. Public health studies in the 1950's demonstrated that smoking cigarettes causes lung cancer. Environmental epidemiologists have been evaluating the evidence that living near power lines may have a high risk for childhood leukemia. Cancer researchers wonder why older women are less likely to be screened for breast cancer than younger women. All of these are examples of epidemiologic research, because they all attempt to describe the relationship between a health outcome and one or more explanations or causes of that outcome. All of these examples share several challenges: they must choose an appropriate study design, they must be careful to avoid bias, and they must use appropriate statistical methods to analyze the data. Epidemiology deals with each of these three challenges.

epidemiology

Health Outcome	Explanation
Heart Attack Status	Aspirin Intake
Lung Cancer	Smoking
Childhood Leukemia	Powerline Exposure
Breast Cancer Screening	Age

Choose Study Design
Be Careful to Avoid Bias
Use Appropriate Statistical Methods

CHAPTER 2
THE BIG PICTURE - WITH EXAMPLES

The field of epidemiology was initially concerned with providing a methodological basis for the study and control of population epidemics. Now, however, epidemiology has a much broader scope, including the study of both acute and chronic diseases, the quality of health care, and mental health problems. As the focus of epidemiologic inquiry has broadened, so has the methodology. In this overview chapter, we describe examples of epidemiologic research and introduce several important methodological issues typically considered in such research.

The Sydney Beach Users Study

Epidemiology *is primarily concerned with identifying the important factors or variables that influence a health outcome of interest. In the Sydney Beach Users Study, the key question was "Is swimming at the beaches in Sydney associated with an increased risk of acute infectious illness?"*

In Sydney, Australia, throughout the 1980s, complaints were expressed in the local news media that the popular public beaches surrounding the city were becoming more and more unsafe for swimming. Much of the concern focused on the suspicion that the beaches were being increasingly polluted by waste disposal.

In 1989, the New South Wales Department of Health decided to undertake a study to investigate the extent to which swimming and possible pollution at 12 popular Sydney beaches affected the public's health, particularly during the s Summer months when the beaches were most crowded. The primary research question of interest was: *are persons who swim at Sydney beaches at increased risk for developing an acute infectious illness?*

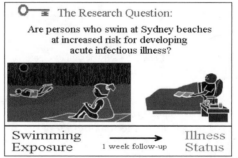

The study was carried out by selecting subjects on the beaches throughout the summer months of 1989-90. Those subjects eligible to participate at this initial interview were then followed-up by phone a week later to determine swimming exposure on the day of the beach interview and subsequent illness status during the week following the interview.

Water quality measurements at the beaches were also taken on each day that subjects were sampled in order to match swimming exposure to pollution levels at the beaches.

Analysis of the study data lead to the overall conclusion that swimming in polluted water carried a statistically significant 33% increased risk for an infectious illness when compared to swimming in non-polluted water. These results were considered by health department officials and the public alike to confirm that swimming in Sydney beaches posed an important health problem. Consequently, the state and local health departments together with other environmental agencies in the Sydney area undertook a program to reduce sources of pollution of beach water that lead to improved water quality at the beaches during the 1990's.

Summary
❖ The Sydney Beach Users Study is an example of the application of epidemiologic principles and methods to investigate a localized public health issue.
❖ The key question in the Sydney Beach Users Study was:
  o Does swimming at the beaches in Sydney, Australia (in 1989-90) pose an increased health risk for acute infectious illnesses?
  o The conclusion was yes, a 33% increased risk.

Important Methodological Issues

We provide a general perspective of epidemiologic research by highlighting several broad issues that arise during the course of most epidemiologic investigations.

There are many issues to worry about when planning an epidemiologic research study (see Box below). In this chapter we will begin to describe a list of broad methodological issues that need to be addressed. We will illustrate each issue using the previously described Sydney Beach Users Study of 1989.

Issues to consider when planning an epidemiologic research study	
Question	Define a question of interest and key variables
Variables	What to measure: exposure (**E**), disease (**D**), and control (**C**) variables
Design	What study design and sampling frame?
Frequency	Measures of disease frequency
Effect	Measures of effect
Bias	Flaws in study design, collection, or analysis
Analysis	Perform appropriate analyses

The first two issues require clearly defining the study **question** of interest, followed by specifying the key **variables** to be measured. Typically, we first should ask: *What is the relationship of one or more hypothesized determinants to a disease or health outcome of interest?*

determinants ▬▬▶ health outcome

A *determinant* is often called an **exposure variable** and is denoted by the letter **E**. The disease or health outcome is often denoted as **D**. Generally, variables other than exposure and disease that are known to predict the health outcome must be taken into account. We often call these variables **control variables** and denote them using the letter **C**.

Next, we must determine how to actually measure these variables. This step requires determining the information-gathering instruments and survey questionnaires to be obtained or developed.

The next issue is to select an appropriate **study design** and devise a sampling plan for enrolling subjects into the study. The choice of study design and sampling plan depends on feasibility and cost as well as a variety of characteristics of the population being studied and the study purpose.

Measures of disease frequency and effect then need to be chosen based on the study design. A measure of **disease frequency** provides quantitative information about how often a health outcome occurs in subgroups of interest. A **measure of effect** allows for a comparison among subgroups.

We must also consider the potential **biases** of a study. Are there any flaws in the study design, the methods of data collection, or the methods of data analysis that could lead to spurious conclusions about the exposure-disease relationship?

Finally, we must perform the appropriate **data analysis**, including stratification and mathematical modeling as appropriate. Analysis of epidemiologic data often includes taking into account other previously known risk factors for the health outcome. Failing to do this can often distort the results and lead to incorrect conclusions.

Summary: Important Methodological Issues

- ❖ What is the study question?
- ❖ How should the study variables be measured?
- ❖ How should the study be designed?
- ❖ What measures of disease frequency should be used?
- ❖ What kinds of bias are likely?
- ❖ How do we analyze the study data?

Data is obtained from:
Surveys
Interviews
Samples
Laboratories
Terms to learn
Study Designs:
Clinical trials
Cross-sectional
Case-control
Cohort
Measures of Disease Frequency
Rate
Proportion
Risk
Odds
Prevalence
Incidence
Measures of Effect
Risk ratio
Odds ratio
Rate ratio
Prevalence ratio
Biases
Selection bias
Information bias
Confounding bias
Data Analysis
Logistic Regression
Risk factors
Confounding
Effect modification

The Study Question

Epidemiology is primarily concerned with identifying the important factors or variables that influence a health outcome of interest. Therefore, an important first step in an epidemiologic research study is to carefully state the key study question of interest.

The study question needs to be stated as clearly and as early as possible, particularly to indicate the variables to be observed or measured. A typical epidemiologic research question describes the relationship between a health outcome variable, **D**, and an exposure variable, **E**, taking into account the effects of other variables already known to predict the outcome (**C**, control variables).

D = health outcome variables
E = exposure variables
C = control variables

A simple situation, which is our primary focus throughout the course, occurs when there is only one **D** and one **E**, and there are several control variables. Then, the typical research question can be expressed as shown below, where the arrow indicates that the variables **E** and the controls (**C**s) on the left are the variables to be evaluated as predictors of the outcome **D**, shown on the right.

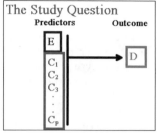

In the Sydney Beach Users Study, the health outcome variable, **D**, of interest is whether or not a person swimming at a beach in Sydney develops an acute infectious illness such as a cough, cold, flu, ear infection, or eye infection, within one week of swimming at the beach.

The study subjects could be classified as either:

D=0 for those did not get ill, or **D**=1 for those became ill.

A logical choice for the exposure variable is the exposure variable *swimming status*, which is set to:

E=0 for non-swimmers and **E**=1 for swimmers during the time period of the study.

(Note that other coding schemes could be used other than 0/1, such as 1/2, Y/N, or +/-, but we will use 0/1).

Control variables might include pollution level at the beach, age of the subject, and duration of swimming. Generally speaking, a study will not be very useful unless a question or hypothesis of some kind can be formulated to justify the time and expense needed to carry out the study.

Thus, the research question of this study example is to describe the relationship of swimming to the development of an infectious illness, while taking into account the effects of relevant control variables such as pollution level, age of subject and duration of swimming.

Because several variables are involved, we can expect that a complicated set of analyses will be required to deal with all the possible relationships among the variables involved.

Summary: The Study Question
❖ An important first step in an epidemiologic research study is to carefully state the key study question of interest.
❖ The general question: To what extent is there an association between one or more exposure variables (**E**s) and a health outcome (**D**), taking into account (i.e., controlling for) the possible influence of other important covariates (**C**s)?
❖ We can expect a complicated set of analyses to be required to deal with all possible relationships among the variables involved.

Quiz (Q2.1)
In the Sydney Beach Users study, exposure was alternatively defined by distinguishing those who swam in polluted water from those who swam in non-polluted water and from those who did not swim at all. Based on this scenario, fill

in the missing information in the following statement:

1. The exposure variable has **???** categories, one of which is **???**
   Choices: **2 3 4 5   did not swim   polluted water   swam   water not polluted**

2. When considering both swimming and pollution together, which of the following choices is appropriate for defining the exposure variable in the Sydney Beach Users study: **???**
   Choices:
   a) E=O if did not swim, E=1 if swam in polluted water
   b) E=O if did not swim, E=1 if swam in non-polluted water
   c) E=O if did not swim, E=1 if swam in polluted water, E=2 if swam in non-polluted water
   d) E=O if did not swim, E=1 if swam

In the Sydney Beach Users study, the illness outcome was whether or not an acute infectious illness developed 1 week after swimming at the beach. Also, in addition to age, another control variable was whether or not a study subject swam on days other than the day he or she was interviewed. Fill in the missing information:

3. The health outcome has **???** categories.
4. There are at least **???** control variables.
5. Which of the following choices is not a control variable: **???**
   a) age b) swimming status on other days c) swimming status on day of interview
   Choices: **2 3 4 5 a b c**

Measuring the Variables

Another important issue is: How do we measure the variables to be studied? Several measurement issues are now introduced.

Once the study question is determined, the investigators must determine how to measure the variables identified for the study and any other information that is needed. For example, how will the exposure variable be measured? If a subject went into the water but never put his head under the water, does that count as swimming? How much time is required to spend in the water to be counted as swimming? Is it feasible to observe each subject's swimming status on the day of initial interview, and if not, how should swimming status be determined?

After considering these questions, the study team defined swimming as *any immersion of the face and head in the water*. It was decided that subject self-reporting of swimming was the only feasible way to obtain swimming information.

> **Measuring Exposure Variables**
> Definition of Swimming
>   Any immersion of face & head in water
> Measuring Swimming Status
>   Subject self-reporting

How will the health outcome be measured? Should illness be determined by a subject's self-report, which might be inaccurate, or by a physician's confirmation, which might not be available? The study team decided to use self-reported symptoms of illness obtained by telephone interview of study subjects 7 to 10 days after the initial interview.

Another measurement issue concerned how to determine water quality at the beach. Do water samples need to be collected? What time of day should they be collected? How will such information be linked to study subjects? The study team decided that health department surveyors would collect morning and evening samples at the midpoint of each of three sectors of the beach.

As nearly as could practicably be achieved, study subjects were to be interviewed during the period in which water samples were taken. A standard protocol was determined for how much water was to be sampled and how samples were to be assessed for water quality.

A final measurement issue concerned what information should be obtained from persons interviewed at the beach for possible inclusion into the study? The study team decided to collect basic demographic data including age, sex, and postcode, to ask whether or not each respondent had been swimming anywhere in the previous 5 days, and had any condition that precluded swimming on the day of the interview.

Interview Variables
Age
Sex
Postcode
Swimming history
Health status

Subjects were excluded from the study if they reported swimming in the previous 5 days or having an illness that prevented them from swimming. Subjects were included if they were at least 15 years old and agreed to both an initial beach interview and a follow-up telephone interview.

All the measurement issues described above must be addressed prior to data collection to ensure standardized information is collected and to provide a study that is both cost and time efficient.

Study Questions (Q2.2)
1. What other variables might you also consider as control variables in the Beach Users Study?
2. How do we decide which variables to measure as control variables?
3. Why should age be considered?
4. How would you deal with subjects who went to the beach on more than one day?

Summary: Measuring the Variables
General measurement issues:
- How to operationalize the way a measurement is carried out?
- Should self-reporting of exposure and/or health outcome be used?
- When should measurements be taken?
- How many measurements should be taken on each variable and how should several measurements be combined?
- How to link environmental measures with individual subjects?

The Study Design, including the Sampling Plan

*Another important issue is: What **study design** should be used and how should we select study subjects? Several study design issues are now introduced.*

There are a variety of study designs used in epidemiology. The Sydney Beach Users study employed a **cohort** design. A key feature of such a design is that subjects without the health outcome are followed-up over time to determine if they develop the outcome. Subjects were selected from 12 popular Sydney beaches over 41 sampling days. An initial interview with the study subjects took place on the beach to obtain consent to participate in the study and to obtain demographic information.

Persons were excluded from the study if they had an illness that prevented them from swimming on that day or if they had been swimming within the previous 5 days. It was not considered feasible to determine swimming exposure status of each subject on the day of initial interview. Consequently, a follow-up telephone interview was conducted 7 to 10 days later to obtain self-reported swimming exposure as well as illness status of each subject.

Study Questions (Q2.3)
1. How might you criticize the choice of using self-reported exposure and illnesses?
2. How might you criticize the decision to determine swimming status from a telephone interview conducted 7 to 10 days after being interviewed on the beach?

A complex sample survey design was used to obtain the nearly 3000 study participants. Six beaches were selected on any given day and included 2 each from the northern, eastern and southern areas of Sydney. Each beach was divided into three sectors, defined by the position of the swimming area flags erected by the lifeguards. Trained interviewers recruited subjects, starting at the center of each sector and moving in a clockwise fashion until a quota for that sector had been reached. Potential subjects had to be at least 3 meters apart.

Study Questions (Q2.4)
1. Why do you think potential subjects in a given sector of the beach were specified to be at least 3 meters apart?
2. Why is the Sydney Beach Users Study a cohort study?
3. A fixed cohort is a group of people identified at the onset of a study and then followed over time to determine if they developed the outcome. Was a fixed cohort used in the Sydney Beach Users Study? Explain.
4. A case-control design starts with subjects with and without an illness and looks back in time to determine prior exposure history for both groups. Why is the Sydney Beach Users study *not* a case-control study?
5. In a cross-sectional study, both exposure and disease status are observed at the same time that subjects are selected into the study. Why is the Sydney Beach Users study not a cross-sectional study?

<u>**Summary: Study Design**</u>
* ❖ Two general design issues:
  * o Which of several alternative forms of **epidemiologic study designs** should be used (e.g., cohort, case-control, cross-sectional)?
  * o What is the **sampling plan** for selecting subjects?

Measures of Disease Frequency and Effect

*Another important issue is: What **measure of disease frequency** and **measure of effect** should be used? These terms are now briefly introduced.*

Once the study design has been determined, appropriate measures of disease frequency and effect can be specified. A measure of disease frequency provides quantitative information about how often the health outcome has occurred in a subgroup of interest.

For example, in the Sydney Beach Users Study, if we want to measure the frequency with which those who swam developed the illness of interest, we could determine the number of subjects who got ill and swam and divide by the total number who swam. The denominator represents the total number of study subjects among

Measure of Disease Frequency
Sydney Beach Users Study
Swimmers: $\dfrac{\text{\# ill swimmers}}{\text{total \# swimmers}}$
Non-Swimmers: $\dfrac{\text{\# ill non-swimmers}}{\text{total \# non-swimmers}}$

swimmers that had the opportunity to become ill. The numerator gives the number of study subjects among swimmers who actually became ill. Similarly, if we want to measure the frequency of illness among those who did *not* swim, we could divide the number of subjects who got ill and did not swim by the total number of non-swimming subjects.

The information required to carry out the above calculations can be described in the form of a two-way table shown below. This table shows the number who became ill among swimmers and non-swimmers. We can calculate the proportion ill among the swimmers to be 0.277 or 27.7 percent. We can also calculate the proportion ill among the non-swimmers as 0.165 or 16.5 percent.

		Swim		
		Yes	No	Total
Ill	Yes	532	151	683
	No	1392	764	2156
	Total	1924	915	2839

proportion ill (swimmers): $\dfrac{532}{1924} = .277$ or 27.7%

proportion ill (non-swimmers): $\dfrac{151}{915} = .165$ or 16.5%

Each proportion is a measure of disease frequency called a **risk**. **R(E)** denotes the risk among the exposed for developing the health outcome. **R(not E)** [or **R($\overline{\text{E}}$)**] denotes the risk among the *un*exposed. There are measures of disease frequency other than risk that will be described in this course. The choice of measure (e.g., risk, odds, prevalence, or rate) primarily depends on the type of study design being used and the goal of the research study.

If we want to compare two measures of disease frequency, such as two risks, we can divide one risk by the other, say, the risk for swimmers divided by the risk for non-swimmers. We find that the ratio of these risks in our study is 1.68; this means that swimmers have a risk for the illness that is 1.68 times the risk for non-swimmers.

Risk
proportion ill (swimmers):   27.7%
proportion ill (non-swimmers): 16.5%
$\dfrac{R(E)}{R(not\ E)} = \dfrac{27.7\%}{16.5\%} = 1.68$
$Risk_{(swimmers)} = 1.68 \times Risk_{(non\text{-}swimmers)}$

Such a measure is called a **measure of effect**. In this example, the effect of interest refers to the effect of one's swimming status on becoming or not becoming ill. If we divide one risk by the other, the measure of effect or association is called a **risk ratio**. There are other measures of effect that will be described in this course (e.g., such as the risk ratio, odds ratio, prevalence ratio, rate ratio, risk difference, and rate difference). As with measures of disease frequency, the choice of effect measure depends on the type of study design and the goal of the research study.

Summary: Measures of Disease Frequency and Effect

❖ A **measure of disease frequency** quantifies how often the health outcome has occurred in a subgroup of interest.

❖ A **measure of effect** quantifies a comparison of measures of disease frequency for two or more subgroups.

❖ The choice of measure of disease frequency and measure of effect depends on the type of study design used and the goal of the research study.

Bias

Another important issue is: What are the potential biases of the study?   The concept of bias is now briefly introduced.

The next methodologic issue concerns the potential biases of a study. Bias is a flaw in the study design, the methods of data collection, or the methods of data analysis that may lead to spurious conclusions about the exposure-disease relationship. Bias may occur because of: the **selection** of study subjects; incorrect information gathered on study subjects; or failure to adjust for variables other

Bias: A flaw in the
- study design
- methods of data collection
- methods of data analysis
… which leads to spurious conclusions.

Sources of bias:
- Selection
- Information
- Confounding

than the exposure variable, commonly called **confounding.**

In the Sydney Beach Users Study, all 3 sources of bias were considered. For example, to avoid **selection bias**, subjects were excluded from the analysis if they were already ill on the day of the interview. This ensured that the sample represented only those healthy enough to go swimming on the day of interview. Sometimes selection bias cannot be avoided. For example, subjects had to be excluded from the study if they did not complete the follow-up interview. This

non-response bias may affect how representative the sample is.

There was also potential for **information bias** since both swimming status and illness status were based on self-reporting by study subjects. Swimming status was determined by self-report at least seven days after the swimming occurred. Also, the report of illness outcome did not involve any clinical confirmation of reported symptoms.

Confounding in the Beach Users Study concerned whether all relevant variables other than swimming status and pollution level exposures were taken into account. Included among such variables were age, sex, duration of swimming for those who swam, and whether or not a person swam on additional days after being interviewed at the beach. The primary reason for taking into account such variables was to ensure that any observed effect of swimming on illness outcome could not be explained away by these other variables.

Summary
- Bias is a flaw in the study design, the methods of data collection, or the methods of data analysis that may lead to spurious conclusions about the exposure-disease relationship.
- Three general sources of bias occur in:
  - Selection of study subjects
  - Incorrect information gathered on study subjects
  - Failure to adjust for variables other than the exposure variable (confounding)

Analyzing the data

Another important issue is: How do we carry out the data analysis? We now briefly introduce some basic ideas about data analysis.

The final methodologic issue concerns the data analysis. We must carry out an appropriate analysis once collection and processing of the study data are complete. Since the data usually come from a sample of subjects, the data analysis typically requires the use of statistical procedures to account for the inherent variability in the data. In epidemiology, data analysis typically begins

Statistics	
Frequency	**Effect**
Risk	risk ratio
Prevalence	prevalence ratio
Odds	odds ratio
Rate	rate ratio
Stratification	
Mathematical modeling	

with the calculation and statistical assessment of simple measures of disease frequency and effect. The analysis often progresses to more advanced techniques such as stratification and mathematical modeling. These latter methods are typically used to control for one or more potential confounders.

Let's consider the data analysis in the Sydney Beach Users Study. We had previously compared swimmers with non-swimmers. Now, we may wish to address the more specific question of whether those who swam in polluted water had a higher risk for illness than those who swam in non-polluted water. We can do this by separating the swimmers into two groups. The non-swimmers represent a baseline comparison group with which the two groups of swimmers can be compared.

Based on the two-way table, we can estimate the risk for illness for each of the three groups by computing the proportion that got ill out of the total for each group. The three risk estimates are 0.357, 0.269 and 0.165, which translates to 35.7 percent, 26.9 percent and 16.5 percent, respectively.

Sydney Beach Users Study				
		Swim		
Ill		Yes-P	Yes-NP	No	Total
	Yes	55	477	151	683
	No	99	1293	764	2156
	Total	154	1770	915	2839
risk for illness:		35.7%	26.9%	16.5%	

The risk ratio that compares the Swam-Polluted (Yes-P) group with the Swam-Nonpolluted (Yes-NP) group is 1.33 indicating that persons who swam in polluted water had a 33 percent increased risk than persons who swam in nonpolluted water.

$$\text{risk ratio:} \quad \frac{35.7\%}{26.9\%} = 1.33$$
(P vs. NP)

Also, the risk ratio estimates obtained by dividing the risks for each group by risk for non-swimmers are 2.16, 1.63, and 1. This suggests what we call a dose-response effect, which means that as exposure increases, the risk increases.

risk ratio: 35.7% 26.9% 16.5%
            16.5% 16.5% 16.5%

2.16   1.63   1.00 (referent)

Dose-response effect

The analysis just described is called a "crude" analysis because it does not take into account the effects of other known factors that may also affect the health outcome being studied. A list of such variables might include age, swimming duration, and whether or not a person swam on additional days. The conclusions found from a crude analysis might be altered drastically after adjusting for these potentially confounding variables.

Several questions arise when considering the control of many variables:

- Which of the variables being considered should actually be controlled?
- What is gained or lost by controlling for too many or too few variables?
- What should we do if we have so many variables to control that we run out of numbers?
- What actually is involved in carrying out a stratified analysis or mathematical modeling to control for several variables?
- How do the different methods for control, such as stratification and mathematical modeling, compare to one another?

These questions will be addressed in later activities.

Study Questions (Q2.5)

1. How do you interpret the risk ratio estimate of 1.33?
2. Does the estimated risk ratio of 1.33 indicate that swimming in polluted water poses a health risk?
3. Given the relatively small number of 154 persons who swam in polluted water, what statistical question would you need to answer about the importance of the estimated risk ratio of 1.33?

Summary: Analyzing the Data

❖ The data analysis typically requires the use of statistical procedures to account for the inherent variability in the data.

❖ In epidemiology, data analysis often begins with assessment and comparison of simple measures of disease frequency and effect.

❖ The analysis often progresses to more advanced techniques such as stratification and mathematical modeling.

Example: Alcohol Consumption and Breast Cancer

The Harvard School of Public Health followed a cohort of about 100,000 nurses from all over the US throughout the 1980s and into the 1990s. The investigators in this Nurses Health Study, were interested in assessing the possible relationship between diet and cancer. One particular question concerned the extent to which alcohol consumption was associated with the development of breast cancer.

Nurses identified as being 'disease free' at enrollment into the study were asked about the amount of alcohol they currently drank. Other relevant factors, such as age and smoking history, were also determined. Subjects were followed for four years, at which time it was determined who developed breast cancer and who did not. A report of these findings was published in the New England Journal of Medicine in 1987.

Recall that the first methodologic issue is to define the **study question**. Which of the study questions stated here best addresses the question of interest in this study?

A. Is there a relationship between drinking alcohol and developing breast cancer?
B. Are alcohol consumption, age, and smoking associated with developing breast cancer?
C. Are age and smoking associated with developing breast cancer, after controlling for alcohol consumption?
D. Is alcohol consumption associated with developing breast cancer, after accounting for other variables related to the development of breast cancer?

The best answer is "D," although "A" is also correct. In stating the study question of interest, we must identify the primary variables to be measured.

Study Questions (Q2.6) Determine whether each of the following is a:
  Health outcome variable (D), Exposure variable (E), or Control variable (C)

1. Smoking history
2. Whether or not a subject develops breast cancer during follow-up
3. Some measure of alcohol consumption
4. Age

Once we have specified the appropriate variables for the study, we must determine how to measure them. The health outcome variable, **D**, in this example is simply *yes* or *no* depending on whether or not a person was clinically diagnosed with breast cancer. The investigators at Harvard interviewed study subjects about their drinking habits, **E**, and came up with a quantitative

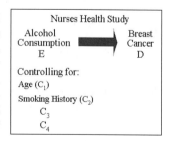

measurement of the amount of alcohol in units of grams per day that were consumed in an average week around the time of enrollment into the study. How to treat this variable for purposes of the analysis of the study data was an important question considered. One approach was to categorize the alcohol measurement into 'high' versus 'low'. Another approach was to categorize alcohol into 4 groups: non-drinkers; less than 5 grams per day; between 5 and 15 grams per day; and 15 or more grams per day.

Age, denoted C_1, is inherently a quantitative variable, although many of the analyses treated age as a categorical variable in three age groups, shown here:

34 to 44 years, 45 to 54 years, 55 to 59 years

Smoking history, C_2, was categorized in several ways; one was *never* smoked versus *ever* smoked.

The research question in the nurse's health study can thus be described as determining if there is a relationship between alcohol consumption, **E**, and breast cancer, **D**, controlling for the effects of age, C_1, and smoking history, C_2, and possibly other variables (C_3, C_4, etc.).

Although a detailed analysis is not described here, the data did provide evidence of a significant association between alcohol use and development of breast cancer. For heavy drinkers, when compared to non-drinkers, there was

	Compared to Non-drinkers:
Heavy drinkers	80% increased risk
Moderate drinkers	50% increased risk
Light drinkers	20% increased risk

about an 80% increase in the risk of developing breast cancer. Moderate drinkers were found to have about a 50% increase in risk, and light drinkers had an increased risk of about 20%.

Note: The Nurses Health Study provides an example in which the exposure variable, alcohol consumption, has several categories rather than simply binary. Also, the control variables age and smoking history can be a mixture of different types of variables. In the Nurses Health Study, age is treated in three categories, and smoking history is treated as a binary variable.

Example: The Bogalusa Outbreak

On October 31, 1989, the Louisiana State Health Department was notified by two physicians in Bogalusa, Louisiana, that over 50 cases of acute pneumonia had occurred within a three-week interval in mid to late October, and that six

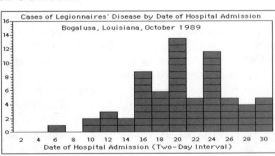

persons had died. Information that the physicians had obtained from several patients suggested that the illness might have been Legionnaires Disease.

In 1989, Bogalusa was a town of about 16,000 persons. The largest employer was a paper mill located in the center of town adjacent to the main street. The paper mill included five prominent cooling towers. The mill also had three paper machines that emitted large volumes of aerosol along the main street of town. Many people suspected that the cooling towers and or the paper mill were the cause of the outbreak, since they were prominent sources of outdoor aerosols where the legionnaire's bacteria could have been located.

Recall that the first methodologic issue is to define the **study question** of interest. Which of the study questions stated here best addresses the question of interest in this study?

A. Was the paper mill the source of the Legionnaires Disease outbreak in Bogalusa?
B. What was the source of the outbreak of Legionnaires Disease in Bogalusa?
C. Why did the paper mill cause the outbreak of Legionnaires Disease in Bogalusa?
D. Was there an outbreak of Legionnaires Disease in Bogalusa?

The most appropriate study question is "B." Even though the paper mill was the suspected source, the study was not limited to that variable only, otherwise, it might have failed to collect information on the true source of the outbreak.

Study Questions (Q2.7) In stating the study question, we identify the primary variables to be considered in the study. Determine whether each of these variables is the health outcome variable, **D**, an exposure variable, **E**, or a control variable, **C**:
1. Exposure to the cooling towers of the paper mill?
2. Exposure to emissions of the paper machines?
3. Age of subject?
4. Visited grocery store A?
5. Visited grocery store B?
6. Diagnosed with Legionnaires Disease?
7. Visited drug store A?
8. Visited drug store B?
9. Ate at restaurant A?

The health outcome variable, **D**, indicates whether or not a study subject was clinically diagnosed with Legionnaires Disease during the three week period from mid to late October. The exposure variable is conceptually whatever variable indicates the main source of the outbreak. Since this variable is essentially unknown at the start of the study, there is a large collection of exposure variables, all of which need to be identified as part of the study design and investigated as candidates for being the primary source of the outbreak. We denote these exposure variables of interest E_1 through E_7. One potential control variable of interest was age, which we denoted as C_1.

The general research question of interest in the Bogalusa outbreak was to evaluate the relationship of one or more of the exposure variables to whether or not a study subject developed Legionnaires Disease, controlling for age.

A **case-control study**, was carried out in which 28 **cases** diagnosed with confirmed Legionnaires Disease were compared with 56 non-cases or **controls**. This investigation led to the hypothesis that a misting machine for vegetables in a grocery store was the source of the outbreak. This misting machine was removed from the grocery store and sent to CDC where laboratory staff was able to isolate Legionella organisms from aerosols produced by the machine. This source was a previously unrecognized vehicle for the transmission of Legionella bacteria.

Note: The Bogalusa study provides an example in which there are several exposure variables that are candidates as the primary source of the health outcome being studied. Hopefully, the investigators will be able to identify at least one exposure variable as being implicated in the occurrence of the outbreak. It is even possible that more than one candidate exposure variable may be identified as a possible source.

The case-control study of this and many other outbreaks can often be viewed as hypothesis generating. Further study, often using laboratory methods, clinical diagnosis, and environmental survey techniques, must often be carried out in order to confirm a suspected exposure as the primary source of the outbreak. The Centers for Disease Control and Prevention has a variety of scientists to provide the different expertise and teamwork that is required, as carried out in the Bogalusa study.

Example: The Rotterdam Study

The Rotterdam study has been investigating the determinants of chronic disabling diseases, including Alzheimer's disease, during the 1990s and beyond.

In the early 1990s, the Department of Epidemiology of the Erasmus University in Rotterdam, the Netherlands, initiated the Rotterdam Study. A cohort of nearly 8000 elderly people was selected. They continue to be followed to this day. The goal of the study is to investigate determinants of chronic disabling diseases, such as Alzheimer's and

> ## Rotterdam Study
>
> Study subjects:
> - free of dementia at 1st exam
> - cognition test- 2 years later
> - neurologist exam (if test +)
> - health outcome: Alzheimer's (D)
> - exposure variable: smoking history (E)
> 3 categories:
> current smokers, previous smokers, never smokers

cardiovascular disease. One particular study question of interest was whether smoking increases the risk of Alzheimer's disease.

Subjects who were free of dementia at a first examination were included in the study. This excluded anyone diagnosed at this exam with Alzheimer's or any other form of dementia due to organic or psychological factors. Approximately two years later, the participants were

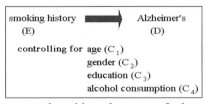

asked to take a brief cognition test. If they scored positive, they were further examined by a neurologist. The investigators could then determine whether or not a participant had developed Alzheimer's disease, the health outcome variable **D** of interest, since the start of follow-up.

The primary exposure variable, **E**, was smoking history. Three categories of smoking were considered: current smokers at the time of the interview; previous but not current smokers; and, never smokers. Control variables considered in this study included age, gender, education, and alcohol consumption.

We define the study question of interest as: *Is there a relationship between smoking history and Alzheimer's disease, controlling for the effects of age, gender, education and alcohol consumption?*

Recall that one important methodologic issue is to determine the study design.

How would you define the design of this study?
1. Cohort design
2. Case-control design
3. Cross-sectional design
4. Clinical trial

This is a cohort design because participants without the health outcome of interest, in this case Alzheimer's disease, are followed up over time to determine if they develop the outcome later in life.

Which of the following is influenced by the design of the study?
A. The assessment of confounding
B. The choice of the measures of disease frequency and effect
C. A decision regarding the use of stratified analysis
D. The analysis is not influenced in any way by the study design used

The answer is B. We determine the appropriate measures of disease frequency and effect based on the study design characteristics. Choices A and C are incorrect because they are typically considered regardless of the study design used.

The investigators found that 105 subjects developed Alzheimer's disease. After taking the control variables into account, the risk of Alzheimer's disease for current smokers was 2.3 times the risk for subjects who had never smoked. For subjects who had smoked in the past but who had given up smoking before the study started, the risk of Alzheimer's disease was 1.3 times the risk for subjects who had never smoked.

Results
• 105 subjects developed Alzheimer's
• risk for current smokers was 2.3 times risk for never smokers
• risk for previous smokers was 1.3 times risk for never smokers

Study Questions (Q2.8) Based on the above results:
1. What is the *percent increase* in the risk for current smokers when compared to the risk for never smokers?
2. What is the *percent increase* in the risk for previous smokers when compared to the risk for never smokers?

Because these results were statistically significant and controlled for previously established predictors of Alzheimer's, the study gave support to the hypothesis that smoking history was a significant risk factor in the development of Alzheimer's disease.

Nomenclature

C	Control variable or covariate
D	Disease or outcome variable
E	Exposure variable
R(E)	Risk among the exposed for developing the health outcome
R(not E) or **R($\overline{E}$)**	Risk among **non**exposed for developing the health outcome
RR	Risk ratio

References

For the Sydney Beach Users Study:
Corbett SJ, Rubin GL, Curry GK, Kleinbaum DG. The health effects of swimming at Sydney Beaches. The Sydney Beach Users Study Advisory Group. Am J Public Health. 1993;83(12): 1701-6.

For the Nurses Health Study:
Willett WC, Stampfer MJ, Colditz GA, Rosner BA, Hennekens CH, Speizer FE. Moderate alcohol consumption and the risk of breast cancer. N Engl J Med. 1987;316(19):1174-80.

For the Bogalusa Outbreak:
Mahoney FJ, Hoge CW, Farley TA, Barbaree JM, Breiman RF, Benson RF, McFarland LM. Communitywide outbreak of Legionnaires' disease associated with a grocery store mist machine. J Infect Dis. 1992;165(4):736-9.

For The Rotterdam Study:
Hofman A, Grobbee DE, de Jong PT, van den Ouweland FA. Determinants of disease and disability in the elderly: the Rotterdam Elderly Study. Eur J Epidemiol. 1991;7(4); 403-22.
Ott A, Slooter AJ, Hofman A, van Harksamp F, Witteman JC, Van Broeckhoven C, van Duijin CM, Breteler MM. Smoking and risk of dementia and Alzheimer's disease in a population-based cohort study: the Rotterdam Study. Lancet. 1998;351(9119):1840-3.

A CDC Website. The Centers for Disease control has a website called **EXCITE**, which stands for **Excellence in Curriculum Integration through Teaching Epidemiology.** The website address is http://www.cdc.gov/excite/
   We suggest that you open up this website on your computer and look over the various features and purposes of the website described on the first page you see. Then click on the item (on menu on left of page) **Disease Detectives at Work** and read the first two articles entitled *Public Health on Front Burner After Sept 11* and *USA's 'Disease Detectives' Track Epidemics Worldwide*. Then click on the item (on menu on left of page) **Classroom Exercises** and go through the exercise on Legionnaires Disease in Bogalusa, Louisiana. The specific website address for this exercise is:
   http://www.cdc.gov/excite/legionnaires.htm

Answers to Study Questions and Quizzes

Q2.1
1.   3, did not swim
2.   C
3.   2
4.   2
5.   C

Q2.2
1.   General health status, smoking status, diet, including what a subject might have eaten at the beach.
2.   Choose variables that are already known determinants of the health outcome. This will be discussed later under the topic of confounding.
3.   Younger subjects might be less likely to get ill than older subjects.
4.   In the actual study, the investigators chose to exclude subjects from the analysis if they visited the beach on days other than the day they were interviewed on the beach.

Q2.3
1.   Self-reported information may be inaccurate and can therefore lead to spurious study results.

2. As with the previous question, the information obtained about exposure much later than when the actual exposure occurred may be inaccurate and can lead to spurious study results.

Q2.4

1. To minimize the inclusion in the study of a family or social groups.
2. Subjects without the health outcome, that is, healthy subjects selected at the beach, were followed-up over time to determine if they developed the outcome.
3. No, the Sydney Beach User's Study did not use a fixed cohort. Study subjects were added over the summer of 1989-90 to form the cohort.
4. Because the study started with exposed and unexposed subjects, rather than ill and not-ill subjects, and went forward rather than backwards in time to determine disease status.
5. Exposure and disease status were observed at different times for different subjects. Also, each subject was selected one week earlier than the time his or her exposure and disease status were determined.

Q2.5

1. The risk of illness for persons who swam in polluted water is estimated to be 1.33 times the risk of illness for

persons who swam in non-polluted water.
2. Not necessarily. The importance of any risk ratio estimate depends on the clinical judgment of the investigators and the size of similar risk ratio estimates that have been found in previous studies.
3. Is the risk ratio of 1.33 significantly different from a risk ratio of 1? That is, could the risk ratio estimate of 1.33 have occurred by chance?

Q2.6

1. C
2. D
3. E
4. C

Q2.7

1. E
2. E
3. E
4. E
5. D
6. E
7. E
8. E

Q2.8

1. The increased risk of 2.3 translates to a 130% increase in the risk of current smokers compared to never smokers.
2. The increased risk of 1.3 translates to a 30% increase in the risk for previous smokers compared to never smokers.

CHAPTER 3

HOW TO SET THINGS UP? STUDY DESIGNS

*A key stage of epidemiologic research is the **study design**. This is defined to be the process of planning an empirical investigation to assess a **conceptual hypothesis** about the relationship between one or more **exposures** and a **health outcome**. The purpose of the study design is to transform the conceptual hypothesis into an **operational hypothesis** that can be empirically tested. Since all study designs are potentially flawed, it is therefore important to understand the specific strengths and limitations of each design. Most serious problems or mistakes at this stage cannot be rectified in subsequent stages of the study.*

Types of Epidemiologic Research

There are two broad types of epidemiologic studies, **experimental** and **observational**. An experimental study uses **randomization** to allocate subjects to different categories of the exposure. An observational study does not use randomization. (For additional information on randomization, please refer to the end of this chapter.) In experimental studies, the investigator, through randomization, determines the exposure status for each subject, then follows them and documents subsequent disease outcome. In an observational study, the subjects themselves, or perhaps their genetics, determine their exposure, for example, whether to smoke or not. The investigator is relegated to the role of simply observing exposure status and subsequent disease outcome.

Experimental studies in epidemiology usually take the form of **clinical trials** and **community intervention trials**. The objective of most *clinical trials* is to test the possible effect, that is, the efficacy, of a therapeutic or preventive treatment such as a new drug, physical therapy or dietary regimen for either treating or preventing the occurrence of a disease. The objective of most *community intervention trials* is to assess the effectiveness of a prevention program. For example, one might study the effectiveness of fluoridation, of sex education, or of needle exchange.

Most epidemiologic studies are observational. Observational studies are broadly identified as two types: **descriptive** and **analytic**. Descriptive studies are performed to describe the natural history of a disease, to determine the allocation of health care resources, and to suggest hypotheses about disease causation. Analytic studies are performed to test hypotheses about the determinants of a disease or other health condition, with the ideal goal of assessing causation. (See the end of this chapter for additional information on disease causation.)

Summary
* There are two broad types of epidemiologic studies: experimental and observational
* Experimental studies use randomization of exposures
* Observational studies do **not** use randomization of exposures

❖ In experimental studies, the investigator pro-actively determines the exposure status for each subject.

❖ In observational studies, the subject determines his/her exposure status.

❖ Experimental studies are usually clinical trials or community intervention trials.

❖ Observational studies are either descriptive or analytic.

Randomization

Randomization is an allocation procedure that assigns subjects into (one of the) the exposure groups being compared so that each subject has the same probability of being in one group as in any other. Randomization tends to make demographic, behavioral, genetic, and other characteristics of the comparison groups similar except for their exposure status. As a result, if the study finds any difference in health outcome between the comparison groups, that difference can only be attributable to their difference in exposure status.

For example, if subjects are randomly allocated to either a new drug or a standard drug for the treatment of hypertension, then it is hoped that other factors such as age and sex might have approximately the same distribution for subjects receiving the new drug as for subjects receiving the standard drug. Actually, there is no guarantee even with randomization that the distribution of, for example age, will be the same for the two treatment groups. The investigator can always check the data to see what has happened regarding any such characteristic, providing the characteristic is measured or observed in the study. If the age distribution is found to be different between the two treatment groups, the investigator can take this into account in the analysis, for example, by stratifying on age.

The advantage of randomization is what it offers with regard to those characteristics not measured in one's study. Variables that are not measured obviously cannot be taken into account in the analysis. Randomization offers insurance, though no guarantee, that such unmeasured variables are evenly distributed among the different exposure groups. In observational studies, on the other hand, the investigator can account for only those variables that are measured, allowing more possibility for spurious conclusions because of unknown effects of important unmeasured variables.

Causation

In any research field involving the conduct of scientific investigations and the analysis of data derived from such investigations to test etiologic hypotheses, the assessment of **causality** is a complicated issue. In particular, the ability to make **causal inferences** in the health sciences typically depends on synthesizing results from several studies, both epidemiologic and non-epidemiologic (e.g., laboratory or clinical findings).

Instigated by a governmental sponsored effort in the United States to assess the health consequences of smoking, health scientists in the late 1950's and 1960's began to consider defining objective criteria for evaluating causality. The particular focus of this effort was how to address causality based on the results of studies that consider exposures that cannot be randomly assigned, i.e., observational studies.

In 1964, a report was published by the US Department of Health, Education and Welfare that reviewed the research findings dealing with the health effects of smoking, with the objective of assessing whether or not smoking could be identified as a "cause" of lung cancer and perhaps other diseases. The type of synthesis carried out in this report has been referred to in the 1990's as a meta analysis, so that this report was in essence, one of the earliest examples of a **meta analysis** conducted in the health sciences.

The 1964 document based much of its conclusions about smoking causation on a list of general criteria that was formalized by Bradford Hill and later incorporated into a famous 1971 textbook by Hill. The criteria are listed as follows:

1. **Strength of the Association**: The stronger the observed association, the less likely the association is due to bias; weaker associations do not provide much support to a causal

interpretation.

2. **Dose-response Effect**: If the disease frequency increases with the dose or level of exposure, this supports a causal interpretation. (Note, however, that the absence of a dose-response effect may not rule out causation from alternative explanations, such as a threshold effect.)

3. **Lack of Temporal Ambiguity**: The hypothesized cause must precede the occurrence of the disease.

4. **Consistency of Findings**: If all studies dealing with a given relationship produce similar results, a causal interpretation is advanced. (Note: Inconsistencies may be due to different study design features, so that perhaps some kind of weighting needs to be given to each study.)

5. **Biological Plausibility of the Hypothesis**: If the hypothesized effect makes sense in the context of current biological knowledge, this supports a causal interpretation. (Note, however, the current state of biological knowledge may be inadequate to determine biological plausibility.)

6. **Coherence of the Evidence**: If the findings do not seriously conflict with our understanding of the natural history of the disease or other accepted facts about disease occurrence, this supports a causal interpretation.

7. **Specificity of the Association**: If the study factor is found to be associated with only one disease, or if the disease is found to be associated with only one factor, a causal interpretation is supported. (However, this criterion cannot rule out a causal hypothesis, since many factors have multiple effects and most diseases have multiple causes.) Examples include vinyl chloride and angiosarcoma of the liver; DES by women and vaginal cancer in offspring.

8. **Experimentation**: use of experimental evidence, such as clinical trials in humans, animal models, and in vitro laboratory experiments. May support causal theories when available, but its absent does not preclude causality.

9. **Analogy**: when similar relationships have been shown with other exposure-disease relationships. For example, the offspring of women given DES during pregnancy were more likely to develop vaginal cancer. By analogy, it would seem possible that other drugs given to pregnant women could cause cancer in their offspring.

Quiz (Q3.1) Fill in the blanks with **<u>Experimental</u>** or **<u>Observational</u>**

1. A strength of the **???** study is the investigator's control in the assignment of individuals to treatment groups.

2. A potential advantage of an **???** study is that they are often carried out in more natural settings, so that the study population is more representative of the target population.

3. The major limitation of **???** studies is that they afford the investigator the least control over the study situation; therefore, results are generally more susceptible to distorting influences.

4. A weakness of an **???** study is that randomization to treatment groups may not be ethical if an arbitrary group of subjects must be denied a treatment that is regarded as beneficial.

5. One community in a state was selected by injury epidemiologists for a media campaign and bicycle helmet discount with any bicycle purchase. A similar community about 50 miles away was identified as a comparison community. The epidemiologists compared the incidence of bicycle-related injuries through emergency room surveillance and telephone survey. This is an example of an **???** study.

6. Researchers administered a questionnaire to all new students at a large state university. The questionnaire included questions about behaviors such as seat belt use, exercise, smoking, and alcohol consumption. The researchers plan to distribute follow-up questionnaires at graduation and every five years thereafter, asking about health events and conditions such as diabetes and heart disease. This is an example of an **???** study.

Directionality

The directionality of a study refers to when the exposure variable is observed relative in time to when the health outcome is observed. In a study with forward directionality, the investigator starts by determining the exposure status for subjects selected from some population of interest and then follows these subjects over time to determine whether or not they develop the health outcome. Cohort studies and clinical trials always have forward directionality.

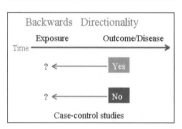

In a backwards design, the investigator selects subjects on the basis of whether or not they have the health outcome of interest, and then obtains information about their previous exposures. Case-control studies always have backwards directionality.

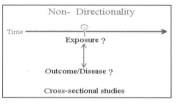

In a non-directional design, the investigator observes both the study factor and the health outcome simultaneously, so that neither variable may be uniquely identified as occurring first. A cross-sectional study is always non-directional.

The directionality of a study affects the researcher's ability to distinguish antecedent from consequent. This is important for evaluating **causality**. Also, the directionality chosen affects the way subjects can be selected into the study. Designs that are backwards or non-directional have more potential for **selection bias** than forward designs. Selection bias will be addressed in more detail in a later chapter.

<u>**Summary**</u>
- ❖ Directionality answers the question: when did you observe the exposure variable relative in time to when you observed health outcome?
- ❖ Directionality can be forward, backward, or non-directional.
- ❖ Directionality affects the researcher's ability to distinguish antecedent from consequent.
- ❖ Directionality also affects whether or not a study will have selection bias.

Timing

Timing concerns the question of whether the health outcome of interest has already occurred before the study actually began. If the health outcome has occurred before the study is initiated, the timing is **retrospective**. For example, let's say a case-control study is initiated to investigate cases of a

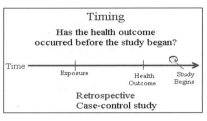

disease that occurred in the previous year; this would be an example of a **retrospective** case control study.

If, on the other hand, the health outcome occurs after the onset of the study, then the timing is **prospective**. Clinical trials are always *prospective*.

Cohort and case-control studies may *either* be retrospective or prospective since the study may begin either before or after the health outcome has occurred. The timing of a study can have important implications for the quality of the data. Retrospective data are often based on personal recall, or on hospital or

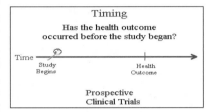

employment records, and are therefore more likely than prospective studies to involve measurement errors. Measurement errors frequently lead to information bias, which we discuss in a later chapter.

Summary
- ❖ Timing answers the question: has the health outcome of interest already occurred before the study actually began?
- ❖ If the health outcome occurs before the study is initiated, the timing is retrospective.
- ❖ If the health outcome occurs after the onset of the study, the timing is prospective.
- ❖ Timing affects measurement error and information bias.

Clinical Trials

A clinical trial is an *experimental study* designed to compare the therapeutic or health benefits of two or more treatments. The major objective of a clinical trial is to test the efficacy of a **preventive** or **therapeutic** intervention. The long-range goal of a preventive trial is to prevent disease; the long-range goal of a therapeutic trial is to cure or control a disease. Examples of preventive trials include studies of vaccine efficacy, use of aspirin to prevent coronary heart disease, smoking cessation, diet modification, and exercise. Therapeutic trials are typically performed by pharmaceutical companies to test new drugs for treating disease.

Key features of any clinical trial are **randomization, blinding, ethical concerns**, and the use of **intention to treat analysis**. **Randomization** is used to allocate subjects to treatment groups so that these groups are comparable on all factors except for exposure status. **Blinding** means that either the patient or the investigator is unaware of the treatment assigned. Single-blinding m eans either the patient or investigator are unaware of the treatment assignment and double blinding means that both the patient and the investigator are unaware of the treatment assignment. Blinding helps eliminate bias. The study must be **ethical,** treatments that may be harmful are not used. Stopping rules are planned that would end a trial early if it becomes clear that one of the treatments is superior. An **intention-to-treat analysis** requires that the investigators "analyze what they randomize", that is, analysis should be compared to the originally randomized treatment groups, even if study subjects switch treatments during the study period.

Summary
* The major objective of a clinical trial is to test the efficacy of a preventive or therapeutic intervention.
* Key features of any clinical trial are:
  Randomization   Ethical concerns
  Blinding   Intention to treat analysis

Clinical Trial Example

A clinical trial involving 726 subjects conducted in 1993 compared *standard* insulin therapy with *intensive* insulin therapy involving more frequent insulin injections and blood glucose monitoring for the treatment of diabetes mellitus. The outcome studied was retinopathy resulting in blindness, defined as either present or absent for each patient.

Subjects were randomized to treatment groups using a computerized random number generator. Double blinding could not be used in this clinical trial since both the patient and their physician would know which treatment group the patient was randomized. However, the individuals who graded the fundus photographs to determine the presence or absence of retinopathy were unaware of treatment-group assignments. The randomization resulted in the standard and intensive therapy groups having very similar distributions of baseline characteristics, such as age and sex.

An intention-to-treat analysis compared the originally randomized treatment groups with regard to the occurrence of retinopathy. It was found that 24% of the 378 subjects on standard

Clinical Trial	
Treatment:	
Standard Therapy Vs. Intensive Therapy	
n=378	n=348
24%	6.7%

therapy developed retinopathy, whereas 6.7% of the 348 subjects on intensive therapy developed retinopathy.

These data and more complicated analyses that controlled for several other important predictors indicated that intensive therapy had a much lower risk than standard therapy for retinopathy.

Summary
* A clinical trial involving 726 subjects conducted in 1993 compared standard insulin therapy with intensive insulin therapy.
* The outcome studied was retinopathy resulting in blindness, defined as either present or absent for each patient.

❖ 24% of subjects on standard therapy developed retinopathy whereas 6.7% of subjects on intensive therapy developed retinopathy.

Quiz (Q3.2) Fill in the Blanks; choices are <u>Preventive</u> or <u>Therapeutic</u>

1. **???** trials are conducted on individuals with a particular disease to assess a possible cure or control for the disease. For example, we may wish to assess to what extent, if at all, a new type of chemotherapy prolongs the life of children with acute lymphatic leukemia.

2. **???** trials can be conducted on either individuals or entire populations. An example is a study in which one community was assigned (at random) to receive sodium fluoride added to the water supply, while the other continued to receive water without supplementation. This study showed significant reductions in the development of tooth decay in the community receiving fluoride.

For each of the following features, choose the option that applies to *clinical trials*:

3. The investigator's role regarding exposure: .   .   **???**
         a. assign   b. observe
4. Subject selection into groups: .   .   .   .   **???**
         a. self-selection   b. randomization
5. Directionality: .   .   .   .   **???**
         a. backwards   b. forwards   c. non-directional
6. Timing: .   .   .   .   .   .   **???**
         a. prospective   b. retrospective   c. either
7. Blinding: .   .   .   .   .   .   **???**
         a. single   b. double   c. either
8. Topic: .   .   .   .   .   .   **???**
         a. medication   b. vaccine   c. either
9. Analysis by: .   .   .   .   **???**
         a. original assignment   b. actual experience

Observational Study Designs

There are three general categories of observational designs:
- Basic Designs: Cohort, Case-Control, Cross-Sectional
- Hybrid Designs: Nested Case-Control, Case-Cohort
- Incomplete Designs: Ecologic, Proportional

Cohort Studies

In 1948, a long-term observational study began in Framingham Massachusetts. Fifty-one hundred subjects without cardiovascular disease (CVD) were selected and examined, and information about potential risk factors for this disease was recorded. Subjects were then re-examined if possible every 2 years over the next 50

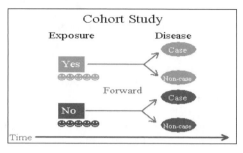

years. This classic study became known as the *Framingham Heart Study* and has been the source of much of our knowledge about risk factors for cardiovascular disease. The Framingham Heart study is an example of a **prospective** cohort study.

A cohort design starts with subjects who do not have a health outcome of interest and are followed forward to determine health outcome status. A key feature of a cohort study is that subjects are grouped on the basis of their exposure characteristics prior to observing the health outcome, that is, the directionality of the study is always forward.

A cohort study may be retrospective or prospective. The Framingham Heart study is an example of a prospective study since the study began before the health outcome occurred.

Summary

- ❖ The Framingham Heart Study is a classic example of a cohort study.
- ❖ The cohort design is always a follow-up study with forward directionality.
- ❖ A cohort study can be prospective or retrospective.
- ❖ The Framingham study is a prospective cohort study because the study began before the health outcome occurred.

Advantages of a Cohort Study

The primary advantage of a cohort study is its forward directionality. The investigator can be reasonably sure that the hypothesized cause preceded the occurrence of disease. In a cohort study, disease status cannot influence the way subjects are selected, so a cohort study is free of certain selection biases that seriously limit other types of studies.

A prospective cohort design is less prone than other observational study designs to obtaining incorrect information on important variables. Cohort studies can be used to study several diseases, since several health outcomes can be determined from follow-up.

Cohort studies are also useful for examining *rare* exposures. Since the investigator selects subjects on the basis of exposure, he can ensure a sufficient number of exposed subjects. A *retrospective* cohort study can be relatively low-cost and quick. Occupational studies that are based on employment records and death certificates or insurance and worker's comp records are an example.

Disadvantages of a Cohort Study

A prospective cohort study is often quite costly and time-consuming. A potential problem in any cohort study is the loss of subjects because of migration, lack of participation, withdrawal, and death. Such attrition of the cohort over the follow-up period can lead to biased results.

A cohort design is statistically and practically inefficient for studying a *rare* disease with long latency because of the long follow-up time and the number of subjects required to identify a sufficient number of cases. However, a retrospective cohort study may find enough cases since the study events of interest have already occurred.

Another problem in cohort studies is that the exposed may be followed more closely than the unexposed; if this happens, the outcome is more likely to be diagnosed in the exposed. This might create an appearance of exposure-disease relationship where none exists.

Summary: Cohort Study +'s (advantages) and –'s (disadvantages)

- ❖ (+) Prospective cohort study: least prone to bias compared with other observational study designs.
- ❖ (+) Can address several diseases in the same study.
- ❖ (+) Retrospective cohort study: can be relatively low-cost and quick; frequently used in occupational studies.
- ❖ (-) Loss to follow-up is a potential source of bias
- ❖ (-) Prospective cohort study: quite costly and time-consuming; may not find enough cases if disease is rare.
- ❖ (-) If exposed are followed more closely than unexposed, the outcome is more likely to be diagnosed in exposed.

Example: Retrospective Cohort Study of Spontaneous Abortions

The relationship between adverse pregnancy outcomes and the use of video display terminals (VDT's) became a public health concern in the 1980's when adverse pregnancy outcomes were reported among several clusters of women who used VDT's. A more comprehensive study of the effect of VDT's was reported in the New England Journal of Medicine in 1991. This study, conducted by the National Institute for Occupational Safety and Health (NIOSH) used a retrospective cohort design to examine the hypothesis that electromagnetic energy produced by VDT's might cause spontaneous abortions.

In the NIOSH study, a cohort of female telephone operators who were employed between 1983 and 1986 was selected from employers' personnel records at two telephone companies in eight southeastern states in the US. In this cohort, there were 882 women who had pregnancies

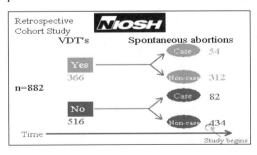

that met the inclusion criteria for the study. Of these women, the pregnancy outcomes of 366 directory assistance operators who used VDT's at work were compared with 516 general telephone operators who did not use VDT's.

The results of the study showed no excess risk of spontaneous abortion among women who used VDT's during their first trimester of pregnancy. No dose-response relation was found from the analysis of the women's hours of VDT use per week either. Also, no excess risk was associated with VDT use when other relevant characteristics of the study subjects were taken into account. The investigators therefore concluded that the use of VDT's and exposure to electromagnetic fields they produce were not associated with an increased risk of spontaneous abortion.

Summary
- ❖ A 1991 study used a retrospective cohort design to examine the hypothesis that electromagnetic energy produced by VDT's might cause spontaneous abortions.
- ❖ The pregnancy outcomes of 366 operators who used VDT's at work were compared with 516 operators who did not use VDT's
- ❖ The results of the study showed no excess risk of spontaneous abortion among women who used VDT's.

Example: Prospective Cohort Study of Alzheimer's Disease

Inflammatory activity in the brain is thought to contribute to the development of Alzheimer's disease. This hypothesis suggests that long-term use of nonsteroidal anti-inflammatory drugs (NSAIDs),may reduce the risk of this disease.

This hypothesis was investigated within the Rotterdam Study, a cohort study of the elderly that started in the Netherlands in 1990. At that time, 7,000 participants did not have Alzheimer's disease. During eight years of follow-up, 293 of the participants developed the disease.

To avoid information bias from measuring NSAIDs, the investigators used computerized pharmacy records instead of interview data to determine the total number of months during which participants had used NSAIDs after the study onset. Controlling for age, gender, and smoking status, the investigators found that the risk of Alzheimer's for participants who had used NSAIDs for more than 24 months was significantly less than the risk of Alzheimer's disease for participants who used NSAIDs for less than or equal to 24 months. The investigators concluded that long-term use of NSAIDs has a beneficial effect on the risk of Alzheimer's disease.

Summary
- ❖ The Rotterdam study examined the hypothesis that long-term use of nonsteriodal anti-inflammatory drugs (NSAIDs) may reduce the risk of Alzheimer's disease.
- ❖ The study used a prospective cohort design that followed 7,000 participants without Alzheimer's disease in 1990 over eight years.
- ❖ The risk of Alzheimer's disease for subjects using NSAIDs for more than 24 months was significantly smaller than for subjects using NSAIDs less than or equal to 24 months.

Quiz (Q3.3)   **Fill in the Blanks.** For each of the following features, choose the option that applies to *cohort studies*:

1. The investigator's role regarding exposure: ???
     a. assign   b. observe
2. Subject selection into groups: ???
     a. self-selection   b. randomization
3. Directionality: ???
     a. backwards   b. forwards   c. non-directional
4. Timing: ???
     a. prospective   b. retrospective   c. either
5. Analysis by: ???
     a. original assignment   b. actual experience

For each of the following characteristics (strengths or weaknesses) of a study, choose the type of cohort study with that characteristic; the choices are:

Both   **Neither**   **Prospective Cohort**   **Retrospective Cohort**

6. Less expensive: .   .   .   .   .   **???**

7. Quicker: .   .   .   .   .   **???**

8. More accurate exposure information: .   .   .   **???**

9. Appropriate for studying rare exposures: .   .   .   **???**

10. Appropriate for studying rare diseases: .   .   **???**

11. Problems with loss to follow-up: .   .   .   **???**

12. Better for diseases with long latency: .   .   .   **???**

Case-Control Studies

In case control studies, subjects are selected based on their disease status. The investigator first selects *cases* of a particular disease and then chooses *controls* from persons without the disease. Ideally, cases are selected from a clearly defined population, often called the **source population**, and controls

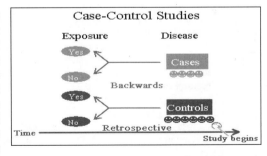

are selected from the same population that yielded the cases. The prior exposure histories of cases and controls are then determined. Thus, in contrast to a cohort study, a case-control study works backwards from disease status to prior exposure status. While case-control studies are always backward in directionality, they can be either prospective or retrospective in timing.

     In addition to being both cheaper and quicker than cohort studies, case-control studies have other **advantages**:

- They are feasible for obtaining sufficient numbers of cases when studying chronic or other rare diseases or diseases with long latency periods.
- They tend to require a smaller sample size than other designs.
- They can evaluate the effect of a variety of different exposures.

There are, nevertheless, several **disadvantages** of case-control studies:

- They do not allow several diseases to be evaluated, in contrast to cohort studies.
- They do not allow disease risk to be estimated directly because they work backwards from disease to exposure
- They are more susceptible to selection bias than other designs since the exposure has already occurred before cases and controls are selected.
- They are more susceptible to information bias than cohort studies because they are always backward in directionality.
- They are not efficient for studying rare exposures

Summary
- ❖ Start with cases and non-cases of a disease or other health outcome and proceed backwards to determine prior exposure history.
- ❖ Popular primarily because cheaper and less time-consuming than cohort studies.
- ❖ Other advantages include providing sufficient numbers of cases for rare diseases with long latencies and allowing several exposures to be evaluated.
- ❖ Disadvantages include being susceptible to both selection and information bias, not allowing estimation of risk, not considering more than one disease, and not feasible for rare exposures.

Incident versus Prevalent Cases in a Case-Control Study?

Cases can be chosen to be either incident or prevalent. Incident cases are new cases of a disease that develop over the time-period covered by the case-control study. When used in case-control studies, incident cases are typically obtained from an institutional or population-based disease registry, such as a cancer registry, or a health maintenance organization that continuously records new illnesses in a specified population.

Prevalent cases are existing cases of a disease at a point in time. When used in case-control studies, prevalent cases are usually obtained from hospital or clinic records.

An advantage of using of incident cases in case-control studies is that an exposure-disease relationship can be tied only to the development rather than the prognosis or duration of the disease.

In contrast, for prevalent cases, the exposure may affect the prognosis or the duration of the illness. If prevalent cases were used, therefore, an estimate of the effect of exposure on disease development could be biased because of failure to include cases that died before case-selection.

Choosing Controls in a Case-Control Study

One must select a comparison or control group carefully when conducting a case-control study. The ideal control group should be representative of the population from which the cases are derived, typically called the **source population**. This ideal is often hard to achieve when choosing controls.

Two common types of controls are **population-based controls** and **hospital-based controls**. In population-based case-control studies, controls are selected from the community. Methods used to select such controls include random telephone dialing, friend or neighborhood, and department of motor vehicle listings. An advantage of a population-based case-control study is that cases and controls come from the same source population, so they are similar in some way. A disadvantage is that it is difficult to obtain population lists and to identify and enroll subjects. Increasing use of unlisted numbers and answering machines increases non-response by potential controls.

In a hospital-based case-control study, controls are selected from hospital patients with illnesses *other than the disease of interest*. Hospital controls are easily accessible and tend to be more cooperative than population-based controls. Hospital-based studies are much less expensive and time-consuming than population-based studies. But, hospital-based controls are not likely to be representative of the source population that produced the cases. Also, hospital-based controls are ill and the exposure of interest may be a determinant of the control illness as well as the disease of interest. If so, a real association of the exposure with the disease of interest would likely be missed.

Summary

- ❖ The ideal control group should be representative of the source population from which the cases are derived.
- ❖ Two common types of controls are population-based controls and hospital-based controls.
- ❖ In population-based case-control studies, cases and controls come from the same source population.
- ❖ Hospital controls are easily accessible, tend to be cooperative, and are inexpensive.
- ❖ Hospital controls do not usually represent the source population but may represent an illness caused by the exposure.

Example: Case-Control Study of Reye's Syndrome

Reye's syndrome is a rare disease affecting the brain and liver that can result in delirium, coma, and death. It usually affects children, and typically occurs following a viral illness. To investigate whether aspirin is a determinant of Reye's Syndrome, investigators in the nineteen seventies and nineteen eighties decided that using a clinical trial would not be ethical.

Why might a clinical trial on aspirin use and Reye's syndrome be unethical? (Choose one of the four choices below)
   A. Children are involved.
   B. Harmful consequences of the use of aspirin.
   C. Double blinding may be used.
   D. Clinical trials are never ethical.

The answer is B, because of the potential harmful consequences of the use of aspirin. A cohort study was also considered inefficient:

Why would a cohort study of aspirin and Reye's syndrome be inefficient? Choose one of the four choices below)
    A. The outcome is rare (would require a lot of subjects).
    B. Requires at least 5 years of follow-up.
    C. The exposure is rare.
    D. Cohort studies are always inefficient

The answer is A, because the outcome is so rare. Consequently, a case-control study was preferred, since such a study could be accomplished over a shorter period, provide a sufficient number of cases, yet require fewer subjects overall than a cohort study.

The original investigation of Reye's Syndrome that identified aspirin as a risk factor was a case-control study conducted in Michigan in 1979 and 1980. This study involved 25 cases and 46 controls. Controls were children who were absent from the same school, in a similar grade, had a similar time of preceding illness, had the same race, the same year of birth, and the same type of preceding illness. A larger 1982 study attempted to confirm or refute the earlier finding. Investigators used a statewide surveillance system to identify all cases with Reye's syndrome in Ohio. This study thus used newly developed, or incident, cases. Population-based controls were selected by identifying and then sampling subjects in the statewide community who had experienced viral illnesses similar to those reported by the cases but had not developed Reye's syndrome. Parents of both cases and controls were asked about their child's use of medication during the illness.

Another study published in 1987 selected cases from children admitted with Reye's syndrome to any of a pre-selected group of tertiary care hospitals. Hospital-based controls were selected from children from these same hospitals who were admitted for a viral illness but did not develop Reye's syndrome. Parents were interviewed to assess previous use of aspirin.

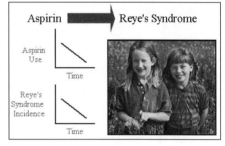

As a result of this case-control research on the relationship between use of aspirin and Reye's syndrome, health professionals recommended that aspirin *not* be used to treat symptoms of a viral illness in children. Subsequently, as the use of aspirin among children declined, so did the occurrence of Reye's syndrome.

Summary
❖ In the 1970s and 1980s, case-control studies were used to assess whether the use of aspirin for the treatment of viral illnesses in children was a determinant of Reye's syndrome.
❖ These studies started with subjects with the disease (i.e., Reye's syndrome) and similar subjects without the disease.
❖ Parents of both cases and controls were asked about their child's use of medication over a comparable time period preceding the child's first symptoms of Reye's syndrome.

❖ Health professionals recommended that aspirin not be used to treat symptoms of viral illnesses in children.

❖ As the use of aspirin among children declined, so did the occurrence of Reye's syndrome.

Example: Case-Control Study on Creutzfeldt-Jakob Disease

Creutzfeldt-Jakob disease (CJD) is a rare disease characterized by rapidly progressive dementia. In the 1990's, a new variant of CJD in humans was discovered in Europe following an epidemic in cattle of mad cow disease, the animal form of CJD. Subsequently, the European Union organized a study to investigate whether a diet containing animal products is a risk factor for CJD.

Because CJD is a very rare disease with a long latency period, the investigators chose a case-control study design. They collected data on 405 cases of CJD that had occurred in the European Union. An equal number of control participants were recruited from the hospitals where the patients with CJD had been diagnosed. Due to the mental deterioration of patients from the disease, diet information on cases had to be collected by interviewing one of the cases' next of kin.

How do you think the investigators collected diet information on control subjects? Even though the control participants were perfectly capable of giving information about their diets themselves, the investigators interviewed one of the control participants' next of kin instead. This way, they tried to avoid information bias by keeping the quality of the data on diet similar for both cases and controls.

Remember that one of the advantages of a case-control study is the opportunity to evaluate the effect of a variety of different exposures. In this study, the investigators examined separately whether consumption of sausage, raw meat, raw fish, animal blood products, milk, cheese, as well as other specified animal products, increased the risk of CJD. None of these food products significantly increased the risk of CJD, so, the investigators concluded that it is unlikely that CJD is transmitted from animals to man via animal products.

Quiz (Q3.4) For each of the following, choose the option that applies to **case-control studies**:

1. The investigator's role regarding exposure: **???**
   a. assign   b. observe
2. Subject selection into groups: **???**
   a. self-selection   b. randomization
3. Directionality: **???**
   a. backwards   b. forwards   c. non-directional
4. Timing: **???**
   a. prospective   b. retrospective   c. either
5. Analysis by: **???**
   a. original assignment   b. actual experience

For each of the following characteristics (strengths or weaknesses) of a study, choose the type of study with that characteristic. The choices are:

Case-control   **Prospective cohort**

6. Less expensive: . . . . . **???**

7. Quicker: . . . . . **???**

8. More accurate exposure information: . . . **???**

9. Appropriate for studying rare exposures: . . . **???**

10. Appropriate for studying rare diseases: . . **???**

11. Can study multiple outcomes: . . . **???**

12. Requires a smaller sample size: . . . . **???**

13. Can estimate risk: . . . . **???**

Determine whether each of the following statements is **true** or **false**:

14. Ideally, controls should be chosen from the same population that gave rise to the cases. . . **???**

15. Ideally, controls should be selected from hospitalized patients **???**

16. Population-based controls include only neighbors and persons identified by calling random telephone numbers. . **???**

Cross-Sectional Studies

In a cross-sectional study, subjects are sampled at a fixed point or within a short period of time. All participating subjects are examined, observed, and questioned about their disease status, their current or past exposures, and other relevant variables. A cross-sectional study provides a snapshot of the health experience of a population at a specified time and is therefore often used to describe patterns of disease occurrence. A cross-sectional sample is usually more representative of the general population being studied than are other study designs. A cross-sectional study is a convenient and inexpensive way to look at the relationships among several exposures and several diseases. If the disease of interest is relatively common and has long duration, a cross-sectional study can provide sufficient numbers of cases to be useful for generating hypotheses about exposure-disease relationships. Other more expensive kinds of studies, particularly cohort and clinical trials, are used to test such hypotheses.

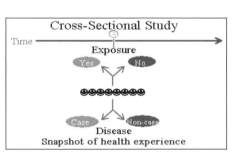

There are some disadvantages to cross-sectional studies. For example, such a study can identify only *existing* or *prevalent* cases at a given time, rather than *new* or *incident* cases over a follow-up time period. Therefore, a cross-sectional study cannot establish whether the exposure preceded the disease or whether the disease influenced the exposure.

Because only existing cases are allowed, a cross-sectional study includes only cases that survive long enough to be available for study. This could lead to a misleading conclusion about an exposure-disease relationship since non-survivors are excluded (see note at the end of this chapter on this issue).

Short-duration diseases, such as the common cold or influenza, especially those that occur during a particular season, may be under-represented by a cross-sectional study that looks at the presence of such a disease at a point in time.

Summary: Cross-Sectional Studies
❖ Subjects are sampled at a fixed point or short period of time: a snapshot.
Advantages
❖ Convenient and inexpensive.
❖ Can consider several exposures and several diseases.
❖ Can generate hypotheses.
❖ Usually represents the general population.
Disadvantages
❖ Cannot establish whether the exposure preceded disease or disease influence exposure.
❖ Possible bias since only survivors are available for study.
❖ May under-represent diseases with short duration.

How Can Bias Occur from Survivors in a Cross-sectional Study?

In a cross-sectional study, bias can result because only cases that survive long enough are available for such a study. To illustrate this point, suppose that everyone with a certain disease who does not do strenuous physical exercise regularly dies very quickly. Suppose, also, that those who have the disease but do strenuous physical exercise regularly survive for several years.

Now consider a cross-sectional study to assess whether regular strenuous physical activity is associated with the disease. Since this type of study would contain only survivors, we would likely find a low proportion of cases among persons not doing strenuous physical exercise. In contrast, we would likely find a relatively higher proportion of cases among persons who do strenuous physical exercise. This would suggest that doing strenuous physical exercise is harmful for the disease, even if, in fact, it were protective.

Example of a Cross-Sectional Study – Peripheral Vascular Disease, Scotland

A 1991 study examined a sample of 5000 Scottish men for the presence of peripheral vascular disease (PVD). Other characteristics, including whether or not a subject ever smoked, were also determined for each subject during the exam.

This was a cross-sectional study since all study subjects were selected

Ever smoked? ▬▬▬▶ PVD

	Smoked		
	Ever	Never	Total
PVD	23	8	31
No PVD	1704	1291	2995
Total	1727	1299	3026

$$\frac{.013}{.006} = 2.2$$

Ever smokers:
2.2 x more likely to have PVD than never-smokers.

and observed at one point in time. Even though physical exams were performed, the study cost and time was much less than that required if disease-free subjects were followed over time to determine future PVD status. The sample was representative of the Scottish male population.

The study found that 1.3 percent of 1727 ever-smokers had PVD whereas only 0.6 percent of 1299 never-smokers had PVD. Dividing .013 by .006, we see that ever-smokers were 2.2 times more likely to have PVD than never-smokers.

These results suggested that smoking may contribute to developing PVD. Yet, the results are just a snapshot of subjects at a point in time, 1991. Subjects without PVD have not been followed over time. So, how do we know from this snapshot whether PVD leads to smoking or smoking leads to PVD? This illustrates one of the problems with cross-sectional studies - they are always **non-directional**. Also, persons who died from PVD prior to the time that subjects were selected are not allowed in the study. Therefore, the study results may be biased because only PVD survivors are being counted.

Summary

* An example of a cross-sectional study is a 1991 study of peripheral vascular disease (PVD) in Scotland.
* Results show that ever-smokers are 2.2 times more likely to have PVD than never-smokers.
* This study was much cheaper and quicker then a cohort study.
* Cannot determine whether PVD leads to smoking or smoking leads to PVD.
* The study results may be biased because only PVD survivors are considered.

Quiz (Q3.5) For each of the following features, choose the option that applies to *cross-sectional* studies:

1. The investigator's role regarding exposure: .   .   **???**
        a. assign   b. observe
2. Subject selection into groups: .   .   .   **???**
        a. self-selection   b. randomization
3. Directionality: .   .   .   .   .   **???**
        a. backwards   b. forwards   c. non-directional
4. Timing: .   .   .   .   .   .   **???**
        a. prospective   b. retrospective   c. either

Determine whether each of the following statements is **true** or **false**:

5. Cross-sectional studies are better suited to generating hypotheses about exposure-disease relationships than to testing such relationships.   **???**
6. Because exposure and disease are assessed at the same time, cross-sectional studies are not subject to survival bias.   .   .   .   **???**
7. Because exposure and disease are assessed at the same time, cross-sectional studies may not be able to establish that exposure preceded onset of the disease process.   .   .   .   .   .   **???**
8. Cross-sectional studies can examine multiple exposures and multiple diseases.   .   .   .   .   .   .   **???**

Hybrid Designs

*Hybrid designs combine the elements of at least two basic designs, or extend the strategy of one basic design through repetition. Two popular hybrid designs are the **case-cohort study** and the **nested case-control study**. Both these designs combine elements of a cohort and case-control study. Another more recently developed hybrid design is called the **case-crossover** design.*

Incomplete Designs

Incomplete designs are studies in which information is missing on one or more relevant factors. An **ecologic study** is an incomplete design for which the unit of analysis is a group, often defined geographically, such as a census tract, a state, or a country. A **proportional morbidity** or **proportional mortality** study only includes observations on cases but lacks information about the candidate population at risk for developing the health outcome. If the design involves incident cases, the study is a proportional morbidity study. If deaths are used, the study is a proportional mortality study.

See Lesson Page 3-3 in the ActivEpi CD ROM for further details on Hybrid and Incomplete Designs

References
Reference for Diabetes Research Group Study (Clinical Trial)
The Diabetes Control and Complications Trial Research Group. The effect of intensive treatment of diabetes on the development and progression of long-term complications in insulin-dependent diabetes mellitus. N Engl J Med 1993; 329(14):977-86.
Reference for Framingham Heart Study (Prospective Cohort Study)
Feinleib M, The Framingham study: sample selection, follow-up, and methods of analysis, in National Cancer Institute Monograph, No. 67, Greenwald P (editor), US Department of Health and Human Services, 1985.
Dorgan JF, Brown C, Barrett M, et al. Physical activity and risk of breast cancer in the Framingham Heart Study, Am J Epidemiol 1994;139(7): 662-9.
Margolis JR, Gillum RF, Feinleib M, et al. Community surveillance for coronary heart disease: the Framingham Cardiovascular Disease Survey. Methods and preliminary results. Am J Epidemiol 1974;100(6):425-36.
Reference for VDT use and Spontaneous Abortion (Retrospective Cohort Study)
Schnorr TM, Grajewski BA, Hornung RW, et al. Video display terminals and the risk of spontaneous abortion. N Engl J Med 1991;324(11):727-33.
Reference for Nonsteroidal anti-inflammatory drugs and Alzheimer's disease (Prospective Cohort Study)
in t' Veld BA, Ruitenberg A, Hofman A, et al. Nonsteroidal antiinflammatory drugs and the risk of Alzheimer's disease. N Engl J Med 2001;345(21):1515-21.
References for Reye's Syndrome (Case-Control Studies)
Waldman RJ, Hall WN, McGee H, Van Amburg G. Aspirin as a risk factor in Reye's syndrome. JAMA 1982;247(22):3089-94.
Halpin TJ, Holtzhauer FJ, Campbell RJ, et al. Reye's syndrome and medication use. JAMA 1982;248(6):687-91.
Daniels SR, Greenberg RS, Ibrahim MA. Scientific uncertainties in the studies of salicylate use and Reye's syndrome. JAMA 1983;249(10):1311-6.
Hurwitz ES, Barrett MJ, Bregman D, et al. Public Health Service study of Reye's syndrome

and medications. Report of the main study. JAMA 1987;257(14):1905-11.

Forsyth BW, Horwitz RI, Acampora D, et al. New epidemiologic evidence confirming that bias does not explain the aspirin/Reye's syndrome association. JAMA 1989;261(17):2517-24

References for Creutzfeldt-Jakob Disease (Case-Control Studies)

van Duijn CM, Delasnerie-Laupretre N, Masullo C, et al. Case-control study of risk factors of Creutzfeldt-Jakob disease in Europe during 1993-95. European Union (EU) Collaborative Study Group of Creutzfeldt-Jakob disease (CJD). Lancet 1998;351(9109):1081-5.

Will RG, Ironside JW, Zeidler M, et al. A new variant of Creutzfeldt-Jakob disease in the UK. Lancet 1996;347(9006):921-5.

General epidemiologic design

Checkoway H, Pearce N, Dement JM. Design and conduct of occupational epidemiology studies: II. Analysis of cohort data. Am J Ind Med 1989;(15(4):375-94.

Greenberg RS, Daniels SR, Flanders WD, et al. Medical Epidemiology (3rd Ed). Lange Medical Books, New York, 2001.

Kleinbaum DG, Kupper LL, Morgenstern H. Epidemiologic Research: Principles and Quantitative Methods. John Wiley and Sons Publishers, New York, 1982.

Example of Cross-Sectional Studies

Smith WCS, Woodward M, Tunstall-Pedoe H. Intermittent claudication in Scotland, in Epidemiology of Peripheral Vascular Disease. (ed FGR Fowkes.), Springer-Verlag, Berlin, 1991

Hybrid designs

Coates RJ, Weiss NS, Daling JR, et al. Cancer risk in relation to serum copper levels. Cancer Res 1989;49(15): 4353-6.

Linn JT, Wang LY, Wang JT, et al. A nested case-control study on the association between Helicobacter pylori infection and gastric cancer risk in a cohort of 9775 men in Taiwan. Anticancer Res 1995;15:603-6.

Maclure M, Mittleman MA. Should we use a case-crossover design? Annu Rev Public Health 2000;21:193-221.

Maclure M. The case-crossover design: a method for studying transient effects on the risk of acute events. Am J Epidemiol 1991;133(2):144-53.

Redelmeier DA, Tibshirani RJ. Association between cellular-telephone calls and motor vehicle collisions. N Eng J Med 1997;336(7):453-8.

Ecologic

CDC. Summary of notifiable diseases in the United States. MMWR Morb Mortal Wkly Rep 1990;38(54):1-59.

Morgenstern H. Ecologic studies in epidemiology: concepts, principles, and methods. Ann Rev Public Health 1995;16:61-81.

Proportional Mortality

Mancuso TF, Stewart A, Kneale G. Radiation exposures of Hanford workers dying from cancer and other causes. Health Phys 1977;33:369-85.

Causation and Meta Analysis

Blalock HM, **Causal Inferences in Nonexperimental Research**, Chapter 1, Norton Publishing, 1964.

Chalmers I, Altman DG (eds.), **Systematic Reviews**, BMJ Publishing Group, London, 1995.

Chalmers TC. Problems induced by meta-analyses. Stat Med 1991;10(6):971-80.

Hill AB, Principles of Medical Statistics, 9th Edition, Chapter 24, Oxford University Press, 1971.

Lipsey MW, Wilson DB. Practical meta-analysis. Applied Social Research Methods Series; Vol. 49. Sage Publications, Inc., Thousand Oaks, CA: 2001.

Mosteller F, Colditz GA. Understanding research synthesis (meta-analysis). Annu Rev

Public Health 1996;17:1-23.

Petitti DB, Meta-analysis Decision Analysis and Cost-Effectiveness Analysis; Methods for Quantitative Synthesis in Medicine, Oxford University Press, 1994.

Popper KR, The Logic of Scientific Discovery, Harper and Row Publishers, 1968.

Rothman KJ. Causes. Am J Epidemiol 1976;104(6): 587-92.

Susser M, Causal Thinking in the Health Sciences, Oxford University Press, 1973.

U.S. Department of Health, Education, and Welfare, Smoking and Health, PHS Publ. No. 1103, Government Printing, Washington DC, 1964.

Weiss NS. Inferring causal relationships: elaboration of the criterion of dose-response. Am J Epidemiol 1981;113(5):487-90.

Answers to Quizzes

Q3.1
1. Experimental
2. Observational
3. Observational
4. Experimental
5. Experimental
6. Observational

Q3.2
1. Therapeutic
2. Preventive
3. a
4. b
5. b
6. a
7. c
8. c
9. a

Q3.3
1. b
2. a
3. b
4. c
5. b
6. Retrospective
7. Retrospective
8. Prospective
9. Both
10. Neither
11. Both
12. Retrospective

Q3.4
1. b
2. a
3. a
4. c
5. b

6. case-control
7. case-control
8. prospective cohort
9. prospective cohort
10. case-control
11. prospective cohort
12. case-control
13. prospective cohort
14. T – If controls are chosen from a different population from which the cases came, there may be selection bias.
15. F – Hospital controls have an illness; such controls are typically not representative of the community from which the cases came.
16. F – Population-based controls can be obtained from random dialing of telephone numbers in the community from which the cases are derived. There is no guarantee that neighbors of cases will be chosen.

Q3.5
1. b
2. a
3. c
4. b
5. T
6. F
7. T – A cross-sectional study includes only cases that survive long enough to be available for study. This could lead to a misleading conclusion about an exposure-disease relationship since non-survivors are excluded.
8. T

CHAPTER 4

HOW OFTEN DOES IT HAPPEN? DISEASE FREQUENCY

*In epidemiologic studies, we use a **measure of disease frequency** to determine how often the disease or other health outcome of interest occurs in various subgroups of interest. We describe two basic types of measures of disease frequency in this chapter, namely, measures of incidence and measures of prevalence. The choice typically depends on the study design being used and the goal of the study.*

Incidence versus Prevalence

There are two general types of measures of disease frequency, **incidence (I)** and **prevalence (P)**. Incidence measures *new* cases of a disease that develop over a period of time. Prevalence measures *existing* cases of a disease at a particular point in time or over a period of time.

To illustrate how incidence and prevalence differ, we consider our experience with AIDS. The number of annual incident cases of AIDS in gay men decreased in the US from the mid-1980s to the late 1990s. This has resulted primarily both from recent anti-retroviral treatment approaches and from prevention strategies for reducing high-risk sexual behavior. In contrast, the annual prevalent cases of AIDS in gay men has greatly increased in the US during the same period because recent treatment approaches for AIDS have been successful in prolonging life of persons with the HIV virus and/or AIDS.

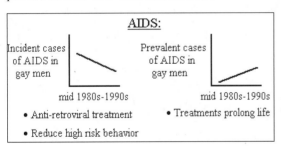

Prevalence can also be viewed as describing a pool of disease in a population, whereas incidence describes the input flow of new cases into the pool, and fatality and recovery reflects the output flow from the pool.

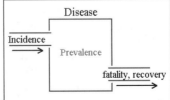

Incidence measures are useful for identifying risk factors and assessing disease etiology. Typically, incidence measures are estimated from clinical trials and from cohort studies, which involve the follow-up of subjects over time.

Prevalence measures are not as useful as incidence measures for assessing etiology because prevalence does not consider persons who die from the disease before the prevalence study begins. Typically, prevalence measures are estimated from cross-sectional studies and from case-control studies that use prevalent rather than incident cases. Since the number of prevalent cases indicates demand for health care, prevalence measures are most useful in the planning of health services.

Summary

❖ Incidence concerns new cases of disease or other health outcome over a period of follow-up.

❖ Prevalence concerns existing cases of a disease at a point in time.

❖ Incidence measures are useful for identifying risk factors and assessing disease etiology

❖ Prevalence measures are most useful in the planning of health services

---

Mortality Might Be Used Instead of Disease Incidence

We discuss incidence and prevalence in terms of new or existing cases of a **disease**, whether or not these cases eventually die or not during or after the period of study. There are many situations, however, when the use of strictly **mortality** information is also worthwhile.

Mortality measures are an important tool for **epidemiologic surveillance**. Today such surveillance programs have been applied to monitor the occurrence of a wide variety of health events, including deaths, in large populations. Mortality statistics are also convenient for **evaluating etiologic hypotheses**, especially when incidence data are not available. In particular, for diseases with a low rate of cure or recovery, such as lung cancer, mortality measures give a reasonable approximation to incidence measures.

Use of mortality information for any of the above purposes has several pragmatic advantages:

• Mortality data are widely collected and virtually complete since registration of deaths is compulsory in most industrialized countries and few deaths are not reported.

• Mortality data are defined using standardized nomenclature. In particular, the International Classification of Diseases (ICD) is used to promote uniformity in reporting causes of death.

• Recording of mortality data is relatively inexpensive.

House Guests Example

Suppose guests arrive at your house at the rate of two per day and stay exactly five days. How many people will be in your house after a week?

Let's see what happens day by day. On the first day, two guests arrive and none depart, so there are 2 guests in your house at the end of the first day. On the second day two more guests arrive, and none depart, so there are now 4 guests in your house after 2 days. Similarly, there are 6 guests after 3 days, 8 after 4 days and 10 guests in your house after five days, with no guests departing up to this point. But, on the sixth day, two new guests arrive, but the two guests that came on day 1, having been there for five days, now depart, leaving you again with 10 guests in the house. At the end of the seventh day, there will still be 10 guests in the house, which answers the question raised at the start of all this.

This scenario illustrates the fundamental difference between incidence and prevalence. In the example, after 5 days, a "steady state" is reached at which point there are 10 houseguests as long as the arrival rate is 2 per day. This steady state of 10 houseguests is a prevalence, which describes the existing count of guests, at any point in time after a steady state has been reached. The arrival rate of 2 guests per day is an incidence, which describes how quickly new guests are arriving. The duration of five days that guests stay in your house is the information needed to link the incidence to the prevalence. Prevalence can be linked to incidence with the following formula: **P = I x D**

In our example, **P** is the number of guests in the house on any day after day five, **I** is the arrival rate of 2 guests per day, and **D** is the duration of 5 days for each guest. The formula works in this example since 2 times 5 equals 10.

We can see from this formula that for a given incidence, the prevalence will increase or decrease as the duration increases or decreases. For example, if guests stayed for 8 days rather than 5 days, with the same arrival rate, the number of guests at the house at steady state would be 2 times 8, which equals 16, rather than 10.

For a given duration, the prevalence will increase or decrease as the incidence increases or decreases. Thus, if the guests arrive at the rate of only 1 guest per day rather than 2, and stay 8 days, the prevalence will be 1 times 8, which equals 8, instead of 16.

Summary

❖ A scenario involving houseguests who arrive at 2 per day and stay five days illustrates the fundamental difference between incidence and prevalence.

❖ A steady state of 10 houseguests illustrates *prevalence*, which describes the existing count of guests at any point in time after steady state is reached.

❖ The arrival of 2 guests per day illustrates *incidence*, which describes how quickly new guests are arriving.

❖ The *duration* of 5 days is the information needed to link how incidence leads to prevalence

❖ Prevalence is obtained as the product of incidence and duration (P = I x D)

The Relationship between Prevalence and Incidence

In the example involving "house guests", the formula $P = (I \times D)$

was used to demonstrate that the steady state number of guests in the house after 7 days was equal to the product of the number of guests arriving each day times the duration that each guest stayed in the house.

The terms **P**, **I**, and **D** in this formula represent the concepts of prevalence, incidence and duration, respectively, but, as used in the example, they each do not strictly conform to the epidemiologic definitions of these terms. As described in later activities in this chapter on measures of disease frequency, the strict definitions of prevalence and incidence require denominators, whereas the "house guest" scenario described here makes use only of numerator information.

Specifically, *prevalence* is estimated using the formula: $P = \dfrac{C}{N}$

and *incidence* uses one of the following two possible formulas depending on whether risk or rate is the incidence measure chosen:

$$CI = \frac{I}{N} \text{ or } IR = \frac{I}{PT}$$

In the above formulae, **P**, **C**, and **N** denote the prevalence, number of existing cases, and steady state population-size, respectively. Also, **CI** denotes cumulative incidence, which estimates risk, **I** denotes the number of new (incident cases), and **N** denotes the size of a disease-free cohort followed over the entire study period. Further, **IR** stands for incidence rate, and **PT** for accumulated person-time information. All these formulae are described and illustrated in later activities.

The important point being made here is that all three of the above formulae have denominators, which were not used in the houseguest example, but are required for computing prevalence and incidence in epidemiology.

The term **D** in the formula at the top of this page was used in the houseguest example to define the duration of stay that was assumed for each houseguest. In the epidemiologic use of this formula, **D** actually denotes the average duration of illness for all subjects in the population under study, rather than being assumed to be the same for each person in the population.

Nevertheless, using the stricter epidemiologic definitions of prevalence and incidence measures and using average duration, the above formula that relates prevalence to incidence and duration still holds, provided the population is in steady state and the disease is rare. By steady state, we mean that even though the population may be dynamic, the number of persons who enter and leave the population for whatever reasons are essentially equal over the study period, so that the population does not change. If the disease is not rare, a modified formula relating prevalence to incidence is required instead, namely:

$$P = \frac{I \times D}{(I \times D) + 1}$$

Quiz (Q4.1) For each of the following scenarios, determine whether it is more closely related to **incidence** or to **prevalence**.

1. Number of campers who developed gastroenteritis within a few days after eating potato salad at the dining hall? **???**
2. Number of persons who reported having with diabetes as part of the National Health Interview Survey? **???**
3. Occurrence of acute myocardial infarction (heart attack) among participants during the first 10 years of follow-up of the Framingham Study? **???**
4. Number of persons who died and whose deaths were attributed to Hurricane Floyd in North Carolina in 1999? **???**
5. Number of children who have immunity to measles, either because they had the disease or because they received the vaccine? **???**

Suppose a surveillance system was able to accurately and completely capture all new occurrences of disease in a community. Suppose also that a survey was conducted on July 1 that asked every member of that community whether they currently had that disease. For each of the following conditions, determine whether **incidence** (per 1,000 persons per year) or **prevalence** (per 1,000 persons on July 1) is *likely to be higher*.

6. Rabies (occurs rarely and has a short duration, e.g., death within one week)?   **???**
7. Multiple sclerosis (rare occurrence, long duration [many years])?   **???**
8. Influenza (common but winter-seasonal occurrence, short duration)?   **???**
9. Poison ivy dermatitis (common spring/summer/fall occurrence, 2-week duration)?   **???**
10. High blood pressure (not uncommon occurrence, lifelong duration)?   **???**

Risk

The term risk is commonly used in everyday life to describe the likelihood, or probability, that some event of interest will occur. We may wonder, for example, what is the risk that the stock market will crash or that we will be involved in a serious auto collision? We may worry about our risk for developing an undesirable health condition, such as a life-threatening illness, even our risk for dying.

In epidemiology, risk is the probability that an individual with certain characteristics, say, age, race, sex, and smoking status, will develop or die from a disease, or even more generally, will experience a health status change of interest over a specified follow-up period. When the health outcome is a disease, this definition assumes that the individual does not have the disease at the start of follow-up and does not die from any other cause during follow-up. Because risk is a probability, it is a number between 0 and 1, or, correspondingly, a percentage.

$$0 \le \text{RISK} \le 1$$
$$(0 \le \text{Percentage} \le 100)$$

When describing risk, it is necessary to specify a period of follow-up, called the **risk period**. For example, to describe the risk that a 45 year-old male will develop prostate cancer, we must state the risk period, say, 10 years of follow-up, over which we want to predict this risk. If the risk period were, for example, 20 years instead of 10 years, we would expect our estimate of risk to be larger than the 10-year risk since more time is being allowed for the disease to develop.

Study Questions (Q4.2)
1. What is the meaning of the following statement? The 10-year risk that a 45-year-old male will develop prostate cancer is 5%? (State your answer in probability terms and be as specific as you can in terms of the assumptions required.)
2. Will the 5-year risk for the same person described in the previous question be larger or smaller than the 10-year risk? Explain briefly.

Summary
❖ Risk is the probability than an individual will develop or die from a given disease or, more generally, will experience a health status change over a specified follow-up period.
❖ Risk assumes that the individual does not have the disease at the start of the follow-up and does not die from any other cause during the follow-up.
❖ Risk must be some value between 0 and 1, or correspondingly, a percentage
❖ When describing risk, it is necessary to give the follow-up period over which the risk is to be predicted.

> **Confusing Risk with Rate**
>
> The term *rate* has often been used incorrectly to describe a measure of *risk*. For example, the term *attack rate* is frequently used in studies of outbreaks to describe an estimate of the probability of developing an infectious illness, when in fact, an estimate of *risk* is computed. Also, the term *death rate* has been confused with *death risk* in mortality studies. In particular, the term *case-fatality rate* has often been misused to describe the proportion of cases that die, i.e., such a proportion is actually estimating a *risk*.
>
> The terms risk and rate have very different meanings, as described in other activities in this chapter. Ideally, the correct term should be applied to the actual measure being used. This does not always happen in the publication of epidemiologic findings. Consequently, when reading the epidemiologic literature, one should be careful to determine the actual measure being reported.

Cumulative Incidence

The most common way to estimate risk is to divide the number of newly detected cases that develop during follow-up by the number of disease-free subjects available at the start of follow-up. Such an estimate is often called *cumulative incidence* or **CI**. When describing cumulative incidence, it is necessary to give the follow-up period over which the risk is estimated.

$$CI = \frac{I}{N} = \frac{\#\text{ of new cases during follow - up}}{\#\text{ of disease - free subjects at start of follow - up}}$$

Technically speaking, cumulative incidence is not equivalent to individual risk, but rather is an estimate of individual risk computed from either an entire population or a sample of a population. However, we often use the terms risk and cumulative incidence interchangeably, as we do throughout this course.

We usually put a hat ("^") over the CI when the estimate of cumulative incidence is based on a sample; we leave off the hat if we have data for the entire population.

$$\hat{CI} = CI \text{ "hat"}$$

The cumulative incidence formula, with or without a "hat", is always a proportion, so its values can vary from 0 to 1. If the cumulative incidence is high, as in an outbreak, the CI is sometimes expressed as a percent.

As a simple example, suppose we followed 1000 men age 45 and found that 50 developed prostate cancer within 10 years of follow-up and that no subject was lost to follow-up or withdrew from the study. Then our estimate of simple cumulative incidence is 50 over 1000, or 0.05, or, 5 %.

$$\hat{CI} = \frac{I}{N} = \frac{50}{1000} = .05 = 5\%$$

In other words, the 10-year risk, technically the cumulative incidence for a 45 year-old male is estimated to be 5%. The formula we have given for computing risk is often referred to as **Simple Cumulative Incidence** because it is a simple proportion that assumes a fixed cohort. Nevertheless, the use of simple cumulative incidence is not always appropriate in all kinds of follow-up studies. Problems with simple cumulative incidence and methods for dealing with such problems are discussed in activities to follow.

Summary

- ❖ Cumulative incidence (CI) is a population-based estimate of individual risk
- ❖ Cumulative incidence is always a proportion
- ❖ When describing cumulative incidence, it is necessary to give the follow-up period over which the risk is estimated.
- ❖ The formula for simple cumulative incidence is CI=I/N, where I denotes the number of new cases of disease that develop over the follow-up period and N denotes the size of the disease-free population at the start of follow-up.
- ❖ The terms cumulative incidence and risk are used interchangeably here, even though technically, they are different.

Shifting the Cohort

The formula for *simple cumulative incidence* implicitly assumes that the cohort is **"fixed"** in the sense that no entries into the cohort are allowed during the follow-up period. What we should do if we do allow new entries into the cohort?

For example, in the Sydney Beach Users study described in Chapter 2, subjects were selected from 12 popular Sydney beaches over 41 sampling days throughout the summer months of 1989-90. Subjects could progressively enter the cohort on different days during the summer, after which self-reported exposure and disease information were obtained one week later.

To illustrate, consider six subjects shown to the right. Each subject is followed for the required 7 days. Subjects 1 and 5 (going from the bottom individual to the top individual) are the only subjects who reported becoming ill.

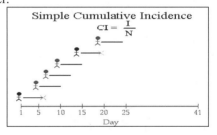

We can restructure these data by shifting the line of follow-up for each person to the left margin so that the horizontal time axis now reflects days of observation from the start of observation for each subject, rather than the actual calendar days at which the observations occurred. This conforms to the follow-up of a fixed cohort, for which the cumulative incidence is estimated to be 2/6 or one-third.

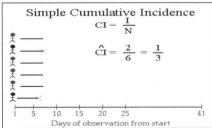

We often have a cohort that allows subjects to progressively enter the study at different calendar times. We can restructure the cohort to be fixed by shifting the data for each subject to reflect the time of observation since initial entry into the study rather than calendar time. We can then use the simple cumulative incidence formula to estimate risk.

<u>Study Questions (Q4.3)</u> Suppose after shifting the cohort, one subject remained disease-free during 4 years of follow-up whereas another subject in the cohort remained disease-free but was only followed for 2 years.
1. Do we have to assume that subjects who became cases were followed for the same amount of time as subjects who remained disease-free?
2. Is there a problem with computing the cumulative incidence that includes both these subjects in the denominator of the CI formula?
3. After we have shifted the cohort, do we have to assume that ALL subjects, including those who became cases, were followed for the same amount of time in order to compute cumulative incidence (CI)?

<u>Summary</u>
❖ If subjects progressively enter the study at different calendar times, the data can be **shifted** to reflect the time of observation since initial entry.
❖ Simple cumulative incidence can be used to estimate risk for a **shifted** cohort.
❖ After shifting the cohort, we can compute cumulative incidence provided all subjects who remained disease-free throughout follow-up are followed for the entire length of follow-up.

Problems with Simple Cumulative Incidence

There are several potential problems with assuming a fixed cohort when using the formula for simple cumulative incidence to estimate risk. One problem occurs because the size of a fixed cohort is likely to be reduced during the follow-up period as a result of deaths or other sources of attrition such as loss to follow-up or withdrawal from the study. We don't know whether a subject lost during follow-up developed the disease of interest.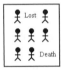

Another problem arises if the population studied is a **dynamic population** rather than a **fixed cohort**. A fixed cohort is a group of subjects identified at some point in time and followed for a given period for detection of new cases. The cohort is "fixed" in the sense that no entries are permitted into the study after the onset of follow-up, although subsequent losses of subjects may occur for various reasons such as withdrawal, migration, and death. But, a dynamic population is continually changing, allowing for both the addition of new members and the loss of previously entered members during the follow-up period.

The denominator in the simple cumulative incidence formula does not reflect the continually changing population size of a dynamic population. And the numerator in the simple cumulative incidence formula does not count new cases that may arise from those persons who entered a dynamic population after the beginning of follow-up.

Another difficulty for either a fixed or dynamic cohort is that subjects may be followed for *different periods of time* so that a cumulative incidence estimate will not make use of differing follow-up periods. This problem can occur when subjects are lost to follow-up or withdraw from the study. It could also occur if subjects enter the study after the study start and are disease-free until the study ends, or if the follow-up time at which a subject develops the disease varies for different subjects.

To illustrate these problems, let's consider a hypothetical example involving 12 initially disease-free subjects who are followed over a 5- year period from 1990 to 1995.

An **X** denotes the time at which a subject was diagnosed with the disease and a **circle (O)** denotes the time of death *that could be due to the disease (circle with an **X** inside) or due to another cause (circle without an **X**).* Those

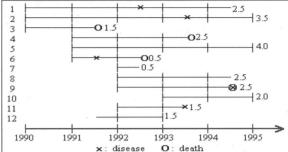

subjects that have no X or circle on their time line either withdrew from the study, or were lost to follow-up, or were followed until the end of the study without the developing the disease. The value to the right of each subject's time line denotes that subject's follow-up time period until either the disease was diagnosed, the subject withdrew or was lost to follow-up, or until the study ended. Based on this information, answer the following questions:

Study Questions (Q4.4) The questions below refer to the figure above:
1. What type of cohort is being studied, **fixed** or **dynamic**?
2a. Which of these subjects was diagnosed with the disease?
    Subject 2 Subject 3 Subject 5 Subject 7
2b. Which of these subjects was lost or withdrawn?
    Subject 2 Subject 3 Subject 5 Subject 7
2c. Which of these subjects died with disease?
    Subject 3 Subject 5 Subject 7 Subject 9
2d. Which of these subjects died with*out* the disease?
    Subject 3 Subject 5 Subject 7 Subject 9
2e. Which one was with*out* the disease and alive at the end?
    Subject 3 Subject 5 Subject 7 Subject 9

Shifted Cohort

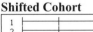

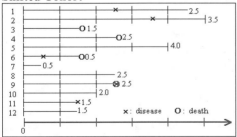

3. If we could shift the cohort, what is your estimate of simple cumulative incidence of disease diagnosis *in percent*?

4. What is your estimate of simple cumulative incidence of death *in percent with no decimal places?*
5. *Using the "unshifted" graph from the previous page,* Subjects 5, 8, 10 and 12 have which of the following in common:
   A. Same amount of observed follow-up time
   B. Entered study at same calendar time
   C. Withdrew from the study
   D. Did not develop disease during follow-up

Computing simple cumulative incidence for the previously shown data is a problem because …

6a. Not all subjects developed the disease	**Yes**	**No**
6b. Not all subjects died	**Yes**	**No**
6c. The cohort is dynamic	**Yes**	**No**
6d. Some subjects died from another cause	**Yes**	**No**
6e. Some subjects were lost or withdrew	**Yes**	**No**

6f. Some subjects developed disease at different follow-up times
Yes   No

6g. Subjects not developing the disease had different follow-up times
Yes   No

Summary
❖ There are problems with assuming a fixed cohort when using the formula for simple cumulative incidence to estimate risk.
❖ If there is attrition of a fixed cohort, we will not know whether a subject lost during follow-up developed the disease.
❖ For a dynamic cohort, the denominator in the simple cumulative incidence formula does not reflect the continually changing population size
❖ Simple cumulative incidence does not allow subjects to be followed for different periods of time.

Quiz (Q4.5)
After the second game of the college football season, 60 members of the 97-person football team developed fever, malaise, loss of appetite, and abdominal discomfort. Within a few days, 30 players became jaundiced. Blood samples were drawn from all members of the team to test for antibodies to hepatitis A (the presumptive diagnosis) and to test for elevation of liver enzymes

1. What is the cumulative incidence of jaundice?   .   **???**
2. If you assume that all persons with symptoms had hepatitis A, even those that did not develop jaundice, what is the presumed cumulative incidence of hepatitis A?   **???**
3. Laboratory testing revealed that 91 had elevated liver enzymes of which 90 had IgM antibody indicative of acute hepatitis A infection. Two players with normal liver enzymes had IgG antibody, indicating that they had previously been exposed to hepatitis A and are now immune. What is the cumulative incidence of hepatitis A?   **???**

Choices

30/60   30/97   60/97   90/91   90/95   90/97   91/95   91/97

Label each of the following statements as **True** or **False**:

4. Cumulative incidence is always a proportion, even for a cohort with staggered entry ("shifted cohort").   **???**
5. Cumulative incidence is a useful measure for diseases with short incubation periods in well-defined populations.   **???**
6. Cumulative incidence is a less-than-ideal measure for diseases with long incubations periods in dynamic populations.   **???**
7. If a fixed population has substantial loss-to-follow-up, cumulative incidence will overestimate the true risk of disease.   **???**

Rate

Rate is a measure of disease frequency that describes how rapidly health events such as new diagnoses of cases or deaths are occurring in a population of interest. Synonyms: **hazard**, **incidence density**.

Concept of a Rate

The concept of a rate is not as easily understood as risk, and is often confused with risk. Loosely speaking, a rate is a measure of how quickly something of interest happens. When we want to know how fast we are traveling in our car, how quickly the stock market prices are increasing, or how steadily the crime rate is decreasing, we are seeking a rate.

Suppose we are taking a trip in a car. We are driving along an expressway and we look at our speedometer and see we are going 65 miles per hour. Does this mean that we will cover exactly 65 miles in the next hour? Of course not. The speedometer reading tells us how fast we are traveling at the moment of time we looked at the reading. If we were able to drive exactly this way for the next hour without stopping for gas or a rest or slowing down for heavy traffic, we would cover 65 miles in the next hour. The reading of 65 miles per hour on our speedometer is the velocity at which we are traveling, and velocity is an example of a rate.

Actually, velocity is an example of an **instantaneous rate**, since it describes how fast we are traveling at a particular instant of time. There is another kind of rate, called an **average rate**, which we can also illustrate by continuing our car trip. If we actually traveled along the highway for the next hour and covered 55 miles during that time, the average rate, often called the speed that we traveled over the one-hour period, would be 55.

In epidemiology, we use a rate to measure how rapidly new cases of a disease are developing, or alternatively, how rapidly persons with a disease of interest are dying. As with velocity or speed, we might want to know either the instantaneous rate or the average rate. With epidemiologic data, it is typically easier to determine an average rate than an instantaneous rate. We could hardly expect to have a speedometer-like device that measures how fast a disease is occurring at a particular moment of time in a cohort of subjects. Consequently, in epidemiologic studies, we typically measure the average rate at which a disease is occurring over a period of time.

Because a rate is a measure of how quickly something is occurring, it is always measured in units of time, say, days, weeks, months, or years. This clarifies its interpretation. If we describe a rate of 50 new cases per 10,000 person-years, we mean that an average of 50 cases occurs for every 10,000 years of disease free follow-up time observed on a cohort of subjects. The 10,000 figure is obtained by adding together the follow-up times for all subjects in the cohort.

If the unit of time was *months* instead of *years*, the interpretation of the rate can be quite different. A rate of 50 new cases per 10,000 person months indicates a much quicker rate than 50 new cases per 10,000 person years.

Study Questions (Q4.6)

1. Which of the following rates is *not* equivalent to a rate of 50 new cases per 10,000 person years?
    - A. 100 new cases per 20,000 person years
    - B. 50 new cases per 120,000 person months
    - C. 50 new cases per 52,000 person weeks

2. Determine whether or not each of the following statements describes a rate:

A.	5 new cases per 100 person days	**Yes**	**No**
B.	40 miles per hour	**Yes**	**No**
C.	10 new cases out of 100 disease-free persons	**Yes**	**No**
D.	60 new murders per year	**Yes**	**No**
E.	60 deaths out of 200 clung cancer patients	**Yes**	**No**

Summary

❖ Generally, a rate is a measure of how quickly something of interest is happening

❖ In epidemiology, a rate is a measure of how rapidly new cases of a disease or other outcome develop.

❖ An **instantaneous rate**, like velocity, describes how rapidly disease or death is occurring at a moment in time

❖ An **average rate**, like speed, describes how rapidly disease or death is occurring as an average over a period of time.

❖ In epidemiology, we typically use average rates rather than instantaneous rates.

❖ Rates must be measured in units of time.

Incidence Density- The Concept

The term incidence density (ID) has been proposed by Miettinen to provide an intuitive interpretation of the concept of an **average incidence rate**. The diagram below illustrates incidence density as the concentration (i.e., **density**) of new case occurrences in an accumulation (or *sea*) of person-time. **Person-time (PT)** is represented by the area under the curve **N(t)** that describes number of disease-free persons at time t during a period of follow-up from time T_0 to T_1. Each new case is denoted by a small circle located within the sea of person-time at the time of disease occurrence. The concentration of circles within the sea represents the **density of cases**. The higher the concentration, the higher is the average rate during the period of follow-up.

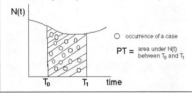

Calculation of a Rate

To calculate a rate, we must follow a cohort of subjects, count the number of new (or incident) cases, **I**, of a disease in that cohort, and compute the total time, called person-time or **PT**, that disease-free individuals in the cohort are observed over the study period. The estimated incidence rate ($\hat{\text{IR}}$) is obtained by dividing **I** by **PT**:

$$\hat{\text{IR}} = \frac{I}{PT}$$

This formula gives an average rate, rather than the more difficult to estimate instantaneous rate. The formula is general enough to be used for any outcome of interest, including death. If the outcome is death instead of disease incidence, the formula gives the **mortality incidence rate** rather than the **disease incidence rate**.

Consider again the following hypothetical cohort of 12 initially disease-free subjects followed over a 5-year period from 1990 to 1995.

From these data, the number of new cases is 5. The total person-time, in this case person-years, is obtained by adding the

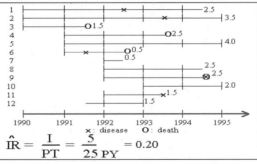

$$\hat{\text{IR}} = \frac{I}{PT} = \frac{5}{25\ PY} = 0.20$$

individual observed disease-free follow-up times this gives a total of 25 person years. The incidence rate is therefore 5 divided by 25 or 0.20, which can be translated as 20 new cases per 100 person years of follow-up.

<u>**Study Questions (Q4.7)**</u>
1. In this example, is the value of 0.20 a proportion?
2. In this example, does the value of 0.20 represent the risk of developing disease?
3. Which of the following rates is not equivalent to a rate of 20 new cases per 100 person years?
   - A. 5 new cases per 25 years
   - B. 40 new cases per 200 person years
   - C. 480 new cases per 2400 person months
   - D. 20 new cases per 1200 person months

Summary
- ❖ A rate is calculated using the formula **I/PT**, where **I** denotes the number of incident cases and **PT** denotes the accumulated person-time of observed follow-up over the study period.
- ❖ This formula gives an average rate, rather than the more difficult to estimate instantaneous rate.
- ❖ A rate is always greater than zero and has no upper bound.
- ❖ The rate is always stated in units of person-time.
- ❖ A rate of .20 cases per person-year is equivalent to 20 cases per 100 person-years as well as 20 cases per 1200 person-months

---

The Big-Mac Assumption about Person-Time

We have seen that the general formula for calculating an **average rate (R)** is:

$$R = \frac{I}{PT}$$

where **I** is the number of new cases and **PT** is the accumulated person-time over a specified period of follow-up. When individually observed follow-up times are available, PT is determined by summing these individual times together for all N subjects in the disease-free cohort.

For example, if 100 persons are each followed for 10 years, then PT=1000 person-years. Also, if 1000 persons are each followed for 1 year, we get PT=1000.

A key assumption about PT is that both of these situations provide equivalent person-time information. In other words, the rate corresponding to a specified value of PT should not be affected by how the total person-time is obtained. We call this assumption the **Big-Mac assumption** because it is similar to assuming that eating 50 fast-food hamburgers costing $2.00 each is equivalent to eating: $100 gourmet meal at the best-rated restaurant in town.

The Big-Mac assumption for PT will not hold, however, if the average time between first exposure and detection of the disease (i.e., the latency) is longer than the average individually observed follow-up time. If so, we would expect the rate to be lower in a large cohort that accumulates the same PT as a smaller cohort with larger individual follow-up times.

For example, if the latency were 2 years, we would expect an extremely low rate for 1000 persons followed for one-year each but a much larger rate for 100 persons followed for two-years each. Individuals in the larger cohort would not be followed long enough to result in many new cases.

Determining Person Time Information

There are a number of ways to determine the person-time denominator in the formula for a rate. As illustrated in the previous section, when individual follow-up times are available on each person in the cohort, the person-time is calculated by summing (Σ) individual follow-up times over the entire disease-free cohort:

$$\hat{IR} = \frac{I}{PT}$$

When individual follow-up times are not available, one method for computing person-time information uses the formula:

$$PT = N^* \times \Delta t$$

where N^* is the average size of the disease-free cohort over the time period of study and Δt is the time length of the study period. This formula is particularly useful if the study cohort is a large population, such as a city, where individual person time information would be very difficult to obtain. For such a large cohort, it would also be difficult to exclude existing cases of the disease at the start of the study period as well as to determine the number of disease-free persons that are not followed for the entire period of study.

Nevertheless, it may be that relatively few persons in the population develop the disease. And, we may be able to assume that the population is a stable dynamic cohort, that is, the population undergoes no major demographic shifts during the time period of interest. If so, the average size of the disease free cohort can be estimated by the size of the entire population based on census data available close to the time period of the study, which is what we have denoted N^* in our person-time formula.

As an example, suppose a stable population of 100,000 men is followed for a period of 5 years, during which time 500 new cases of bladder cancer are detected. The accumulated person-years for this cohort can then be estimated as 100,000 times 5, or 500,000 person-years. Consequently, the average incidence rate for the 5-year period is given by 500 divided by 500,000, or 0.001 per year, or equivalently 1 new case per 1000 person years.

Example
$\hat{IR} = \dfrac{I}{PT} = \dfrac{500}{500,000} = 0.001$ per year
$PT = N^* \times \Delta t$ $= 100,000 \times 5 = 500,000$ person-years
$N^* = 100,000$ men
$\Delta t = 5$ years
$I = 500$ cases

Summary

❖ There are alternative ways to determine person-time information required in the denominator of a rate when individual follow-up times are not available.

❖ One method uses the formula $PT = N^* \times \Delta t$, where N^* denotes the average size of a stable dynamic cohort based on census data available close to the chronological time of the study, and Δt is the time period of the study.

❖ This formula is useful if the study cohort is a large population for which individual person time information would be difficult to obtain.

Incidence Rate of Parkinson's Disease

Parkinson's disease is a seriously disabling disease characterized by a resting tremor, rigidity, slow movements, and disturbed reflexes. A cohort of more than 6,500 Dutch elderly people who did not have Parkinson's disease at the start of the study was followed for six years to determine the incidence rate at which new cases of Parkinson's disease develop. During the follow-up period, 66 participants were diagnosed with Parkinson's disease.

Because Parkinson's disease has a subtle onset, it was difficult to determine exactly when the disease process had begun. Therefore, the investigators calculated the time of onset as the midpoint between the time of diagnosis and the time at which a participant was last known to be free of Parkinson's. They could then calculate the total number of disease-free person-years in this study by adding up the number of person-years that each of the 6,500 participants had contributed to the study until he or she either:

1. Developed Parkinson's disease
2. Died
3. Reached the end of the study period alive without having developed Parkinson's disease.

This resulted in a total of 38,458 disease-free person-years. In this study, the average incidence rate of Parkinson's disease for the 6-year study period is:

66 / 38,458 = 0.0017 cases per person-year

This means that, 1.7 new cases of Parkinson's disease develop per 1,000 person-years.

Study Questions (Q4.8)

1. Using the formula $PT = N^* \times (\Delta t)$, how many person-years would have been computed for this study population had no detailed information on each individual's contribution to the total amount of person-years been available?
2. Using the number of person-years from the previous question, what is the incidence rate?

Summary

❖ A cohort of more than 6,500 Dutch elderly people who did not have Parkinson's disease at the start of the study was followed for six years to determine the rate at which new cases develop.
❖ The results indicate that 1.7 new cases of Parkinson's disease develop for every 1,000 person-years of follow-up.
❖ The person-years calculation used the formula $PT = N^* \times \Delta t$ since there was no detailed information on each individual's person-years.

Quiz (Q4.9) Label each of the following statements as **True** or **False**.

1. Rate is not a proportion   ???
2. Rate has units of 1/person-time, and varies from zero to one.   ???
3. A rate can only be calculated if every person in a cohort is followed individually to count and add up the person-time.   ???
4. Rate can be calculated for a dynamic cohort, but not for a fixed, stable cohort.
                                                                                                          ???

Risk versus Rate

*Incidence can be measured as either **risk** or **rate**. Which of these types to use is an important choice when planning an epidemiologic study.*

We have seen two distinct measures for quantifying disease frequency, risk and rate. **Risk** is a probability, lying between 0 and 1 that gives the likelihood of a change in health status for an individual over a specified period of follow-up.

Rate describes how rapidly new events are occurring in a population. An **instantaneous rate**, which is rarely calculated, applies to a fixed point in time whereas an **average rate** applies to a period of time. A rate is *not* a probability, is always non-negative, has no upper bound (i.e. $0 \leq \text{Rate} \leq \infty$) and is defined in units of time, such as years, months, or days.

When planning an epidemiologic study, which measure do we want to use, risk or rate? The choice depends on the objective of the study, the type of disease condition being considered, the nature of the population of interest, and the information available.

If the study objective is to predict a change in health status for an individual, then risk is required. In particular, risk is relevant for assessing the prognosis of a patient, for selecting an appropriate treatment strategy, and for making personal decisions about health-related behaviors such as smoking, exercise, and diet. By contrast, a rate has no useful interpretation at the individual level.

If the study objective is to test a specific hypothesis about disease etiology, the choice can be either risk or rate depending on the nature of the disease and the way we observe new cases. If the disease is a chronic disease that requires a long period of follow-up to obtain sufficient case numbers, there will typically be considerable loss to follow-up or withdrawals from the study. Consequently, individual observed follow-up times tend to vary considerably. A rate, rather than a risk, can address this problem.

However, if an acute disease is considered, such as an outbreak due to an infectious agent, there is likely to be minimal loss to follow-up, so that risk can be estimated directly. With an acute illness, we are not so much interested in how rapidly the disease is occurring, since the study period is relatively short. Rather, we are interested in identifying the source factor chiefly responsible for increasing individual risk.

If the population studied is a large dynamic population, individual follow-up times, whether obtainable or not, will vary considerably for different subjects, so rate must be preferred to risk. However, if individual follow-up times are not available, even a rate cannot be estimated unless it is assumed that the population size is stable, the disease is rare, and a recent census estimate of the population is available.

Risk is often preferred to rate because it is easier to interpret. Nevertheless, rate must often be the measure of choice because of the problems associated with estimating risk.

Summary

❖ Risk is the probability that an individual will develop a given disease over a specified follow-up period.

❖ Rate describes how rapidly new events are occurring in a population.
❖ Risk must be between 0 and 1 whereas rate is always non-negative with no upper bound, and is defined in units of time.
❖ Risk is often preferred to rate because it is easier to interpret.
❖ Rate must often be the measure of choice because of problems with estimating risk.
❖ The choice of risk versus rate depends on the study objective, the type of disease, the type of population, and the information available.

Quiz (Q4.10) Do the following statements define a **rate**, **risk**, or **both**?

1. More useful for individual decision-making.	???
2. Numerator is number of new cases during a period of follow-up.	???
3. Lowest possible value is zero.	???
4. No upper bound.	???
5. Can be expressed as a percentage.	???
6. Better for studies with variable periods of follow-up.	???
7. Traditionally calculated in the acute outbreak (short follow-up) setting.	???
8. Measures how quickly illness or death occurs in a population.	???
9. Cumulative incidence.	???
10. Measure of disease occurrence in a population.	???

Prevalence

*Prevalence measures existing cases of a health condition and is the primary design feature of a **cross-sectional study**. There are two types of prevalence, **point prevalence**, which is most commonly used, and **period prevalence**.*

In epidemiology, prevalence typically concerns the identification of existing cases of a disease in a population and is the primary design feature of cross-sectional studies. Prevalence can also more broadly concern identifying persons with any characteristic of interest, not necessarily a disease. For example, we may wish to consider the prevalence of smoking, immunity status, or high cholesterol in a population.

The most common measure of prevalence is **point prevalence**, which is defined as the probability that an individual in a population is a case at time **t**, i.e.,

$$\hat{P} = \frac{C}{N} = \frac{(\text{\# of observed cases at time t})}{(\text{Population size at time t})}$$

Point prevalence is estimated as the proportion of persons in a study population that have a disease at a particular point in time (**C**). For example, if there are 150 individuals in a population and, on a certain day, 15 are ill with the flu, the estimated prevalence for this population is 10%, i.e.,

$$\hat{P} = \frac{15}{150} = 10\ \%$$

Study Questions (Q4.11)
1. Is point prevalence a proportion?
2. A study with a large denominator, or one involving rare events, may result in very low prevalence. For example, suppose that 13 people from a population of size 406,245 had a particular disease at time **t**. What is the point prevalence

of this disease at time **t**?

      A. 0.0032   B. 32% C. 0.000032   D. 0.0000032

3. Which of the following expressions is equivalent to the point prevalence estimate of 0.000032?

      A. 3.2 per 1,000   B. 3.2 per 100,000   C. 32 per 100,000

When measuring point prevalence, it is essential to indicate *when* the cases were enumerated by specifying a point calendar time or a fixed point in a time sequence, such as the third post-operative day. Prevalence measures are very useful for assessing the health status of a population and for planning health services. This is because the number of existing cases at any time is a determinant of the demand for healthcare.

However, prevalence measures are not as well suited as incidence measures, such as risk or rate, for identifying risk factors. This is because prevalence concerns only survivors, so that cases that died prior to the time that prevalence is measured are ignored.

PREVALENCE
Useful for:
Assessing the health status of a population.
Planning health services.
Not useful for:
Identifying risk factors.

Summary

❖ Prevalence concerns existing cases of a disease at a point or period of time.

❖ Prevalence measures are primarily estimated from cross-sectional surveys.

❖ Point prevalence is the probability that an individual in a population is a case at time **t**.

❖ Point prevalence is estimated using the formula **P = C/N**, where **C** is the number of existing cases at time **t**, and **N** is the size of the population at time **t**.

❖ Prevalence measures are useful for assessing the health status of a population and for planning health services.

❖ Prevalence measures concern survivors, so they are not well suited for identifying risk factors.

Period Prevalence

An alternative measure to **point prevalence** is **period prevalence (PP)**, which requires the assumption of a stable dynamic population for estimation. **PP** is estimated as the ratio of the number of persons **C*** who were observed to have the health condition (e.g., disease) anytime during a specified follow-up period, say from times T_0 to T_1, to the size **N** of the population for this same period, i.e., the formula for period prevalence is:

$$PP = \frac{C^*}{N} = \frac{C + I}{N}$$

where **C** denotes the number of prevalent cases at time T_0 and **I** denotes the number of incident cases that develop during the period. For example, if we followed a population of 150 persons for one year, and 25 had a disease of interest at the start of follow-up and another 15 new cases developed during the year, the period prevalence for the year would be:

  PP = (25 + 15)/ 150 = .27, or 27%,

whereas the estimated point prevalence at the start of the period is:

  P = 25/150 = .17, or 17%

and the estimated cumulative incidence for the one year period is:

  CI = 15/125 = .12, or 12%

Quiz (Q4.12) Label each of the following statements as **True** or **False**
1. Prevalence is a more useful measure for health planning than for etiologic research.   **???**
2. Like cumulative incidence, prevalence is a proportion that may range from zero to one.   **???**
3. Prevalence measures are most commonly derived from follow-up studies. **???**
4. Whereas incidence usually refers to occurrence of illness, injury, or death, prevalence may refer to illness, disability, behaviors, exposures, and genetic risk factors.   **???**
5. The formula for point prevalence is:
   a. # new cases / # persons in population
   b. # new cases / # persons who did not have the disease at the starting point of observation
   c. # new cases / # person-time of follow-up
   d. # current cases / # persons in population
   e. # current cases / # persons who did not have the disease at the starting point of observation
   f. # current cases / # person-time of follow-up

Mortality

As with incidence measures of disease frequency, incidence measures of mortality frequency can take the form of **risk** or **rate** depending on the study design and the study goals. Mortality risk can be measured in a number of ways, including **disease-specific mortality risk, all-causes mortality risk,** and **case-fatality risk.** For each measure, the formula for simple cumulative incidence can be used. Here, **I** denotes the number of deaths observed over a specific study period in an initial cohort of size **N.**

Mortality Risk
Disease-Specific Mortality Risk
All-Causes Mortality risk
Case-Fatality Risk
$CI = \dfrac{I \;\text{(number of deaths)}}{N \;\text{(size of cohort)}}$

Study Questions (Q4.13)
1. For a **disease-specific mortality risk**, what does the **I** in the formula **CI=I/N** represent. **???**
   A. The number of deaths from all causes
   B. The number of deaths due to the specific disease of interest
   C. The number of persons with a specific disease
   D. The size of the initial cohort regardless of disease status

Answer: For estimating disease-specific mortality risk, **I** is the number of deaths due to the specific disease of interest, and **N** is the size of the initial cohort regardless of disease status.

Study Questions (Q4.13) continued

2. For **all-causes mortality risk**, what does the **I** in the formula **CI=I/N** represent. **???**
   A. The number of deaths from all causes
   B. The number of deaths due to the specific disease of interest
   C. The number of persons with a specific disease
   D. The size of the initial cohort regardless of disease status

Answer: **I** is the number of deaths from all causes, and **N** is the size of the initial cohort, regardless of disease status.

Case-fatality risk is the proportion of people with a disease who die from that disease during the study period.

Study Questions (Q4.13) continued

3. For *case-fatality* risk, what does the **I** in the formula **CI=I/N** represent. **???**
   A. The number of deaths from all causes
   B. The number of deaths due to the specific disease of interest
   C. The number of persons with a specific disease
   D. The size of the initial cohort regardless of disease status

Answer: **I** is the number of persons who die from the given disease, and **N** is the number of persons with this disease in the initial cohort.

In a similar way, **mortality rate** can be measured using the general formula for average rate: **IR = I/ PT.** Here, **I** denotes the number of deaths observed over a specified study period in an initial cohort that accumulates person-time **PT.** For estimating disease-specific mortality rate, **PT** is the person-time for the initial cohort, regardless of disease condition. For estimating **all-cause mortality rate**, **PT** again is the person-time for initial cohort, regardless of disease condition.

For estimating **case-fatality rate**, **PT** is the person time for an initial cohort of persons *with the specific disease of interest* that is followed to observe mortality status.

As an example of the calculation of mortality risk estimates, suppose you observe an initial cohort of 1000 persons aged 65 or older for three years. One hundred out of the 1000 had lung cancer at the start of follow-up, and 40 out of these 100 died from their lung cancer. In addition, 15 persons developed lung cancer during the follow-up period and 10

Mortality		
Start	Follow-up	Died
100 LC ————		————40
1000 persons	15 LC ————	——10
Age: 65+ 900 no LC ——<		
3 years	885 no LC	——150
Total 1000		200

Lung-cancer specific mortality risk $= \dfrac{40+10}{1000} = 5\%$

All-cause mortality risk $= \dfrac{200}{1000} = 20\%$

Case-fatality risk $= \dfrac{40}{100} = 40\%$

died. Of the remaining 885 persons without lung cancer, 150 also died.

- The lung-cancer specific mortality risk for this cohort is 50/1000 or 5%.
- The all-cause mortality risk is 200/1000 or 20%, and
- The case-fatality risk for the 100 lung cancer patients in the initial cohort is 40/100 or 40%.

Study Questions (Q4.14) For the lung cancer example just presented, answer the following questions:
1. From the data, what is the estimated risk for the incidence of lung cancer over the three-year period?
2. Why is the estimated incidence of lung cancer (LC) different from the estimated LC mortality of 5%?
3. Under what circumstances would you expect the LC incidence and LC mortality risk to be approximately equal?

Summary
❖ Incidence measures of mortality frequency can take the form of risk or rate depending on the study design and the study goals.
❖ Mortality risk or rate can be measured in a number of ways, including disease-specific mortality risk or rate, all-causes mortality risk or rate, and case-fatality risk or rate.
❖ For measuring mortality risk, the formula used for simple cumulative incidence, namely, $CI = I / N$, can be used.
❖ Similarly, mortality rate can be measured using the general formula for average rate, namely $IR = I / PT$.

Quiz (Q4.15)
During the past two years, a total of exactly 2,000 residents died in a retirement community with a stable, dynamic population of 10,000 persons.
1. Given these data, the best choice for measure of mortality is the mortality rate. **???**
2. Since mortality is often expressed per 1,000, one could express this mortality measure as 200 per 1,000 per year. **???**
3. The disease-specific mortality risk is the number of deaths attributable to a particular disease, divided by the number of persons with that disease. **???**
4. The denominator for the all-cause mortality risk and the cause-specific mortality risk is the same. **???**
5. The denominator for case-fatality risk is the numerator of the prevalence of the disease. **???**

Age-adjusted rate

Most epidemiologic studies involve a comparison of measures of disease frequency among two or more groups. For example, to study the effect of climate conditions on mortality, we might compare mortality risks or rates in two or more locations with different climates. Let's focus on two U.S. states, Arizona and Alaska. This would allow a comparison of mortality in a cold, damp climate with mortality in a hot dry climate.

The crude mortality rates for these two states for the year 1996 were:
Alaska   426.57 deaths per 100,000 population
Arizona   824.21 deaths per 100,000 population

You might be surprised, particularly considering the climates of the two states, that Arizona's death rate is almost twice as high as Alaska's. Does that mean that it's far more hazardous to live in Arizona than Alaska?

Study Question (Q4.16)
1. What do you think? Is if far more hazardous to live in Arizona than Alaska?

A little knowledge of the demographic make-up of these two states might cause you to question such an interpretation. Look at the age distribution of the two states:

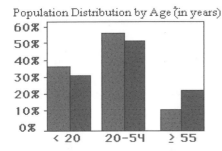

(Note: Alaska is the left bar for each of the clustered bars, Arizona the right bar.)

Study Questions (Q4.16) continued
2. Which population is older?
3. Why should we expect relatively more deaths in Arizona than in Alaska?

The variable age in this situation is called a **confounder** because it distorts the comparison of interest. We should correct for such a potentially misleading effect. One popular method for making such a correction is **rate adjustment**. If the confounding factor is age, this method is generally called **age-adjustment**, and the corrected rates are called **age-adjusted rates**.

The goal of age adjustment is to modify the crude rates so that any difference in mortality rates of Alaska and Arizona cannot be explained by the age differences in the two states. The most popular method of rate adjustment is the **direct method**. This method forces the comparison of the two populations to be made on a **common age distribution**. The confounding factor age is removed by re-computing the rates substituting a common age distribution for the separate age distributions. The two populations are then compared as if they had the same age structure.

The common age distribution is determined by identifying a **standard population**. A logical choice here would be the 1996 total United States population. Other choices for the standard are also possible and usually won't make a meaningful difference in the comparison of adjusted rates.

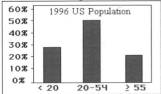

(**Note:** The actual calculation of the age-adjusted rates is not shown here. For details on the calculation of the age-adjusted rates for this example, click on the asterisk on Lesson page 4-4 of the CD-ROM or see the example at the end of this chapter.)

The age-adjusted death rates obtained from using the direct adjustment method with the 1996 US population as the standard are shown here together with the crude rates:

	Alaska	Arizona
Age-adjusted rates	856.00 / 100,000	832.21 / 100,000
Crude rates	426.57 / 100,000	824.21 / 100,000

When we remove age as a factor, the age-adjusted death rate in Arizona is actually lower than in Alaska.

Study Questions (Q4.17)

1. How do we interpret these new age-adjusted results?
2. Based on these results, how do you think the age distribution of Alaska compares to that of the 1996 US population?
3. How do you think the age distribution of Arizona compares to that of the 1996 US population?

Summary

❖ Comparing crude rates for two or more groups may be misleading because such rates do not account for the effects of confounding factors.
❖ If the confounding factor is age, this method is called age-adjustment, and the corrected rates are called age-adjusted rates.
❖ The goal of age adjustment is to modify the crude rates so that any difference in rates cannot be explained by age distribution of the comparison groups.
❖ The direct method of age-adjustment re-computes the rates by substituting a common age distribution for the separate age distributions of the groups being compared.
❖ The common age distribution is determined by identifying a standard population.

Terminology about Adjustment

The rates described for Alaska and Arizona are actually **risks**. We have purposely used the term **rates** in this example to conform to the terminology typically used in published reports/papers that carry out **age adjustment**. In any case, the procedure used for (age) adjustment can be applied to any measure of disease frequency: risk, rate and/or prevalence.

Moreover, potential confounding factors of interest other than age, e.g., race and sex, can also be adjusted, both individually and simultaneously. We generally use the term **rate adjustment** to describe adjustment involving any type or number of confounding factors and any type of measure of disease frequency, whether a risk, rate, or prevalence.

Age-Adjustment – The Steps

The method of direct **age-adjustment** involves the following steps:

1. Select a **standard population** whose age structure is known. By convention, the standard distribution used for age-adjustment of mortality rates in the United States is the US age distribution in the year closest to the year of the rates being compared.
2. Multiply the age-specific mortality rates for each group being compared by the corresponding age-specific numbers of persons in the standard population. The result is the expected number of deaths in each group.
3. Sum the expected numbers of deaths within each age group to yield a total number of expected deaths for each group being compared.
4. Divide the total number of expected deaths in each group by the total size of the standard population to yield summary **age-adjusted mortality rates**.

An asterisk on lesson page 4-4 of the ActivEpi CD ROM provides a worked example of direct adjustment by comparing mortality rates for Alaska and Arizona in 1996.

Quiz (Q4.18)   Label each of the following statements as **True** or **False**
1. Age-adjustment is a method to eliminate disparities in age between two populations.   **???**
2. Age-adjustment always brings two disparate rates closer together   **???**
3. When age-adjusting, one should use the U.S. population as the standard population.   **???**
4. Age-adjustment can be used for one rate, two rates, or many rates.   **???**
5. If the age distributions of two populations are very similar, their age-adjusted rates will also be similar.   **???**
6. If the age distributions of two populations are very similar, the comparison of the age-adjusted rates will not be very different from the comparison of the crude rates.   **???**

In the early 1990s, 7,983 elderly Dutch men and women were included in a prospective cohort study. The investigators computed how many person-years each participant had contributed to the study until January 2000. The total was 52,137 person-years. During follow-up, 2,294 of the participants died, and of these, 477 were due to coronary heart disease.
7. What is the all-cause mortality rate in this population? **???** per 1000 person-years.
8. What is the coronary heart disease-specific mortality rate? **???** per 1000 person-years

Choices   2294   44   477   9.1

The crude all-cause mortality rate for men was 47.4 per 1000 person-years (PY) and for women was 41.9 per 1000 person-years. After making the age distribution in the women comparable to the age distribution in men (by standardizing the rates using the age distribution of the men), the mortality rate for women was only 27.8 per 1000 PY.

9. Based on these figures, the women must be considerably **???** than the men in this population.

Choices   older   younger

Nomenclature

C	Number of prevalent cases at time T
C*	C + I (number of prevalence cases at time T plus incident cases during study period)
CI	Cumulative incidence ("risk"): CI=I/N
D	Duration of disease
I	Incidence
IR	Incidence rate ("rate"): IR=I/PT
N	Size of population under study
P	Prevalence: P=C/N
PP	Period prevalence: PP=C*/N
PT	Person-time
R	Average rate
T or t	Time

References

General References

Greenberg RS, Daniels SR, Flanders WD, Eley JW, Boring JR. Medical Epidemiology (3rd Ed). Lange Medical Books, New York, 2001.

Kleinbaum DG, Kupper LL, Morgenstern H. Epidemiologic Research: Principles and Quantitative Methods. John Wiley and Sons Publishers, New York, 1982.

Ulm K. A simple method to calculate the confidence interval of a standardized mortality ratio (SMR). Am J Epidemiol 1990;131(2):373-5.

References on Rates

Miettinen O. Estimability and estimation in case-referent studies. Am J Epidemiol 1976;103(2):226-35

Giesbergen PCLM, de Rijk MC, van Swieten JC, et al. Incidence of parkinsonism and parkinson's disease in a general population: the Rotterdam Study. Am J Epidemiol (in press).

References on Age-Adjustment

Dawson-Saunders B, Trapp RG. Basic and Clinical Biostatistics, 2nd ed., Appleton and Lange, Stamford, CN, 1994.

Woodward M. Epidemiology: Study Design and Analysis, Chapter 4, pp. 157-167, Chapman and Hall, Boca Raton, FL, 1999.

Reference for Prevalence and Incidence of HIV:

Horsburgh CR, Jarvis JQ, McArthur T, Ignacio T, Stock P. Serconversion to human immunodeficiency virus in prison inmates. Am J Public Hlth 1990;80(2):209-210.

Answers to Study Questions and Quizzes

Q4.1

1. Incidence – Here we are interested in the number of new cases after eating the potato salad.
2. Prevalence – Here we are interested in the number of existing cases.
3. Incidence – Here we are interested in the number of new cases that occur during the follow-up.
4. Incidence – Here we are interested in the number of new deaths attributed to the hurricane.
5. Prevalence – Here we are interested in the existing number of children who have immunity to measles.
6. Incidence – Since rabies has a short duration, we would expect the prevalence on a particular day to be low relative to the incidence.
7. Prevalence – The incidence of multiple sclerosis would be low, but since it has a long duration, we would expect the prevalence to be higher.
8. Incidence – The incidence of influenza would be high, but since it is of short duration the prevalence would be low.
9. Incidence – Since the duration of poison ivy is relatively short the prevalence would be low, and since it is a common occurrence, the incidence would be high.
10. Prevalence – Since high blood pressure is common and of long duration, both incidence and prevalence are high, but the prevalence would be higher.

Q4.2

1. The statement means that a 45-year-old male free of prostate cancer has a probability of .05 of developing prostate cancer over the next 10 years if he does not die from any other cause during the follow-up period.
2. Smaller, because the 5-year risk involves a shorter time period for the same person to develop prostate cancer.

Q4.3

1. No, subjects should be counted as new cases if they were disease-free at the start of follow-up and became a case at any time during the follow-up period specified.
2. Yes, there is a problem, since a subject followed for 2 years does not have the same opportunity for developing the

disease as a subject followed for 4 years.
3. No, but we must assume that subjects who do not develop the disease have the same follow-up time. Otherwise, we can get a misleading estimate of CI because not all subjects will have the same opportunity to develop the disease over the follow-up period.

Q4.4
1. Dynamic
2. Subject 2
3. Subject 7
4. Subject 9
5. Subject 3
6. Subject 5
7. 5/12=42%
8. 4/12=33%
9. D
10. No
11. No
12. Yes
13. Yes
14. Yes
15. No
16. Yes

Q4.5
1. 30/97
2. 60/97
3. 90/95
4. True – The numerator of the CI formula is a subset of the denominator.
5. True – Because the incubation period is short, subjects are not likely to be lost to follow-up.
6. True – The long incubation period means subjects are likely to be lost to follow-up, and hence cases may not be detected. For a dynamic cohort, the denominator in the CI formula does not reflect the continually changing population size.
7. False – the estimated CI will underestimate the true risk of disease.

Q4.6
1. C
2. a. Yes
   b. No
   c. Yes
   d. No

Q4.7
1. No, the denominator of 25 does not describe 25 persons, but rather the accumulated follow-up time for 12 persons.
2. No, the risk in this example would be calculated as 5/12 or 0.42. However, using risk would be questionable here because different subjects have different follow-up times.
3. C

Q4.8
1. N* is the average size of the disease-free cohort and Δt is the time length of the study period. Therefore, a rough estimate of the total amount of person-years contributed by the study is 6,500 *6 = 39,000 person-years.
2. The incidence rate is 66/39,000 = 0.0017, or 1.7 per 1,000 person-years.

Q4.9
1. True – For questions 1 & 2: a rate can range from 0 to infinity, whereas a risk (which is a proportion) ranges from 0 to 1 (or 0% to 100%).
2. False
3. False – There are alternative ways to calculate person-time information when individual follow-up time is unavailable.
4. False – A rate can be calculated for either a dynamic cohort or fixed cohort, depending on the person-time information available.

Q4.10
1. Risk
2. Both
3. Both
4. Rate
5. Risk
6. Rate
7. Risk
8. Rate
9. Risk
10. Both

Q4.11
1. Yes, its value can range from 0 to 1 and it is often expressed as a percentage
2. C. The prevalence of disease is 13/406,245 = 0.000032
3. B. 3.2 per 100,000 is an equivalent expression and is easier to interpret

Q4.12
1. True – Prevalence considers existing cases rather than incident cases.

2. True – Since the numerator is contained in the denominator, prevalence is a proportion and must range from 0 to 1 (or 0% to 100%).
3. False – Cross-sectional studies are carried out at essentially a single (or short) point in time.
4. True – Prevalence may concern a health outcome or any other characteristic of a subject.
5. d

Q4.13
1. B   2. A   3. B

Q4.14
1. The estimate of LC incidence is calculated as CI = 15/900 = .017 or 1.7%
2. The 5% mortality estimate counts the 40 prevalent LC cases and does not count the 5 new LC cases that did not die. Furthermore, the denominators are different.
3. The LC incidence and mortality risks would be about equal if the disease was quickly fatal, so that there would be few if any prevalent cases in the initial cohort and all new cases would have died before the end of follow-up.

Q4.15
1. True   2. True
3. False – The denominator of a disease-specific mortality risk is the size of the initial cohort regardless of disease status.
4. True   5.True

Q4.16
1. The two rates are crude rates because they represent the overall mortality experience in 1996 for the entire population of each state. Crude rates do not account for any differences in these populations on factors such as age, race, or sex that might have some influence on mortality. Without consideration of such factors, it would be premature to make such a conclusion.
2. Arizona. The dry, warm climate of Arizona attracts many older persons than does Alaska.
3. There are relatively older persons living in Arizona, and older persons are at high risk of dying.

Q4.17
1. Controlling for any age differences in the two populations, the overall mortality rate is higher in Alaska with a cold, damp climate, then in Arizona where the climate is warm and dry.
2. The population of Alaska must be much younger than the US population since the age-adjusted rate was so much higher than the crude rate.
3. The rate for Arizona did not change much from crude to adjusted because Arizona's age distribution was only slightly younger than that of the entire US in 1996.

Q4.18
1. True – If age-adjustment is not used, then a difference in risk or rates between two populations may be primarily due to age differences in the two populations.
2. False – There is no guarantee that two adjusted measures will be either closer or further from each other than were corresponding crude measures.
3. False – The choice of standard population depends on the characteristics of the populations being considered.
4. True – There is no limitation on the number populations that could be age-adjusted.
5. False – For questions 5 & 6: If the crude rates are quite different whereas the age distributions are similar, then the adjusted rates are likely to be quite different.
6. True
7. 44
8. 9.1
9. older – Women must be older than men in this case. The mortality rate drops substantially in women when we standardize the rate using the age distribution of men. In other words, if we take age out of the picture, the rates for women drop. If the women were younger we would expect to see the adjusted rate increase once we remove age as a factor.

CHAPTER 5

WHAT'S THE ANSWER? MEASURES OF EFFECT

*In epidemiologic studies, we compare disease frequencies of two or more groups using a **measure of effect**. We will describe several types of measures of effect in this chapter. The choice of measure typically depends on the study design being used.*

Ratio Versus Difference Measures of Effect

Our focus in Chapter 5 is on ratio measures of effect, which are of the form M_1/M_0, where M_1 and M_0 are two measures of disease frequency, e.g., risks, rates, or prevalences that are being compared.

We consider difference measures of effect, which are of the form M_1-M_0, in Chapter 6 on "Measures of Potential Impact". Difference measures are also called measures of attributable risk.

Ratio measures are typically used in epidemiologic studies that address the etiology of a disease/health outcome, whereas difference measures are used to quantify the public health importance of factors that are determinants of a disease/health outcome.

Smoking and Lung Cancer

Cigarette smoking became increasingly popular in America after World War I when cigarettes were handed out to soldiers as a way to boost morale. But along with the rise in smoking, came a disturbing rise in the lung cancer rate and some early warnings from a handful of doctors about possible dangers of smoking. Early studies in the 1930s and 1940s of the possible relationship between smoking and lung cancer were **case-control studies**. It became quite apparent that lung cancer patients smoked much more than controls. In one study in particular, lung cancer patients were 17 times more likely than controls to be two-pack-a-day smokers.

In the early 1950s, doctors Horn and Hammond of the American Cancer Society conducted one of the first **cohort studies** on the harmful effects of smoking. About 200,000 people were given a smoking questionnaire and then followed for four years. Death rates and cause of death for smokers and for non-smokers were compared. The preliminary study published in 1958 caused quite a sensation. It was the largest study on smoking that had been done, and it showed that smokers were ten times more likely than nonsmokers to get lung cancer.

Both the cohort and case-control studies attempted to assess the proposed relationship between smoking and lung cancer by deriving a measure of effect that quantified the extent of this relationship. The measure described in the **case-control study** is called an **odds ratio**. The measure described in the **cohort study** is called a **risk ratio**. The activities that follow discuss these two fundamental measures of effect.

Summary
❖ The odds ratio and the risk ratio are two fundamental measures of effect.
❖ These measures were used in epidemiologic studies of the relationship between smoking and lung cancer.

❖ The odds ratio is typically the measure of effect used in case-control studies.
❖ The risk ratio is typically the measure of effect used in cohort studies.

The Risk Ratio

The table below summarizes the results of a five-year follow-up study to determine whether or not smokers who have had a heart attack will reduce their risk for dying by quitting smoking. A cohort of 156 heart attack patients was studied, all of whom were regular smokers up to the time of their heart attack. Seventy-five of these patients continued to smoke after their attack. The other 81 patients quit smoking during their recovery period. Of the 75 patients that continued smoking, 27 died, so the proportion of these patients that died is 0.36.
Of the 81 patients who quit smoking, 14 died, so the corresponding proportion is 0.17. These proportions estimate the five-year risks of dying for these two groups of patients. We may wonder whether those heart attack patients who continue smoking are more likely to die within 5 years after their first heart attack than those who quit.

Heart Attack Patients			
	Smoke	**Quit**	**Total**
Death	27	14	41
Survival	48	67	115
Total	75	81	156

5-year risks of dying

continuing smokers: $27/75 = 0.36$

smokers who quit: $14/81 = 0.17$

A measure of effect gives a numerical answer to this question. Such a measure allows us to make a comparison of two or more groups, in this case, continuing smokers and smokers who quit. For follow-up studies such as described here, the typical measure of effect is a **risk ratio**. To calculate a risk ratio, we take the ratio of the two risks being compared, that is, we simply divide one risk by the other. Actually, we are getting an "estimate" of the risk ratio, which we indicate by putting a "hat" symbol over the RR notation. $\hat{R}R$ is an estimate because we are using two estimates of risk based on samples from the two groups being compared. In our example, therefore, we divide 0.36 by 0.17 to get 2.1.

$$\text{Estimated } \hat{R}R = \frac{\text{Estimated Risk for continuing smokers}}{\text{Estimated Risk for smokers who quit}} = \frac{0.36}{0.17} = 2.1$$

The estimated risk ratio of 2.1 tells us that continuing smokers are about twice as likely to die as smokers who quit. In other words, for heart attack patients the five-year risk for continuing smokers is about twice the corresponding risk for smokers who quit.

Study Questions (Q5.1) Using the five-year follow-up study comparing mortality between smokers and quitters example:
1. How would you interpret a Risk Ratio of 4.5?
2. What if the Risk Ratio was 1.1?
3. How about if the Risk Ratio was less than 1, say 0.5?
4. How would you interpret a value of 0.25?

If our estimated risk ratio had been 1.1, we would have evidence that the risk for continuing smokers was essentially equal to the risk for smokers who quit. We call a risk ratio of 1 the **null value** of the risk ratio. This is the value that we get for the risk ratio when there is no effect, that is, the effect is null.

Summary
❖ The risk ratio (RR) is the ratio of the risk for one group, say group 1, to the risk for another group, say group 0.
❖ The value of RR can be greater than one, equal to one, or less than one.
❖ If the RR is greater than one, the risk for group 1 is larger than the risk for group 0.
❖ If the RR is below one, the risk for group 1 is less than the risk for group 0.
❖ And, if the RR is equal to 1, the risks for group 1 and 0 are equal, so that there is no effect of being in one group when compared to the other.

Risk Ratio Numerator and Denominator

In general, the risk ratio that compares two groups is defined to be the risk for one group divided by the risk for the other group. It is important to clearly specify which group is in the numerator and which group is in the denominator.

If, for example, the two groups are labeled group 1 and group 0, and the risk for group 1 is in the numerator, then we say that the risk ratio compares group 1 to group 0. On the other hand, if the risk for group 0 is in the numerator, then we say that the risk ratio compares group 0 to group 1.

Quiz (Q5.2) For heart attack patients, the risk ratio is defined to be the risk for continuing smokers divided by the risk for smokers who quit. For the following scenarios what would be the risk ratio?

1. Continuing smokers are twice as likely to die as smokers who quit. <u>???</u>
2. Continuing smokers are just as likely to die as smokers who quit. <u>???</u>
3. Smokers who quit are twice as likely to die as continuing smokers. <u>???</u>

Choices   <u>0</u>   <u>0.1</u>   <u>0.2</u>   <u>0.5</u>   <u>1</u>   <u>2</u>

Let's consider the data from a randomized clinical trial to assess whether or not taking aspirin reduces the risk for heart disease. The exposed group received aspirin every other day whereas the comparison group received a placebo. A table of the results is shown below.

		Aspirin		Placebo		Total
		n	Column %	n	Column %	
Developed	Yes	104	(1.04)	189	(2.36)	293
Heart Disease	No	9,896	(98.96)	7,811	(97.64)	17,707
	Total	10,000	(100.00)	8,000	(100.00)	18,000

4. The estimated risk for the aspirin group is   <u>???</u>
5. The estimated risk for the placebo group is   <u>???</u>
6. The estimated risk ratio that compares the aspirin group to the placebo group is given by   <u>???</u>

Choices   <u>0.0104</u> <u>0.0236</u> <u>0.44</u>   <u>104/189</u>   <u>2.269</u>   <u>98.96/97.64</u>

The Odds Ratio

Epidemiologists in the Division of Bacterial Diseases at CDC, the Centers for Disease Control and Prevention in Atlanta, investigate the sources of outbreaks caused by eating contaminated foods. For example, a case-control study was carried out to determine the source of an outbreak of diarrheal disease at a Haitian Resort Club from November 30 to December 8, 1984.

The investigators wondered whether eating raw hamburger was a primary source of the outbreak. Because this is a **case-control study** rather than a follow-up study, the study design starts with **cases**, here, persons at the resort who had diarrhea during the time period of interest. The **controls** were a random sample of 33 persons who stayed at the resort but

	Raw Hamburger Ate	Did not eat	Total
Cases	17	20	37
Controls	7	26	33
Total	24	46	70

Proportion of cases: $17/37 = 0.46$
Proportions of controls: $7/33 = 0.21$

did not get diarrhea during the same time period. There were a total of 37 cases during the study period. All 37 cases and the 33 controls were interviewed by a team of investigators as to what foods they ate during their stay at the resort.

Of the 37 cases, 17 persons ate raw hamburger, so that the proportion of the cases that ate raw hamburger is 0.46. Of the 33 controls, 7 ate raw hamburger, so the corresponding proportion is 0.21. We may wonder, then, whether these data suggest that eating raw hamburger was the source of the outbreak.

Because this is a case-control study rather than a follow-up study, these proportions do not estimate risks for cases and controls. Therefore, we can**not** compute a risk ratio. So, then, what measure of effect should be used in case-control studies? The answer is the **odds ratio (OR)**, which is described in the next section.

Summary

❖ A case-control study was used to investigate a foodborne outbreak at a Caribbean resort.
❖ In a case-control study, we cannot estimate risks for cases and controls.
❖ Consequently, we cannot use the risk ratio (RR) as a measure of effect, but must use the odds ratio (OR) instead.

Why can't we use a risk ratio in case-control studies?

In a case-control study, we cannot estimate risk, but rather, we estimate **exposure probabilities** for cases and controls. The exposure probability for a case is the probability that a subject is exposed given that he/she is a case; this is not equivalent to the probability that a subject is a case given that he/she is exposed, which is the risk for exposed.

In other words, using conditional probability notation:
Pr(exposed | case) ≠ Pr(case | **exposed**), where "|" denotes "given".
Similarly the exposure probability for a control is not equivalent to 1 minus the risk for exposed. That is,
Pr(**exposed** | control) ≠ 1 - Pr(case | **exposed**).
The ratio of two exposure probabilities is, unfortunately, not a risk ratio. Therefore, in case-control studies we must use a different measure of effect, namely the odds ratio.

The Odds Ratio (continued)

To understand odds ratios, we must start with the concept of an **odds**. The term **odds** is commonly used in sporting events. We may read that the odds are 3 to 1 against a particular horse winning a race, or that the odds are 20 to 1 against Spain winning the next World Cup, or that the odds are 1 to 2 that the New York Yankees will reach the World Series this year. When we say that the odds against a given horse are 3 to 1, what we mean is that the horse is 3 times more likely to lose than to win.

The odds of an event are easily calculated from its probability of occurrence. The odds can be expressed as **P**, the probability that the event will occur, divided by 1 - P, the probability that the event will not occur.

$$\text{Odds} = \frac{P}{1 - P} = \frac{P(\text{Event will occur})}{P(\text{Event will not occur})}$$

In our horse race example, if P denotes the probability that the horse will lose, then 1 - P denotes the opposite probability that the horse will win. So, if the probability that the horse will lose is 0.75, then the probability that the horse will win is 0.25, and the odds are 3, or 3 to 1.

$$\text{Odds} = \frac{P}{1 - P} = \frac{P(\text{horse will lose})}{P(\text{horse will win})} = \frac{0.75}{0.25} = 3 \text{ or } \frac{3}{1}$$

In the Haitian resort case-control study, recall that the event of interest occurs if a study subject ate raw hamburger, and, if so, we say this subject is **exposed**. The estimated probability of exposure for the cases was 0.46, so the estimated **odds of being exposed for cases** is 0.46 divided by 1 - 0.46:

$$\hat{\text{Odds}}_{\text{Cases}} = \frac{0.46}{1 - 0.46} = .85$$

Similarly, the estimated probability of exposure for controls was 0.21, so the estimated odds for controls is 0.21 divided by 1 - 0.21:

$$\hat{\text{Odds}}_{\text{Controls}} = \frac{0.21}{1 - 0.21} = .27$$

The **estimated odds ratio** for these data is the ratio of the odds for cases divided by the odds for controls, which equals 3.2.

$$\text{Odds Ratio} (\hat{\text{OR}}) = \frac{\hat{\text{Odds}}_{\text{Cases}}}{\hat{\text{Odds}}_{\text{Controls}}} = \frac{.85}{.27} = 3.2$$

How do we interpret this odds ratio estimate? One interpretation is that the **exposure odds for cases** is about 3.2 times the **exposure odds for controls**. Since those who ate raw hamburger are the exposed subjects, the odds that a case ate raw hamburger appear to be about 3.2 times the odds that a control subject ate raw hamburger.

Study Questions (Q5.3)

Using the Haiti case-control study example:
1. How would you interpret an odds ratio of 2.5?
2. What if the odds ratio was 1.1?

3. How about if the odds ratio less than 1, say 0.5?
4. How would you interpret a value of 0.25?

Odds ratios, like risk ratios, can be greater than one, equal to one, or less than one. An odds ratio greater than one says that the exposure odds for cases is **larger** than the exposure odds for controls. An odds ratio below one says that the exposure odds for cases is **less** than the exposure odds for controls. An odds ratio equal to 1 says that the exposure odds for cases and controls are equal.

Summary
❖ The odds of an event can be calculated as P/(1-P) where P is the probability of the event.
❖ The odds ratio (OR) is the ratio of two odds.
❖ In case-control studies, the OR is given by the exposure odds for the cases divided by the exposure odds for controls.
❖ Odds ratios, like risk ratios, can be greater than 1, equal to 1, or less than 1, where 1 is the null value.

Quiz (Q5.4) A causal relationship between cigarette smoking and lung cancer was first suspected in the 1920s on the basis of clinical observations. To test this apparent association, numerous studies were conducted between 1930 and 1960. A classic **case-control study** was done in 1947 to compare the smoking habits of lung cancer patients with the smoking habits of other patients.

1. In this case-control study, it is **???** to calculate the risk of lung cancer among smokers, and thus, the appropriate measure of association is the **???**.

Choices   Not possible odds ratiopossible   risk ratio
Let's consider the data below from this classic case-control study to assess the relationship between smoking and lung cancer. Cases were hospitalized patients newly diagnosed with lung cancer. Controls were patients with other disorders. This 2 x 2 table compares smoking habits for the male cases and controls.

2. The probability of being a smoker among cases is   **???**
3. The probability of being a smoker among controls is   **???**
4. The odds of smoking among cases is   **???**
5. The odds of smoking among controls is   **???**
6. The odds ratio is   **???**

Choices   0.11   1.04   10.50 1296/1357   1350/1357 1350/2646   192.86
            21.25 7/68   9.08

	Cigarette Smoker	Non-Smoker	Total
Cases	1350	7	1357
Controls	1296	61	1357
Total	2646	68	2714

In a case-control study to find the source of an outbreak, the odds ratio for eating coleslaw is defined to be the odds for cases divided by the odds for controls. For the following scenarios what would be the odds ratio?

7. Cases have an odds for eating coleslaw three times higher than controls   **???**
8. Cases have the same odds for eating coleslaw as controls   **???**
9. Controls have three times the odds for eating coleslaw as cases   **???**

Choices   **0**   **0.25**   **0.333**   **1**   **3**   **4**

Calculating the Odds Ratio

This layout for a two by two table provides a more convenient way to calculate the odds ratio. The formula is *a* times *d* over *b* times *c*. It is called the **cross product ratio** formula because it is the ratio of one product that crosses the table divided by the other product that crosses the table.

General Form of the 2 by 2 Table

	Exposure Status		
	Yes	No	Total
Cases	a	b	m_1
Controls	c	d	m_0
Total	n_1	n_0	m

Cross Product Ratio

$$\hat{OR} = \frac{a \times d}{b \times c}$$

To illustrate this formula consider the data from the Haitian resort outbreak. The cross product formula gives us the same result, 3.2, as we obtained originally from the ratio of exposure odds for cases and controls.

Case-control Study: Outbreak of Diarrheal Disease at a Haitian Resort Club

Raw Hamburger

	Yes	No	Total
Cases	a=17	b=20	m_1=37
Controls	c=7	d=26	m_0=33
Total	n_1=24	n_0=46	m=70

Cross Product Ratio

$$\hat{OR} = \frac{a \times d}{b \times c} = \frac{(17)(26)}{(20)(7)} = 3.2$$

$$= \frac{\hat{Odds}_{Cases}}{\hat{Odds}_{Controls}}$$

Study Question (Q5.5)

1. Should we calculate the OR for other foods eaten during the outbreak before we blame raw hamburger as the source?

Although the odds ratio must be computed in case-control studies for which the risk ratio cannot be estimated, the odds ratio can also be computed in follow-up studies. (Note that the OR and RR can also be calculated in randomized clinical trials that have cumulative incidence measures.)

	OR	RR
Case-Control Studies	✓	☒
Follow-up (Cohort)	✓	✓

For example, let us consider the "quit smoking" study for heart attack patients. The study design here is a follow-up study. We previously estimated that the risk for patients who continued to smoke was 2.1 times greater than the risk for those who quit.

Using the cross product formula on these follow-up data

Follow-up (Cohort) Study

	Smoke	Quit	Total
Death	27	14	41
Survival	48	67	115
Total	75	81	156

$$\hat{RR} = \frac{\hat{Risk\ for\ continuing\ smokers}}{\hat{Risk\ for\ smokers\ who\ quit}} = \frac{27/75}{14/81} = \frac{0.36}{0.17} = 2.1$$

$$\hat{OR} = \frac{a \times d}{b \times c} = \frac{(27)(67)}{(14)(48)} = 2.7$$

yields 2.7. The fact that these two numbers (the risk ratio and odds ratio) are not equal should not be surprising, since the risk ratio and odds ratio are two different measures. But the values in this example are not very different. In fact, these two estimates have similar interpretations since they both suggest that there is a moderate relationship between quit smoking status and survival status.

Summary
❖ A convenient formula for the OR is the cross product ratio: (ad)/(bc)
❖ The OR can be estimated in both case-control and follow-up studies using the cross-product formula.

(See below for discussion of how the risk ratio can be approximated by the odds ratio.)

Quiz (Q5.6) To study the relationship between oral contraceptive use and ovarian cancer, CDC initiated the Cancer and Steroid Hormone Study in 1980 (see table below). It was a case-control study.

1. Using the cross product ratio formula, the OR comparing the exposure status of cases versus controls is (93) * (**???**) / (**???**) * (959) which equals **???**.
2. This means that the **???** of **???** among the cases was **???** the **???** of exposure among the **???**.

**Choices 0.23   0.77   1.3   683   86   cases   controls   disease
exposed   exposure   greater than   less than   non-exposed   odds   risk**

	Ever Used OCs	Never Used OCs	Total
Cases	93	86	179
Controls	959	683	1642
Total	1052	769	1821

The Odds Ratio in Different Study Designs

The odds ratio can be computed for both case-control and follow-up (cohort) studies. Because a case-control study requires us to estimate exposure probabilities rather than risks, we often call the odds ratio computed in case-control studies the **exposure odds ratio (EOR)**. In contrast, because a follow-up study allows us to estimate risks, we often call the odds ratio computed from follow-up studies the **risk odds ratio (ROR)**.

Odds Ratio

Case-control studies (exposure probabilities):
Exposure odds ratio (EOR)

Follow-up (Cohort) studies (risks):
Risk odds ratio (ROR)

Cross-sectional studies (prevalences):
Prevalence odds ratio (POR)

The odds ratio can also be computed for cross-sectional studies. Since a cross-sectional study measures prevalence or existing conditions at a point in time, we usually call an odds ratio computed from a cross-sectional study a **prevalence odds ratio (POR)**.

As an example of the computation of a prevalence odds ratio for cross-sectional data, consider these data that were collected from a cross-sectional survey designed to assess the relationship between coronary heart disease and various risk factors, one of which was personality type. For these cross-sectional data, we can use the general cross product ratio formula to compute a prevalence odds ratio. The odds of having a type A personality among those with coronary heart disease is 5 times the odds of those without the disease.

Cross-sectional data (POR):

		Personality Type A	B	Total
CHD	Yes	93	36	129
	No	46	89	135
	Total	139	125	264

Prevalence odds ratio (POR) = ad/bc

$$\hat{POR} = \frac{(93)(89)}{(46)(36)} = 5.0$$

Odds of Type A$_{CHD}$ = 5x Odds of Type A$_{NO\text{-}CHD}$

In general we can use the cross product ratio formula to compute an exposure odds ratio, a risk odds ratio, or a prevalence odds ratio depending on the study design used.

Summary
❖ The OR computed from a case-control study is called the exposure odds ratio (EOR).
❖ The OR computed from a follow-up study is called the risk odds ratio (ROR)
❖ The OR computed from a cross-sectional study is called the prevalence odds ratio (POR)
❖ We can use the general cross-product ratio formula to calculate the EOR, ROR, or POR depending on the study design used.

Does ROR = EOR = POR?
Not necessarily. Although the calculation formula (i.e., ad/bc) is the same regardless of the study design, different values of the estimated odds ratio from a 2 x 2 table might be obtained for different study designs. This is because of the possibility of selection bias (described in Chapter 8). For example, a case-control study that uses prevalent cases could yield a different odds ratio estimate than a follow-up study involving only incident cases.

Quiz (Q5.7) Data is shown below for a cross-sectional study to assess whether maternal cigarette smoking is a risk factor for low birth weight.

1. Calculate the odds ratio that measures whether smokers are more likely than non-smokers to deliver low birth weight babies. OR=**???**
2. This odds ratio estimate suggests that smokers are **???** than non-smokers to have low birth weight babies.
3. This odds ratio is an example of a(n) **???** odds ratio.

Choices   **0.48**   **2.04 2.18**   **exposure**   **less likely**   **more likely**
              prevalence   **risk**

	Smokers	Non-Smokers	Total
Low Birth weight	1,556	14,974	16,530
High Birth weight	694	14,532	15,226
Total	2,250	29,506	31,756

Comparing the Risk Ratio and the Odds Ratio in Follow-up Studies

We have described two widely used measures of effect, the risk ratio and the odds ratio. Risk ratios are often preferred because they are easier to interpret. But, as we have seen, in case-control studies, we cannot estimate risks and must work instead with an exposure odds ratio (EOR). In follow-up studies, however, we have the option of computing both a risk ratio and a risk odds ratio (ROR). Which should we prefer?

It can be shown mathematically that if a risk ratio estimate is equal to or greater than one, then the corresponding risk odds ratio is at least as large as the risk ratio. For example, using the follow-up data for the quit smoking study of heart attack patients, we saw that the estimated risk ratio was 2.1, which is greater than one; the corresponding odds ratio was 2.7, which is larger than 2.1.

Follow-up (Cohort) Studies: RR vs. ROR
If $\hat{RR} \geq 1$, then $\hat{ROR} \geq \hat{RR}$

Quit Smoking Data for Heart Attack Patients

	Smoke	Quit	Total	
Death	27	14	41	$\hat{RR} = 2.1$
Survival	48	67	115	$\hat{ROR} = 2.7$
Total	75	81	156	

$$\text{If } \hat{RR} \geq 1, \text{ then } \hat{ROR} \geq \hat{RR}$$

Similarly if the risk ratio is less than one, the corresponding odds ratio is as small or smaller than the risk ratio. For example, if we switch the columns of the quit smoking table, then the risk ratio is 0.48, which is less than one, and the corresponding odds ratio is 0.37, which is less than 0.48.

If $\hat{RR} \leq 1$, then $\hat{ROR} \leq \hat{RR}$

Quit Smoking Data for Heart Attack Patients

	Quit	Smoke	Total	
Death	14	27	41	$\hat{RR} = 0.48$
Survival	67	48	115	$\hat{ROR} = 0.37$
Total	81	75	156	

$$\text{If } \hat{RR} \leq 1, \text{ then } \hat{ROR} \leq \hat{RR}$$

It can also be shown that if a disease is "rare", then the risk odds ratio will closely approximate the risk ratio. For follow-up studies, this *rare disease assumption* means that the risk that any study subject will develop the disease is small enough so that the corresponding odds ratio and risk ratio estimates give essentially the same interpretation of the effect of exposure on the disease.

Typically a rare "disease", is considered to be a disease that occurs so infrequently in the population of interest that the risk for any study subject is approximately zero. For example, if one out of every 100,000 persons develops the disease, the risk for this population is zero to 4 decimal places. Now that's really rare!

Study Questions (Q5.8)
1. Is a risk of .01 rare?
2. Suppose that for a given follow-up study, the true risk is not considered to be rare. Is it possible for the ROR and RR to be approximately the same?

We can write a formula that expresses the risk odds ratio in terms of the risk ratio:

$$ROR = RR \times f \text{ where } f = \frac{(1 - R_0)}{(1 - R_1)}$$

and R_0 is the risk for the unexposed, R_1 is the risk for the exposed, and $RR = R_1/R_0$

This formula says that the risk odds ratio is equal to the risk ratio multiplied by the factor f, where f is defined as 1 minus the risk for the unexposed group (R_0) divided by 1 minus the risk for the exposed group (R_1). You can see from this equation that if both R_1 and R_0 are approximately 0, then f is approximately equal to one, and the risk odds ratio is approximately equal to the risk ratio.

Study Questions (Q5.9)
1. In the quit smoking example, where R_0 is 0.17 and R_1 equals 0.36, what is f?
2. For this value of f, is the ROR close to the RR?
3. What happens to f if the risks are halved, i.e., $R_0 = 0.17/2 = 0.085$ and $R_1 = 0.36/2 = 0.180$?
4. Are the ROR and RR estimates close for this f?
5. What happens to f if we again halve the risks, so that $R_0 = 0.0425$ and $R_1 = 0.09$?
6. Is the approximation better?
7. Based on your answers to the above questions, how "rare" do the risks have to be for the odds and risk ratios to be approximately equal?

Summary
❖ If an estimate of RR $\geq$ 1, then the corresponding estimate of ROR is at least as large as the estimate of the RR.
❖ If an estimate of RR $\leq$ 1, then the corresponding estimate of ROR is as small or smaller than the estimate of RR.
❖ In follow-up (cohort) studies, the "rare disease assumption" says that the risk for any study subject is approximately zero.
❖ Under the rare disease assumption, the risk odds ratio (ROR) computed in a follow-up study approximates the risk ratio (RR) computed from the same study.

Comparing the RR and the OR in the Rotterdam Study

Osteoporosis is a common disease in the elderly, and leads to an increased risk of bone fractures. To study this disease, a cohort consisting of nearly 1800 postmenopausal women living in Rotterdam, the Netherlands, was followed for four years. The Rotterdam Study investigators wanted to know which genetic factors determine the risk of fractures from osteoporosis. They focused on a gene coding for one of the collagens that are involved in bone formation. Each person's genetic make-up consists of two alleles of this gene, and each allele can have one of two alternative forms, called allele A or allele B. The investigators showed that women with two A alleles had a higher bone mass than women with at least one B allele. They therefore hypothesized that the risk of fractures would be higher in women with allele B.

Of the 1194 women with two A alleles, 64, or 5.36%, had a fracture during follow-up. Of the 584 women with at least one B allele, 47, or 8.05%, had a fracture.

Study Questions (Q5.10)
1. Calculate the risk ratio for the occurrence of fractures in women with at least one B allele compared to women with two A alleles.

Because the risk ratio estimate is greater than 1, we expect the risk odds ratio to be at least as large as the risk ratio.

Study Questions (Q5.10) continued
2. Calculate the risk odds ratio for the occurrence of fractures in women with at least one B allele compared to women with two A alleles.

Note that the risk of fractures is relatively rare in this population; therefore the risk odds ratio is approximately equal to the risk ratio. Recall the formula ROR = RR * f. Here, f is defined as 1 minus the risk in women with two A alleles divided by 1 minus the risk in women with at least one B allele.

$$ROR = RR \times \frac{1 - R(2\ A\ alleles)}{1 - R(1\ B\ allele)}$$

Study Questions (Q5.10) continued
3. Using the formula ROR = RR x f, can you show that we computed the correct risk odds ratio?

In this study, both the risk ratio and the risk odds ratio lead to the same conclusion: women with at least one B allele have a 50% higher chance of fractures than women with two A alleles. The Rotterdam Study investigators concluded that genetic make-up can predispose women to osteoporotic fractures.

Quiz (Q5.11): RR versus OR in follow-up studies A questionnaire was administered to persons attending a social event in which 39 of the 87 participants became ill with a condition diagnosed as salmonellosis. The 2 x 2 table below summarizes the relationship between consumption of potato salad and illness.

1. The risk ratio comparing the exposed to the non-exposed is   ???
2. The odds ratio is   ???
3. Does the odds ratio closely approximate the risk ratio?   ???
4. Do you consider this illness to be "rare"?   ???

Choices   **0.25**   **1.7**   **3.7**   **36.0**   **9.8**   **no**   **yes**

	Exposed	**Non-Exposed**	**Total**
Ill	36	3	39
Well	12	36	48
Total	48	39	87

Let's consider data from a classic study of pellagra. Pellagra is a disease caused by dietary deficiency of niacin and characterized by dermatitis, diarrhea, and dementia. Data comparing cases by gender are shown below.

5. The risk ratio of pellagra for females versus males is (1 decimal place)   <u>???</u>
6. The odds ratio is (to one decimal place)   <u>???</u>
7. Does the odds ratio closely approximate the risk ratio?   <u>???</u>
8. Do you consider this illness to be "rare"?   <u>???</u>

Choices   <u>**1.4**</u>   <u>**2.4**</u>   <u>**2.5**</u>   <u>**24.2**</u>   <u>**no**</u>   <u>**yes**</u>

	Females	Males	Total
Ill	46	18	64
Well	1438	1401	2839
Total	1484	1419	2903

Comparing the RR and OR in Case-Control Studies

We have already seen that, for follow-up studies, if the disease is "rare", then the risk odds ratio will be a close approximation to the risk ratio computed from the same follow-up data. However, in case-control studies, a risk ratio estimate cannot be computed, and an exposure odds ratio must be used instead. So, for case-control data, if the disease is "rare", does the exposure odds ratio approximate the risk ratio that would have resulted from a comparable follow-up study? The answer is yes, depending on certain conditions that must be satisfied, as we will now describe.

This two-way table categorizes lung cancer and smoking status for a cohort of physicians in a large metropolitan city that are followed for 7 years. Forty smokers and twenty non-smokers developed lung cancer. The risk ratio is 2. Also, for this population, the risk odds ratio is equal to 2.02, essentially the same as the risk ratio. Since these are

Cohort of Physicians (7-year follow-up)

	Smoker ?		
	Yes	No	Total
LC	40	20	60
No LC	1960	1980	3940
Total	2000	2000	4000

population measures

$$RR = \frac{40/2000}{20/2000} = 2$$

$$ROR = \frac{40 \times 1980}{1960 \times 20} = 2.02$$

measures of effect for a population, we have not put the hat symbol over the risk ratio and risk odds ratio terms.

We now consider the results that we would expect to obtain if we carried out a case-control study using this cohort as our source population. We will assume that the 7-year follow-up has occurred.

Case-Control Study

	E	not E	Total
(incident) Cases	40	20	60
Controls	30	30	60
Total	70	50	120

We also assume that there exists a comprehensive cancer registry, so that we were able to find all 60 incident cases that developed over the 7year period. These would be our cases in our case-control study. Now suppose we randomly select 60 controls from the source population as our comparison group. Since half of the entire cohort of 4000 physicians was exposed and half was unexposed, we would expect 30 exposed and 30 unexposed out of the 60 controls.

We can use the cross product ratio formula to compute the expected exposure odds ratio, which turns

$$\hat{EOR} = 2.0 \approx \hat{RR} = 2$$

out to be 2. This value for the exposure odds ratio obtained from case-control data is the same that we would have obtained from the risk ratio and the risk odds ratio if we had carried out the follow-up study on this population cohort. In other words, the expected EOR from this case-control study would closely approximate the RR from a corresponding follow-up study, even if the follow-up study was never done!

We may wonder whether the EOR would approximate the RR even if the 60 controls did not split equally into exposed and unexposed groups as expected. This can occur by chance from random selection or if we do a poor job of picking controls. For

$$\hat{EOR} = 1.0 \neq \hat{RR} = 2$$

Case-Control Study

		E	not E	Total
(incident)	Cases	40	20	60
	Controls	40	20	60
	Total	80	40	120

$$\hat{EOR} = 1.0$$

example, suppose there were 40 exposed and 20 unexposed among the controls. Then the estimated exposure odds ratio would equal 1 instead of 2, so in this situation, the EOR would be quite different from the RR obtained from a comparable follow-up study.

What we have shown by example actually reflects an important caveat when applying the rare disease assumption to case-control data. The choice of controls in a case-control study must be representative of the source population from which the cases developed. If not, either by chance or a poor choice of controls, then the exposure odds ratio will not necessarily approximate the risk ratio even if the disease is rare. There is another important caveat for applying the rare disease assumption in a case-control study. The cases must be incident cases, that is, the cases need to include all new cases that developed over the time-period considered for determining exposure status. If the cases consisted only of prevalent cases at the time of case-ascertainment, then a biased estimate may result because the measure of effect would be estimating prevalence rather than incidence.

Summary
❖ In case-control studies, the EOR approximates an RR when the following 3 conditions are satisfied:
1) The rare disease assumption holds
2) The choice of controls in the case-control study must be representative of the source population from which the cases developed.
3) The cases must be incident cases.

Quiz (Q5.12): Understanding Risk Ratio In a case-control study, if the rare disease assumption is satisfied, then:

1. The **???** approximates the **???** provided that there is no **???** in the selection of **???**, and the cases are **???** rather than **???** cases.

Choices	**EOR**	**ROR**	**RR**	**bias**	**cases**	**controls**
	incidence	**prevalent**	**randomness**			

In a community of 1 million persons, 100 cases of a disease were reported, distributed by exposure according to the table below.

2. Calculate the RR. **???**
3. Calculate the ROR **???**
4. Is this a rare disease? **???**

	Exposed	**Non-Exposed**	**Total**
Ill	90	10	100
Well	499,910	499,990	999,900
Total	500,000	500,000	1,000,000

If the exposure status of all one million persons in the study population had not been available, the investigator may have conducted a case-control study. Suppose a random sample of 100 controls were selected.

5. Approximately what percentage of these controls would you expect to be exposed? **???**
6. What is the expected EOR in the case-control study? **???**

Choices   **0.11**   **10**   **50**   **9.00**   **90**   **no**   **yes**

Note: On Lesson Page 5-3 of the ActivEpi CD-ROM, there is an activity (and corresponding asterisk) that provides a mathematical proof of the odds ratio approximation to the risk ratio in case control studies. This proof makes use of conditional probability statements and Bayes Theorem.

The Rate Ratio

A **rate ratio** is a ratio of two average rates. It is sometimes called an **incidence density ratio** or a **hazard ratio**. Recall the general formula for an average rate: **I** denotes the number of new cases of the health outcome, and **PT** denotes the accumulation of person-time over the follow-up.

The general data layout for computing a rate ratio is shown below. I_1 and I_0 denote the number of new cases in the exposed and unexposed groups, and PT_1 and PT_0 denote the corresponding person time accumulation for these two groups. The formula for the **rate ratio** or the **incidence density ratio (IDR)** is also provided. We have used the notation IDR instead of RR to denote the rate ratio in order to avoid confusion with our previous use of RR to denote the risk ratio.

Average Rate: $\dfrac{I}{PT}$

Layout for computing a Rate Ratio (i.e., IDR)

	Exposed	Unexposed	Total
New Cases	I_1	I_0	I
Person Time	PT_1	PT_0	PT

Rate Ratio:

$$IDR = \frac{\frac{I_1}{PT_1}}{\frac{I_0}{PT_0}}$$

As with both the risk ratio and odds ratio measures, the rate ratio can be >1, <1, or =1. If the rate ratio is equal to 1, it means that there is no relationship between the exposure and disease using this measure of effect.

To illustrate the calculation of a rate ratio, we consider data on the relationship between serum cholesterol level and mortality from a 1992 study of almost 40,000 persons from the Chicago area. The

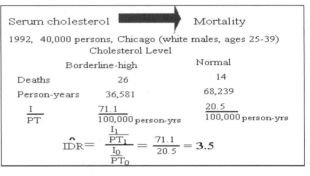

data shown compares white males with borderline-high cholesterol levels and white males with normal cholesterol levels. Subjects, including persons from other race and sex categories, were enrolled into the study between 1967 and 1973, screened for cardiovascular disease (CVD) risk factors, and then followed for an average of 14 to 15 years. There were a total of 26 CHD-related deaths based on 36,581 person-years of follow-up among white males aged 25 to 39 with borderline-high cholesterol at entry into the study. This yields a rate of 71.1 deaths per 100,000 person-years. Among the comparison group there were 14 CHD-related deaths based on 68,239 person-years of follow-up, this yields a rate of 20.5 deaths per 100,000 person-years. Thus, white males aged 25-39 with borderline high cholesterol have 3.5 times the mortality rate as those with normal cholesterol, indicating that persons with even moderately high cholesterol carry an increased risk for CHD mortality.

Summary: Rate Ratio
❖ A ratio of two average rates is called a rate ratio (i.e., an incidence density ratio, hazard ratio)
❖ The formula for the rate ratio (IDR) is given by:

$$IDR = \frac{\dfrac{I_1}{PT_1}}{\dfrac{I_0}{PT_0}}$$

where I_1 and I_0 are the number of new cases and PT_1 and PT_0 are the accumulated person-time for groups 1 and 0, respectively.

❖ As with the RR and the OR, the IDR can be >1, <1, or =1.

Quiz (Q5.13) Data is shown on the next page for a follow-up study to compare mortality rates among diabetics and non-diabetics.

1. The mortality rate for diabetics is   ???
2. The mortality rate for non-diabetics is   ???
3. The rate ratio is   ???

Choices   **13.9   13.9 per 1000 person-years   2.8**
                2.8 per 1000 person-years   38.7   38.7 per 1000 person-years

	Diabetic	Non-diabetic	Total
Dead	72	511	583
Alive	146	3,312	3,458
Person-Years	1,862.4	36,532.2	38,394.6

4. The rate ratio comparing the mortality rates of diabetics with non-diabetics is
   2.8. Which of the following is the correct interpretation of this measure?
   A. Those with diabetes are 2.8 times more likely to die than those without.
   B. People are 2.8 times more likely to die of diabetes than any other illness
   C. Death among diabetics is occurring at a rate 2.8 times that of non-diabetics

Nomenclature

Table setup for cohort, case-control, and prevalence studies:

	Exposed	Not Exposed	Total
Disease/cases	a	b	m_1
No Disease/controls	c	d	m_0
Total	n_1	n_0	n

Table setup for cohort data with person-time:

	Exposed	Not Exposed	Total
Disease (New cases)	I_1	I_0	I
No Disease	-	-	-
Total disease-free person-time	PT_1	PT_0	PT

Δt	Change in time
EOR	Exposure odds ratio; odds of exposure in diseased divided by the odds of exposure in nondiseased
I	Average incidence or total number of new cases
I_0	Number of new cases in nonexposed
I_1	Number of new cases in exposed
IDR	Incidence density ratio; rate in exposed/rate in nonexposed (also called the rate ratio)
N	Size of population under study
N_0	Size of population under study in nonexposed at time zero
N_1	Size of population under study in exposed at time zero
OR	Odds ratio: ad/bc
P	Probability of an event
P(D | E)	Probability of disease given exposed
P(D | not E)	Probability of disease given not exposed
P(E | D)	Probability of exposure given diseased
P(E | not D)	Probability of exposure given not diseased
POR	Prevalence odds ratio; an odds ratio calculated with prevalence data
PT	Disease-free person-time
PT_0	Disease-free person-time in nonexposed
PT_1	Disease-free person-time in exposed
R_0	Risk in unexposed
R_1	Risk in exposed

ROR   Risk odds ratio; an odds ratio calculated from cohort risk data
RR   Risk ratio: risk in exposed divided risk in unexposed
T or t   Time

Formulae

$RR = R_1 / R_0$
$Odds = P / (1-P)$
$Odds\ ratio = ad/bc$
$ROR = RR * f$ where $f=(1-R_0)/(1-R_1)$
$IDR = (I_1/PT_1) / (I_0/PT_0)$

References

Doll R, and Hill AB. Smoking and carcinoma of lungs: preliminary report. Br Med J 1950;2:739-48.

Dyer AR, Stamler J, Shekelle RB. Serum cholesterol and mortality from coronary heart disease in young, middle-aged, and older men and women in three Chicago epidemiologic studies. Ann of Epidemiol 1992;2(1-2): 51-7.

Greenberg RS, Daniels SR, Flanders WD, Eley JW, Boring JR. Medical Epidemiology (3rd Ed). Lange Medical Books, New York, 2001.

Hammond EC, Horn D. The relationship between human smoking habits and death rates. JAMA 1958;155:1316-28.

Johansson S, Bergstrand R, Pennert K, Ulvenstam G, Vedin A, Wedel H, Wilhelmsson C, Wilhemsen L, Aberg A. Cessation of smoking after myocardial infarction in women. Effects on mortality and reinfarctions. Am J Epidemiol 1985;121(6): 823-31.

Kleinbaum DG, Kupper LL, Morgenstern H. Epidemiologic Research: Principles and Quantitative Methods. John Wiley and Sons Publishers, New York, 1982.

Spika JS, Dabis F, Hargett-Bean N, Salcedo J, Veillard S, Blake PA. Shigellosis at a Caribbean Resort. Hamburger and North American origin as risk factors. Am J Epidemiol 1987;126 (6): 1173-80.

Steenland K (ed.). Case studies in occupational epidemiology. Oxford University Press, New York, NY: 1993.

Uitterlinden AG, Burger H, Huang Q, Yue F, McGuigan FE, Grant SF, Hofman A, van Leeuwen JP, Pols HA, Ralson SH. Relation of alleles of the collagen type I alpha1 gene to bone density and the risk of osteoporotic fractures in postmenopausal women. N Engl J Med 1998;338(15):1016-21.

Wynder EL, Graham EA. Tobacco smoking as a possible etiologic factor in bronchogenic carcinoma: a study of six hundred and eighty-four proved cases. JAMA 1950;143:329-36.

Answers to Study Questions and Quizzes

Q5.1

1. The five-year risk for continuing smokers is 4½ times greater than the risk for smokers who quit.
2. The risk ratio is very close to 1.0, which indicates no meaningful difference between the risks for the two groups.
3. Think of an inverse situation.
4. You should have the hang of this by now.

Q5.2

1. 2 2. 1 3. 0.5 4. 0.0104
5. . 0.0236
6. 0.44 – In general, the risk ratio that compares two groups is defined to be the risk for one group divided by the risk for the other group. It is important to clearly specify which group is in the numerator and which group is in the denominator. If, for example, the two groups are labeled *group 1* and *group 0*, and the risk for group 1 is in the numerator, then we say the risk ratio compares group 1 to group 0.

Q5.3
1. The odds that a case ate raw hamburger is about two ½ times the odds that a control subject ate raw hamburger.
2. Because the odds ratio is so close to being equal to one, this would be considered a null case, meaning that the odds that a case ate raw hamburger is about the same as the odds that a control subject age raw hamburger.
3. An odds ratio less than one means that the odds that a case subject ate raw hamburger is less than the odds that a control subject ate raw hamburger.
4. You should have the hang of this by now.

Q5.4
1. Not possible, odds ratio – The risk of disease is defined as the proportion of initially disease-free population who develop the disease during a specified period of time. In a case-control study, the risk cannot be determined.
2. 1350/1357
3. 1296/1357
4. 192.86
5. 21.25
6. 9.08 – In general, the odds ratio that compares two groups is defined to be the odds for the cases divided by the odds for the controls. The odds for each group can be calculated by the formula $P/(1-P)$, where P is the probability of exposure.
7. 3
8. 1
9. 0.333

Q5.5
1. Of course! It is possible, for example, that mayonnaise actually contained the outbreak-causing bacteria and maybe most of the cases that ate raw hamburger used mayonnaise.

Q5.6
1. 683, 86, 0.77
2. odds, exposure, less than, odds, controls – If the estimated odds ratio is less than 1, then the odds of exposure for cases is less than the odds of exposure for controls. If the estimated odds ratio is greater than 1, then the

odds of exposure for cases is greater than the odds of exposure for controls.

Q5.7
1. 2.18
2. more likely
3. prevalence

Q5.8
1. That depends on the disease being considered and on the time-period of follow-up over which the risk is computed. However, for most chronic diseases and short time periods, a risk of .01 is not rare.
2. Yes, because even though the risk may not be rare, it may be small enough so that the ROR and the RR are approximately the same.

Q5.9
1. $f = (1 – 0.17) / (1 – 0.36) = 1.30$
2. No, since for these data, the estimated RR equals 2.1 whereas the estimate ROR equals 2.7.
3. $f = (1 – 0.085) / (1 – 0.180) = 1.12$
4. Yes, since the estimated RR is again 2.1, (0.180/0.085), but the estimated ROR is 2.4.
5. $f=1.05$
6. Yes, since the estimated ROR is now 2.2.
7. In the context of the quit smoking example, risks below 0.10 for both groups indicate a "rare" disease.

Q5.10
1. The risk ratio in this study is 0.0805 divided by 0.0536, which equals 1.50.
2. The risk odds ratio is 47/537 divided by 64/1130 equals 1.54.
3. $f=(1-0.0536) / (1-0.0805) = 1.03$. The ROR = 1.03*RR = 1.03*1.50=1.54.

Q5.11
1. 9.8
2. 36.0
3. No
4. No – The risk ratio that compares two groups is defined to be the risk for one group divided by the risk for the other group. The odds ratio can be calculated by the cross product formula ad/bc. In general, a disease is considered "rare" when the OR closely approximates the RR.
5. 2.44
6. 2.49

7. Yes
8. Yes

Q5.12

1. EOR, RR, bias, controls, incident, prevalent
2. 9
3. 9
4. Yes – A disease is considered rare when the ROR closely approximates the RR.
5. 50
6. 9.00

Q5.13

1. 38.7 per 1000 person-years – The mortality rate for diabetics equals 72/1,862.4 person-years = 38.7 per 1000 person-years.
2. 13.9 per 1000 person-years – The mortality rate for non-diabetics equals 511/36,653.2 person-years = 13.9 per 1000 person-years.
3. 2.8 – The rate ratio is 38.7 per 1000 person-years/13.9 per 1000 person-years = 2.8.
4. C

CHAPTER 6

WHAT IS THE PUBLIC HEALTH IMPACT?

*In the previous chapter on Measures of Effect, we focused exclusively on **ratio measures of effect**. In this chapter, we consider **difference measures of effect** and other related measures that allow the investigator to consider the **potential public health impact** of the results obtained from an epidemiologic study.*

The Risk Difference – An Example

*The **risk difference** is the difference between two estimates of risk, whereas the **risk ratio** is the ratio of two risk estimates. We illustrate a risk difference using a cohort study of heart attack patients who either continue or quit smoking after their heart attack.*

Consider again the results of a five-year follow-up study to determine whether or not smokers who have had a heart attack will reduce their risk for dying by quitting smoking. The estimated risk ratio is 2.1, which means that the risk for continuing smokers was 2.1 times the risk for smokers who quit.

The Risk Difference			
Heart Attack Patients	Smoke	Quit	Total
Death	27	14	41
Survival	48	67	115
Total	75	81	156

Five-year risks of dying
continuing smokers: $27/75 = 0.36$
smokers who quit: $14/81 = 0.17$

Risk Ratio $= 0.36/ 0.17 = 2.1$
Risk Difference $= 0.36 - 0.17 = .19$

We now focus on the difference between the two estimates of risk, rather than their ratio. What kind of interpretation can we give to this difference estimate? The **risk difference (RD)** of 0.19 gives the **excess risk** associated with continuing to smoke after a heart attack. The estimated risk, 0.17, of dying in the quit smoking group is the background or "expected" level to which the risk of 0.36 in the continuing smokers group, is compared.

Study Questions (Q6.1)
1. How many deaths would have occurred among the 75 patients who continued to smoke after their heart attack if these 75 patients had quit smoking instead?
2. How many excess deaths were there among the 75 patients who continued to smoke after their heart attack?
3. What is the proportion of excess deaths among continuing smokers?

The null value that describes "no excess risk" is 0. There would be no excess risk if the two estimated risks were equal. Because the risk difference describes excess risk, it is also called the **attributable risk**. It estimates the additional risk "attributable" to the exposure.

The risk difference, therefore, can be interpreted as the probability that an exposed person will develop the disease because of the additional influence of exposure over the baseline risk. In this example, the five-year attributable risk of 0.19 estimates the probability that continuing smokers will die because they have continued to smoke.

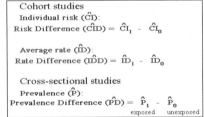

Risk Difference — Prob. that exposed person (Attributable Risk) develops D because of added influence of exposure

Additional Risk from exposure

Baseline Risk - Unexposed

Study Questions (Q6.1) continued
4. If the study involved 1,000 heart attack patients who continued to smoke after their heart attack, how many deaths could be avoided (i.e., attributable to exposure) for a risk difference of 0.19 if all patients quit smoking?
5. How might you evaluate whether the excess risk of 0.19 is clinically (not statistically) excessive
6. Can you think of a reference value to compare with the excess risk? If so, how would you interpret this relative comparison?

Summary
❖ The risk difference is the difference between two estimates of risk.
❖ The null value of the risk difference is 0, whereas the null value of the risk ratio is 1.
❖ The risk difference reflects an **excess risk** attributable to exposure.
❖ Excess risk describes the proportion of cases that could be avoided among exposed subjects if exposed subjects had the same risk as unexposed subjects.
❖ The risk difference is also called the **attributable risk**.

Difference Measures of Effect

Difference measures of effect can be computed in randomized clinical trial, cohort, and cross-sectional studies, but *not* in case-control studies. In cohort studies that estimate individual risk using cumulative incidence measures, the difference measure of interest is called the **risk difference**. It is estimated as the difference between $\hat{CI}_1$, the estimated cumulative incidence for the exposed group, and $\hat{CI}_0$, the estimated cumulative incidence for the unexposed group

In cohort studies that estimate average rate using person-time information, the difference measure is the **rate difference**. It can be estimated as the difference between two estimated rates, or incidence densities, $\hat{ID}_1$ and $\hat{ID}_0$.

Cohort studies
Individual risk ($\hat{CI}$):
Risk Difference ($\hat{CID}$) = $\hat{CI}_1$ - $\hat{CI}_0$

Average rate ($\hat{ID}$):
Rate Difference ($\hat{IDD}$) = $\hat{ID}_1$ - $\hat{ID}_0$

Cross-sectional studies
Prevalence ($\hat{P}$):
Prevalence Difference ($\hat{PD}$) = $\hat{P}_1$ - $\hat{P}_0$
exposed   unexposed

In cross-sectional studies, the difference measure is called the **prevalence difference**, and is estimated as the difference between two prevalence estimates.

Difference measures of effect cannot be estimated in case-control studies because in such studies neither risk, rate, nor prevalence can be appropriately estimated.

We'll illustrate the calculation of the rate difference. We again consider data on the relationship between serum cholesterol level and mortality from a 1992 study of almost 40,000 persons

1992, 40,000 persons, Chicago (white males, ages 25-39)		
Cholesterol Level		
	Borderline-high	Normal
Deaths	26	14
Person-years	36,581	68,239
	$\hat{ID}_1 = \dfrac{71.1}{100,000 \text{ PY}}$	$\hat{ID}_0 = \dfrac{20.5}{100,000 \text{ PY}}$

in Chicago, Illinois. Among white males ages 25-39 with borderline-high cholesterol, there were 71.1 deaths per 100,000 person-years. Among the comparison group, there were 20.5 deaths per 100,000 person-years.

The estimated rate ratio that compares these two groups is 3.5. The estimated rate difference, or IDD, is 50.6 deaths per 100,000 person years. What kind of interpretation can we give to this rate difference?

$$\hat{IDR} = \frac{\dfrac{71.1}{100,000 \text{ PY}}}{\dfrac{20.5}{100,000 \text{ PY}}} = 3.5 \qquad \hat{IDD} = \frac{71.1}{100,000 \text{ PY}} - \frac{20.5}{100,000 \text{ PY}} = \frac{50.6}{100,000 \text{ PY}}$$

The rate difference indicates an excess rate of 50.6 deaths per 100,000 person years associated with having a borderline-high cholesterol when compared to normal cholesterol. Here, we are using the estimated rate of CHD-related deaths in the unexposed group as the *background* or *expected* level to which the rate in the exposed group is compared. The rate difference is also called the **attributable rate** since it gives the additional rate attributable to the exposure.

Study Questions (Q6.2)

1. How many CHD-related deaths per 100,000 person years (i.e., py) could be avoided (i.e., attributable to exposure) among persons with borderline-high cholesterol if these persons could lower their cholesterol level to normal values?
2. What is the excess rate of CHD-related deaths per 100,000 py among persons with borderline-high cholesterol?
3. How might you evaluate whether the excess rate of 50.6 is clinically (not statistically) excessive?
4. Can you think of a reference value to compare with the excess rate? If so, how would you interpret this relative comparison?

Summary

❖ Difference measures can be computed in cohort and cross-sectional studies, but not in case-control studies.
❖ If **risk** is estimated, the difference measure is the **risk difference**.
❖ If **rate** is estimated, the difference measure is the **rate difference**.
❖ If **prevalence** is estimated, the difference measure is the **prevalence difference**.
❖ Difference measures of effect allow you to estimate the (excess) risk attributable to exposure over the background risk provided by the unexposed.

Quiz (Q6.3) Which of the following terms are synonymous with risk difference?

Choices   No Yes

1. Absolute risk   ???
2. Attributable risk   ???
3. Excess risk   ???
4. Relative risk   ???

During the 1999 outbreak of West Nile encephalitis in New York, incidence varied by location. The reported rates were:

Queens	16.4 per million	Bronx	7.5 per million
Brooklyn	1.3 per million	Manhattan	0.7 per million
Staten Island	0.0 per million	Total NYC	6.1 per million

To calculate the rate difference for residents of Queens, which location(s) could be used for the baseline or expected rate? **Choices   No   Yes**

5. Queens   ???
6. Bronx   ???
7. Brooklyn   ???
8. Manhattan   ???
9. Staten Island   ???
10. Total NYC   ???
11. Bronx+Brooklyn+Manhattan+Staten Island   ???

12. Calculate the rate difference between Queens and Manhattan. **???**

Choices   15.7   15.7 per million   23.4   23.4 per million

Investigators interviewed all persons who had attended the Smith-Jones wedding two days earlier, comparing the proportion who developed gastroenteritis among those who did and those who did not eat certain foods. They now want to determine the impact of eating potato salad on gastroenteritis.

13. The appropriate measure of potential impact is **???**.

Investigators conducted a cross-sectional survey, identified respondents who had been diagnosed with diabetes, and calculated an index of obesity using reported heights and weights. They now want to determine the impact of obesity on diabetes.

14. The appropriate measure of potential impact is **???**.

Investigators enrolled matriculating college freshmen into a follow-up study. The investigators administered questionnaires and drew blood each year to identify risk factors for and seroconversion to Epstein-Barr virus (the etiologic agent of mononucleosis). Using person-years of observation, the investigators now want to determine the impact of residing in a co-ed dormitory on EBV seroconversion.

15. The appropriate measure of potential impact is **???**.

Choices   <u>not calculable</u>   <u>odds difference</u>   <u>prevalence difference</u>
                   <u>rate difference</u>   <u>risk difference</u>

Difference versus Ratio Measures of Effect

Consider this table of hypothetical information describing the separate relationships of four different exposures to the same disease.

LOCATION	CHEWT	COFFEE	ALCOHOL
$CI_1 = 0.010$	$CI_1 = 0.005$	$CI_1 = 0.050$	$CI_1 = 0.050$
$CI_0 = 0.010$	$CI_0 = 0.001$	$CI_0 = 0.046$	$CI_0 = 0.010$
$RR = 1.000$	$RR = 5.000$	$RR = 1.087$	$RR = 5.000$
$RD = 0.000$	$RD = 0.004$	$RD = 0.004$	$RD = 0.040$

First focus on location, rural versus urban, for which the risk ratio is one and the risk difference is 0. There is no evidence of an effect of location on the disease, whether we consider the risk ratio or the risk difference. In fact, if the risk ratio is exactly 1, then the risk difference must be exactly 0, and vice versa.

    Location: Rural vs. Urban: RR=1.000 RD = 0.000; No Effect

  Now, let's look at the effect of chewing tobacco on disease. The risk ratio for chewing tobacco is 5; this indicates a very strong relationship between chewing tobacco and the disease. But, the risk difference of .004 seems quite close to zero, which suggests no effect of chewing tobacco.

    Chewing Tobacco: RR = 5.000   RD = 0.004;
                      Strong Effect Small Effect

    Thus, it is possible to arrive at a different conclusion depending on whether we use the risk ratio or the risk difference. Does only one of these two measures of effect give the correct conclusion, or are they both correct in some way? Actually, both measures give meaningful information about two different aspects of the relationship between exposure and disease.

    Let's now compare the effect of chewing tobacco with the effect of coffee drinking.

    Coffee Drinking: RR = 1.087   RD = 0.004

    The risk ratios for these two exposures are very different, yet the risk differences are exactly the same and close to zero. There appears to be little, if any, effect of coffee drinking. So, is there or is there not an effect of tobacco chewing?

    If we ask whether or not we would consider chewing tobacco to be a strong risk factor for the disease, our answer would be yes, since a chewer has 5 times the risk of a non-chewer for getting the disease. That is, chewing tobacco appears to be associated with the etiology of the disease, since it is such a strong risk factor.

    However, if we ask whether chewing tobacco poses a public health burden in providing a large case-load of patients to be treated, our answer would be no. To see the public health implications, recall that the risk difference of .004 for chewing tobacco gives the excess risk that would result if chewing tobacco were completely eliminated in the study population. Thus, out of, say, 1000 chewers, an excess of 1000 times 0.004, or only 4 chewers would develop the disease from their tobacco chewing habit. This is not a lot of patients to have to treat relative to the 1000 chewers at risk for the disease.

Study Questions (Q6.4)
1. Compare the effect of chewing tobacco with the effect of alcohol consumption on the disease. Do they both have the same effect in terms of the etiology of the disease?
2. Do chewing tobacco and alcohol use have the same public health implications on the treatment of disease?
3. Explain your answer to the previous question in terms of the idea of excess risk.

Summary
❖ If the risk ratio is exactly 1, then the risk difference is exactly 0, and vice versa, and there is no effect of exposure on the health outcome.
❖ If the risk ratio is very different from 1, it is still possible that the risk difference will be close to zero.
❖ If the risk difference is close but not exactly equal to 0, it is possible that the risk difference will be large enough to indicate a public health problem for treating the disease.
❖ Ratio measures are primarily used to learn about the etiology of a disease or other health outcome.
❖ Difference measures are used to determine the public health importance of a disease or other health outcome.

Quiz (Q6.5) During the 1999 outbreak of West Nile virus (WSV) encephalitis in New York City, the reported rates were:

Queens	16.4 per million population
Rest of NYC	2.4 per million
Total NYC	6.1 per million

Label each of the following statements as **True** or **False**.

1. If Queens had experienced the same WNV rate as the rest of NYC, 10.3 fewer cases per million would have occurred there, i.e., the rate difference is 10.3 per million. **???**
2. The excess rate in Queens was 14.0 cases per million (compared to the rest of NYC) **???**
3. The attributable rate (i.e., rate difference) in Queens was 16.4 cases per million. **???**
4. The most common measure of effect for comparing Queens to the rest of NYC is 6.8. **???**

Determine whether each of the following statements is more consistent with **risk difference, risk ratio, both,** or **neither.**

5. More of a measure of public health burden . . . . . **???**
6. More of a measure of etiology . . . . **???**

7. Null value is 0.0 . . . .   **???**
8. Can be a negative number . . . .   **???**
9. Can be a number between 0.0 and 1.0 . . . . . .   **???**
10. Can be calculated from most follow-up studies . . . .   **???**
11. Can be calculated from most case-control studies . . .   **???**
12. Has no units . . . .   **???**
13. A value very close to 0.0 indicates a strong effect . . .   **???**
14. Synonymous with attributable risk . . . .   **???**

Consider the data in the table below and the following estimates of risk on smoking and incidence of lung cancer and coronary heart disease (CHD).

	Lung Cancer	**CHD**
Rate Ratio	12.9	2.1
Rate Difference	79.0/100k/yr	190.4/100k/yr

15. Which disease is most strongly associated with smoking?   **???**
16. Elimination of smoking would reduce the most cases of which disease?   **???**

Incidence of lung cancer

	Smokers	**Nonsmokers**	**Total**
New Lung Cancer cases	60,000	10,000	70,000
Estimated person-years	70,000,000	150,000,000	220,000,000
Estimated incidence density per 100,000 person-years	$\hat{ID}_1 = 85.7$	$\hat{ID}_0 = 6.7$	$\hat{ID} = 31.8$

Incidence of coronary heart disease (CHD)

	Smokers	**Nonsmokers**	**Total**
New CHD cases	250,000	250,000	500,000
Estimated person-years	70,000,000	150,000,000	220,000,000
Estimated incidence density per 100,000 person-years	$\hat{ID}_1 = 357.1$	$\hat{ID}_0 = 166.7$	$\hat{ID} = 227.3$

Potential Impact – The Concept

A measure of potential impact provides a public health perspective on an exposure-disease relationship being studied. More specifically, a measure of potential impact attempts to answer the question, by how much would the disease load of a particular population be reduced if the distribution of an exposure variable were changed? By disease load, we mean the number of persons with a disease of interest that would require health care at a particular point in time.

The typical measure of potential impact is a proportion, often expressed as a percentage, of the number of cases that would not have become cases if all persons being studied had the same exposure status. For example, when determining the potential impact of smoking on the development of lung cancer, the potential impact of smoking gives the proportion of new lung cancer cases that would not have developed lung cancer if no one in the population smoked.

Or, one might determine the potential impact of a vaccine on the prevention of a disease, say, HIV, in high-risk persons. The potential impact of the vaccine gives the proportion of all the potential cases of HIV prevented by the vaccine if there had been no vaccine, all of these cases would have occurred.

These examples illustrate two kinds of potential impact measures. A measure of the impact of smoking on lung cancer considers an exposure that is associated with an increased risk of the disease and is called an **etiologic fraction**. A measure of the impact of a vaccine to prevent HIV considers an exposure that is associated with a decreased risk of disease and is called a **prevented fraction**.

The remainder of this chapter will consider the various formulae and the interpretation of the etiologic fraction. *See Lesson Page 6-3 in the ActivEpi CD ROM for details about the prevented fraction.*

Summary

❖ A measure of potential impact gives a public health perspective about the effect of an exposure-disease relationship.

❖ In general, measures of potential impact ascertain what proportion of cases developed the disease as a result of the purported influence of the exposure.

❖ The etiologic fraction is a measure of potential impact that considers an exposure that is a potential cause of disease.

❖ The prevented fraction is a measure of potential impact that considers an exposure that is preventive of the disease.

Etiologic Fraction

The **etiologic fraction** answers the question: what proportion of new cases that occur during a certain time period of follow-up are attributable to the exposure of interest? Other names for this measure are the **etiologic fraction** *in the population*, **attributable fraction** *in the population*, the **population attributable risk**, and the **population attributable risk percent**.

In mathematical terms, the etiologic fraction is given by the formula $I*$ divided by I, where $I*$ denotes the number of new cases attributable to the exposure and I denotes the number of new cases that actually occur. The numerator, $I*$ can be found as the difference between the actual number of new cases and the number of new cases that would have occurred in the absence of exposure, i.e., $EF = I* / I$.

To illustrate the calculation of the etiologic fraction, consider once again the results of a five-year follow-up study to determine whether or not smokers who have had a heart attack will reduce their risk for dying by quilting smoking The estimated risk ratio here is 2.1 and the estimated risk difference is 0.19.

Heart Attack Patients	Smoke	Quit	Total
Death	27	14	41
Survival	48	67	115
Total	75	81	156

Risks { continuing smokers: 0.36   Risk Ratio 2.1
       { smokers who quit: 0.17   Risk Difference .19

$$\hat{EF} = \frac{\hat{CI} - \hat{CI}_0}{\hat{CI}} = \frac{0.263 - 0.17}{0.263} \approx 0.35$$

A computational formula for the etiologic fraction is given here, where $\hat{CI}$ denotes the estimated cumulative incidence or risk for all subjects, exposed and unexposed combined, in the study. And $\hat{CI}_0$ denotes the estimated cumulative incidence for unexposed subjects. Notice that the numerator in this formula is ***not*** the risk difference, which would involve $\hat{CI}_1$, the estimated risk for exposed persons, rather than $\hat{CI}$, the overall estimated risk.

To calculate the etiologic fraction using our data then, we first must compute $\hat{CI}$, which equals .263, or roughly 26%. We already know that $\hat{CI}_0$ is .173 or roughly 17%. Substituting these values into the formula, we find that the etiologic fraction is .35, or 35%.

How do we interpret this result? The etiologic fraction of .35 tells us that 35% of all cases that actually occurred are due to continuing smoking. In other words, if we could have gotten all patients to quit smoking after their heart attack, there would have been a 35% reduction in the total number of deaths. This is why the etiologic fraction is often referred to as the population attributable risk percent. It gives the percent of all cases in the population that are attributable, in the sense of contributing excess risk, to the exposure.

Study Questions (Q6.6) Based on the smoking example from the previous page:
1. How many cases would have been expected if all subjects had been unexposed?
2. What is the excess number of total cases expected in the absence of exposure?
3. What is I*/I for these data?

Summary
❖ The etiologic fraction is given by the formula I*/I, where I denotes the number of new cases that actually occur and I* denotes the number of new cases attributable to the exposure.
❖ The numerator, I*, can be quantified as the difference between the actual number of new cases and the number of new cases that would have occurred in the absence of exposure.
❖ A computational formula for the etiologic fraction is EF = (CI – CI0) / CI, where CI denotes cumulative incidence.
❖ EF is often referred to as the population attributable risk percent, because it gives the percent of all cases in the population that are attributable to exposure.

Alternative Formula for Etiologic Fraction

In a cohort study that estimates risk, the etiologic fraction can be calculated from estimates of cumulative incidence for the overall cohort and for unexposed persons. An equivalent formula can be written in terms of the

Alternative Formula/ Etiologic Fraction
$\hat{EF} = \dfrac{\hat{CI} - \hat{CI}_0}{\hat{CI}} = \dfrac{p\,(\hat{RR} - 1)}{p(\hat{RR} - 1) + 1}$
p = proportion exposed

risk ratio and the proportion (p) of exposed persons in the cohort.

To illustrate this alternative formula, consider once again the results of a five-year follow-up study to determine whether or not smokers who have had a heart attack will reduce their risk for dying by quitting smoking. Using the first formula, we previously computed the etiologic fraction to be .35, or 35%. Thus, 35% of all cases that actually occurred are due to those who continued to smoke.

5 Year Follow-up Study				
	Smoke	Quit	Total	
Death	27	14	41	$\hat{RR} = 2.1$
Survival	48	67	115	
Total	75	81	156	$\hat{RD} = .19$

To use the second formula, we first calculate the proportion of the cohort exposed, which is

$$p = 75/156 = .481.$$

We now substitute this value and the estimated risk ratio of 2.1 into the second formula. The result is .35, which is exactly the same as previously obtained because both formulas are equivalent.

$$\hat{EF} = \frac{.481\,(\,2.1 - 1\,)}{.481\,(\,2.1 - 1\,) + 1} = 0.35$$

The second formula gives us some additional insight into the meaning of the etiologic fraction. This formula tells us that the size of the etiologic fraction depends on the size of the risk ratio and the proportion exposed. In particular, the potential impact for a strong determinant of the disease, that is, when the risk ratio is high, may be small if relatively few persons in the population are exposed.

Suppose in our example, that only 10% instead of 48% of the cohort were exposed so that p equals .10. Then the etiologic fraction would be reduced to

$$\hat{EF} = \frac{0.10\,(2.1 - 1)}{0.10\,(2.1 - 1) + 1} = 0.10 < 0.35$$

0.10 or 10%, which indicates a much smaller impact of exposure than 35%. Furthermore, if the entire cohort were unexposed, then the etiologic fraction would be zero.

Now suppose that 90%, instead of 48%, of the cohort were exposed, so that p equals .90. Then the etiologic fraction

$$\hat{EF} = \frac{0.90\,(2.1 - 1)}{0.90\,(2.1 - 1) + 1} = 0.50$$

increases to 0.50 or 50%. If the entire cohort were exposed the etiologic fraction would increase to its maximum possible value of .52 or 52% for a risk ratio estimate of 2.1.

In general, for a fixed value of the risk ratio, the etiologic fraction can range between zero, if the entire cohort were unexposed, to a maximum value of RR minus one over RR if the entire cohort were exposed.

For fixed $\hat{RR}$:
$$0 \le \hat{EF} \le \frac{\hat{RR} - 1}{\hat{RR}}$$

$p = 0$	$p = 1$
(all unexposed)	(all exposed)

Study Questions (Q6.7)

1. Use the formula (RR − 1)/RR to compute the maximum value possible EF when the RR is 2.1
2. What is the maximum value possible for EF when RR is 10?
3. As RR increases towards infinity, what does the maximum possible value of the EF approach?
4. If the RR is very large, say 100, can the EF still be relatively small? Explain.

Summary

❖ An alternative formula for the etiologic fraction is $EF = p(RR-1) / [p(RR-1)+1]$, where RR is the risk ratio and p is the proportion in the entire cohort that is exposed.

❖ The size of the etiologic fraction depends on the size of the risk ratio and the proportion exposed.

❖ For a fixed value of the risk ratio, the etiologic fraction can range between zero to a maximum value of $(RR - 1)/RR$.

❖ The potential impact for a strong determinant of the disease (i.e., high risk ratio) may be small if relatively few persons in the population are exposed.

Etiologic Fraction among the Exposed

There are two conceptual formulations of the etiologic fraction. One, which we have previously described, focuses on the potential impact of exposure on the total number of cases, shown below as **I**. A second focuses on the potential impact of the exposure on the number of exposed cases, which we denote as I_1. This measure is called the **etiologic fraction** *among the exposed*, **attributable fraction** *among the exposed*, or the **attributable risk percent** *among the exposed*. In mathematical terms, the etiologic fraction among the exposed, is given by the formula **I*** divided by I_1, where **I*** denotes the number of exposed cases attributable to the exposure and I_1 denotes the

1. Potential Impact on total # of cases (I)

$$EF = \frac{I^*}{I} = \frac{\hat{CI} - \hat{CI_0}}{\hat{CI}} = \frac{p(\hat{RR} - 1)}{[p(\hat{RR} - 1) + 1]}$$

2. Potential Impact on the # of exposed cases (I_1)

$$EF_e = \frac{I^* \longrightarrow \text{\# exposed cases attributable to exposure}}{I_1 \longrightarrow \text{\# exposed cases}}$$

number of exposed cases that actually occur.

The denominator (in the **EFe** formula) is the number of exposed cases. This is different from the denominator in **EF**. That's because the referent group for **EFe** is the number of exposed cases that occur in the cohort rather than the total number of cases in **EF**. The numerator in both formulas is the same, namely **I***. In particular, the **I*** in both **EF** and **EFe** can be quantified as the difference between the actual number of cases and the number of cases that would have occurred in the absence of exposure

To illustrate the calculation of the etiologic fraction among the exposed, consider once again the results of a five-year follow-up study to determine whether or not smokers who have had a heart attack will reduce their risk of dying by quitting smoking. The

Heart Attack Patients	Smoke	Quit	Total
Death	27	14	41
Survival	48	67	115
Total	75	81	156

Risks $\{$ continuing smokers: 0.36 / smokers who quit: 0.17

Risk Ratio 2.1
Risk Difference .19

$$\hat{EF} = \frac{\hat{CI} - \hat{CI_0}}{\hat{CI}} = 35\%$$

$$\hat{EF}_e = \frac{\hat{CI_1} - \hat{CI_0}}{\hat{CI_1}} = \frac{.19}{.36} = \mathbf{53\%}$$

previously computed etiologic fraction, or equivalently, the population attributable risk percent computed for these data was 35%.

The etiologic fraction among the exposed (**EFe**) can be calculated for these same data using the formula shown above. The term $\hat{CI}_1$ denotes the estimated cumulative incidence or risk for exposed subjects in the study and $\hat{CI}_0$ denotes the estimated cumulative incidence for unexposed subjects. The numerator in this formula is the estimated risk difference ($\hat{RD}$). Since the estimated risk difference is .19 and the risk for exposed persons is .36, we can substitute these values into the formula for EFe to obtain .53, or 53%. How do we interpret this result?

The etiologic fraction of .53 tells us that 53% of all deaths among continuing smokers are due to continuing smoking. In other words, if we could have gotten the continuing smokers who died to quit smoking after their heart attack, there would have been a 53% reduction in deaths among these persons.

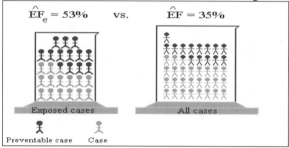

$$\hat{EF}_e = 53\% \quad \text{vs.} \quad \hat{EF} = 35\%$$

Exposed cases | All cases

Preventable case | Case

Study Questions (Q6.8)

Heart Attack Patients	Smoke	Quit	Total
Death	27	14	41
Survival	48	67	115
Total	75	81	156

Risks { continuing smokers: 0.36   Risk Ratio   2.1
Risks { smokers who quit: 0.17   Risk Difference .19

1. What is the excess number of exposed cases (i.e., deaths among continuing smokers) expected in the absence of exposure?
2. Fill in the blanks: In this example, _____ of the _____ deaths among continuing smokers could have been avoided.
3. Use the formula $I*/I_1$ to compute EFe for these data.
4. An alternative formula for the etiologic fraction among exposed is EFe=(RR-1)/RR, where RR is the risk ratio. Use this formula to compute EFe for the heart attack study data.
5. The population attributable risk percent (EF) computed for these data is 35% whereas the attributable risk percent among the exposed (EFe) is 53%. How do you explain these differences?
6. For cohort studies that use person-time information, state a formula for the etiologic fraction among the exposed that involves incidence densities in exposed and unexposed groups.
7. As in the previous question, state an alternative formula for EFe that involves the incidence density ratio.
8. For case-control studies, which cannot estimate risk or rate, can you suggest

formulae for EF and EFe?

Summary

❖ The etiologic fraction among the exposed, EFe, focuses on the potential impact of the exposure on the number of exposed cases, rather than the total number of cases.

❖ EFe is defined as I^*/I_1, where I^* is the excess number of exposed cases due to exposure and I_1 is the actual number of exposed cases.

❖ For cohort studies that estimate risk: $\hat{E}Fe = \dfrac{(\hat{CI}_1 - \hat{CI}_0)}{\hat{CI}_1} = \dfrac{\hat{RR}-1}{\hat{RR}}$

❖ For cohort studies that estimate rate: $\hat{E}Fe = \dfrac{(\hat{ID}_1 - \hat{ID}_0)}{\hat{ID}_1} = \dfrac{\hat{IDR}-1}{\hat{IDR}}$

Etiologic Fraction – An Example

Hypothyroidism, a disease state in which the production of thyroid hormone is decreased, is known to increase the risk of cardiovascular disease. In elderly women, the subclinical form of hypothyroidism is highly prevalent. The Rotterdam Study investigators therefore examined the potential impact of subclinical hypothyroidism on the incidence of myocardial infarction.

In this study of nearly 1,000 women aged 55 and over, the prevalence of subclinical hypothyroidism was 10.8%. Consider the two-by-two table depicted here. The cumulative incidence of myocardial infarction is 2.9% (3/103) in women with subclinical hypothyroidism, 1.2% (10/854) in women without hypothyroidism, and 1.4% (13/957) overall.

	Subclinical Hypothyroidism	No Subclinical Hypothyroidism	Total
MI	3	10	13
No MI	100	844	944
Total	103	854	957
	$\hat{CI}_1$=2.9%	$\hat{CI}_0$=1.2%	$\hat{CI}$=1.4%

Study Questions (Q6.9)
1. Using these data, can you calculate the etiologic fraction?

Answer: The etiologic fraction is: EF = (1.4 - 1.2) / 1.4 = 14%. This indicates that of all myocardial infarctions that occur in elderly women, 14% are due to the presence of subclinical hypothyroidism. In other words, if subclinical hypothyroidism could be prevented, there would be 14% less myocardial infarctions in this population.

2. Can you calculate the etiologic fraction using the alternative formula: EF = [p(RR-1)]/[p(RR-1) + 1] ?
3. Can you calculate the etiologic fraction in the exposed?

Answer to 3: The etiologic fraction in the exposed (EFe) is (2.9-1.2), which is equal to the risk difference, divided by 2.9, which is 60%. Thus, among the women that are affected, 60% of the myocardial infarctions can be attributed to the presence of subclinical hypothyroidism.

Summary
* ❖ The Rotterdam Study investigators examined the potential impact of subclinical hypothyroidism on the incidence of myocardial infarction.
* ❖ Of all myocardial infarctions that occur in elderly women, 14% is due to the presence of subclinical hypothyroidism.
* ❖ Among women that are affected, 60% of the myocardial infarctions can be attributed to the presence of subclinical hypothyroidism.

Quiz (Q6.10) Consider data in the table below on smoking and incidence of lung cancer and cardiovascular disease (CHD).

Incidence of lung cancer

	Smokers	Nonsmokers	Total
New Lung Cancer cases	60,000	10,000	70,000
Estimated person-years	70,000,000	150,000,000	220,000,000
Estimated incidence density per 100,000 person-years	$\hat{ID}_1 = 85.7$	$\hat{ID}_0 = 6.7$	$\hat{ID} = 31.8$

Incidence of coronary heart disease (CHD)

	Smokers	Nonsmokers	Total
New CHD cases	250,000	250,000	500,000
Estimated person-years	70,000,000	150,000,000	220,000,000
Estimated incidence density per 100,000 person-years	$\hat{ID}_1 = 357.1$	$\hat{ID}_0 = 166.7$	$\hat{ID} = 227.3$

1. The prevalence of smoking in this population is   ???
2. The etiologic fraction for lung cancer is   ???
3. The etiologic fraction for coronary heart disease is   ???
4. The etiologic fraction among the exposed for lung cancer is   ???
5. The etiologic fraction among the exposed for CHD is   ???
6. The proportion of lung cancer among smokers attributable to smoking is   ???

Choices   **0.0%**   **26.7%**   **31.8%**   **53.3%**   **79.0%**   **92.2%**

Label each of the following as either a **Risk/Rate Difference**, an **Etiologic Fraction** or an **Etiologic Fraction Among the Exposed**.

7. Attributable risk percent among the exposed   ???
8. Population attributable risk   ???
9. Excess risk   ???
10. Influenced by prevalence of the exposure in the population   ???
11. Has same units as measure of occurrence   ???
12. Can be a negative number   ???

---

13. **???** can never be larger than **???**

Choices (for Q.13)   **Etiologic Fraction**   **Etiologic Fraction Among the Exposed**

Nomenclature:

Table setup for cohort, case-control, and prevalence studies:

	Exposed	Not Exposed	Total
Disease/cases	a	b	n_1
No Disease/controls	c	d	n_0
Total	m_1	m_0	n

Table setup for cohort data with person-time:

	Exposed	Not Exposed	Total
Disease (New cases)	I_1	I_0	I
No Disease	-	-	-
Total disease-free person-time	PT_1 or L_1	PT_0 or L_0	PT

Formulae for difference measures of effect

Risk Data	**Rate Data**	**Prevalence Data**
$\hat{CID} = \hat{CI}_1 - \hat{CI}_0$	$\hat{IDD} = \hat{ID}_1 - \hat{ID}_0$	$\hat{PD} = \hat{P}_1 - \hat{P}_0$

Formulae for etiologic fraction and for the etiologic fraction in the exposed based on risk data, rate data, and case-control data.

	Risk Data	**Rate Data**	**Case-Control***
EF	$\hat{EF} = \dfrac{I^*}{I}$	$\hat{EF} = \dfrac{I^*}{I}$	$\hat{EF} = \dfrac{(p')(\hat{OR} - 1)}{(p')(\hat{OR} - 1) + 1}$
	$\hat{EF} = \dfrac{\hat{CI} - \hat{CI}_0}{\hat{CI}}$	$\hat{EF} = \dfrac{\hat{ID} - \hat{ID}_0}{\hat{ID}}$	
	$\hat{EF} = \dfrac{(p)(\hat{RR} - 1)}{(p)(\hat{RR} - 1) + 1}$	$\hat{EF} = \dfrac{(p^*)(\hat{IDR} - 1)}{(p^*)(\hat{IDR} - 1) + 1}$	
EFe	$\hat{EF}_e = \dfrac{I^*}{I_1}$	$\hat{EF}_e = \dfrac{I^*}{I_1}$	$\hat{EFe} = \dfrac{\hat{OR} - 1}{\hat{OR}}$
	$\hat{EF}_e = \dfrac{\hat{CI}_1 - \hat{CI}_0}{\hat{CI}_1}$	$\hat{EFe} = \dfrac{\hat{ID}_1 - \hat{ID}_0}{\hat{ID}_1}$	
	$\hat{EF}_e = \dfrac{\hat{RD}}{\hat{CI}_1}$	$\hat{EFe} = \dfrac{\hat{IDD}}{\hat{ID}_1}$	
	$\hat{EFe} = \dfrac{\hat{RR} - 1}{\hat{RR}}$	$\hat{EFe} = \dfrac{\hat{IDR} - 1}{\hat{IDR}}$	
where	$p = \dfrac{m_1}{n}$	$p^* = \dfrac{L_1}{L_1 + L_0}$	$p' = \dfrac{c}{n_0}$

*In case-control studies, the EF, EFe, PF, PFe based on the odds ratio will be a good estimates when the OR is a good estimate of the RR (e.g., rare disease assumption)

References

Benichou J, Chow WH, McLaughlin JK, Mandel JS, and Fraumeni JF Jr. Population attributable risk of renal cell cancer in Minnesota. Am J Epidemiol 1988;148(5):424-30.

Cook RJ, Sackett DL. The number needed to treat: a clinically useful measure of treatment effect. BMJ 1995;310(6977):452-4.

Greenberg RS, Daniels SR, Flanders WD, Eley JW, Boring JR. Medical Epidemiology (3rd Ed). Lange Medical Books, New York, 2001.

Hak AE, Pols HA, Visser TJ, Drexhage HA, Hofman A, Witteman JC. Subclinical hypothyroidism is an independent risk factor for atherosclerosis and myocardial infarction in elderly women: the Rotterdam Study. Ann Intern Med 2000;132(4):270-8.

Kleinbaum DG, Kupper LL, Morgenstern H. Epidemiologic Research: Principles and Quantitative Methods. John Wiley and Sons Publishers, New York, 1982.

Landrigan PJ, Epidemic measles in a divided city. JAMA 1972;221(6):567-70.

Medical Research Council trial of treatment of mild hypertension: principal results. MRC Working Party. BMJ 1985;291;97-104.

Morgenstern H and Bursic ES,. A method for using epidemiologic data to estimate the potential impact of an intervention on the health status of a target population. J Community Health 1982;7(4):292-309.

Spirtas R, Heineman EF, Bernstein L, Beebe GW, Keehn RJ, Stark A, Harlow BL, Benichou J. Malignant mesothelioma: attributable risk of asbestos exposure. Occup Environ Med 1994;51(12):804-11.

Wacholder S, Benichou J, Heineman EF, Hartge P, Hoover RN. Attributable risk: advantages of a broad definition of exposure. Am J Epidemiol 1994;140(4):303-9..

Walter SD. Calculation of attributable risks from epidemiological data. Int J Epidemiol 1978;7(2):175-82.

Walter SD. Prevention for multifactorial diseases. Am J Epidemiol 1980;112(3):409-16.

Walter SD. Attributable risk in practice. Am J Epidemiol 1998;148(5):411-3.

Walter SD. Number needed to treat (NNT): estimation of a measure of clinical benefit. Stat Med 2001;20(24);3947-62.

Wilson PD, Loffredo CA, Correa-Villasenor A, Ferencz C. Attributable fraction for cardiac malformations. Am J Epidemiol 1998;148(5):414-23.

Answers to Study Questions and Quizzes

Q6.1

1. 75 * .17 = 12.75 deaths would have occurred if the 75 patients had quit smoking.
2. 27 – 12.75 = 14.25 excess deaths among those who continued to smoke
3. p(excess deaths among continuing smokers) = 14.25 / 75 = .19 = risk difference
4. 1,000 x 0.19 = 190 excess deaths could be avoided.
5. The largest possible risk difference is either plus or minus one. Nevertheless, this doesn't mean that 0.19 is small relative to a clinically meaningful reference value, which would be desirable.
6. One choice for a reference value is the risk for the exposed, i.e., 0.36. The ratio 0.19/0.36 = 0.53 indicates that 53% of the risk for the group of continuing smokers would be reduced if this group had quit smoking.

Q6.2

1. 100,000 x 14 / 68,239 = 20.5 is the expected number of CHD-related deaths per 100,000 py if persons with borderline-high cholesterol had their cholesterol lowered to normal values. Thus 71.1 – 20.5 = 50.6 CHD-related deaths per 100,000 py could be avoided could have been avoided.
2. 50.6 (71.1-20.5) excess CHD-related deaths per 100,000 person years. This value of 50.6 per 100,000 is the rate difference or attributable rate.
3. The largest possible rate difference is infinite. Nevertheless, this does not

mean that 50.6 is small relative to a clinically meaningful reference value.

4. One choice for a reference is 71.1, the rate for the exposed. The ratio 50.6 / 71.1 = .72 indicates that the rate in borderline-high cholesterol group would be reduces by 72% if this group could lower their cholesterol to normal levels.

Q6.3

1. No – Absolute risk describes the risk in a particular group rather than the difference in risk from two groups.
2. Yes
3. Yes
4. No – Relative risk is the *ratio* of (rather than the *difference* between) risk among two groups.
5. No – for questions 5-11: Any location that does not include Queens itself could be used for a baseline or expected rate. So, Queens and New York City would not be good choices since they both include Queens.
6. Yes
7. Yes
8. Yes
9. Yes
10. No
11. Yes
12. 15.7 per million – Since the individual rates are in units of *per million*, the difference in the rates will have the same unit of measurement.
13. Risk difference – In an outbreak such as this, the investigators are comparing two risks. The appropriate measure of impact here is the risk difference.
14. Prevalence difference – In a prevalence study, the appropriate measure of disease frequency is prevalence. A corresponding measure of impact is the prevalence difference.
15. Rate difference – In a follow-up study we can use person-years of observation to calculate a rate. The appropriate measure of potential impact here is the rate difference.

Q6.4

1. Yes, because both chewing tobacco and alcohol use have the same value (5) for the risk ratio.

2. No. Chewing tobacco has little public health effect, whereas alcohol consumption has a much stronger public health effect.
3. Out of 1000 heavy drinkers (i.e., high alcohol consumption), 40 persons would develop the disease because of their drinking. In contract, only 4 tobacco chewers out of 1000 tobacco chewers would develop the disease from chewing tobacco.

Q6.5

1. False – The rate difference between Queens and the rest of NYC is 16.4 per million – 2.4 per million = 14.0 per million. The excess rate (i.e., rate difference) in Queens is therefore 14.0 cases per million population.
2. True – see above for answer
3. False – 16.4 cases per million in not the attributable rate (i.e., rate difference), but the absolute rake of West Nile encephalitis in Queens. The rate difference is 16.4 – 2.4 = 14.0 per million population.
4. True – The most common measure of effect for comparing Queens to the rest of NYC is 6.8 and this is the rate ratio calculated as 16.4/2.4.
5. Risk difference – a measure of public health burden.
6. Risk ratio – a measure of disease etiology.
7. Risk difference – the null value for the risk difference is 0.0; the null value for the risk ratio is 1.0.
8. Risk difference – The risk difference can be negative if the baseline risk is higher than the risk in the group of interest. The risk ratio can never be negative because it is a ratio of two positive numbers.
9. Both – it is *possible* to have a risk difference and a risk ratio in the range of 0.0 to 1.0. Note that the CD states the correct answer is Neither with the rationale that neither the risk ratio or risk difference is restricted to values between 0.0 to 1.0.
10. Both – Since risk can be calculated from most follow-up studies, then both a risk ratio and risk difference can be calculated.

11. Neither – Since risk cannot be calculated from case-control studies, neither a risk difference nor a risk ratio can be calculated.
12. Risk ratio – The risk ratio has no units since it is a ratio of risks that has the same units.
13. Risk ratio – A risk ratio close to zero would indicate a strong protective effect. A risk difference close to zero would indicate no effect
14. Risk difference
15. Lung cancer – The rate ratio is much higher for lung cancer than for CHD
16. CHD – elimination of smoking would reduce the number of CHD by 190.4 cases per 100,000 per year.

Q6.6
1. 156 x .173 = 27, where .173 is the risk for the unexposed subjects.
2. $41 - 27 = 14 = I^*$
3. $I^*/I = 14/41 = .35 = EF$

Q6.7
1. $(2.1 - 1) / 2.1 = .52$
2. $(RR - 1) / RR = (10 - 1) / 10 = .90$
3. The maximum possible value for the EF approaches 1 as RR approaches infinity.
4. Yes, even if RR is very large, the EF can be small, even close to zero, if the proportion exposed in the population is very small.

Q6.8
1. 75 x .19 = 14.25 = I^*, where 75 is the number of exposed subjects and .19 is the risk difference.
2. In this example, 14 of the 27 deaths among continuing smokers could have been avoided.
3. $I^*/I_1 = 14.25 / 27 = .53 = EFe$.
4. $EFe = (2.1 - 1) / 2.1 = .52$. This is the same as the .53 previously obtained, other than round-off error.

5. The EF considers the potential impact of exposure on 'all cases' in the cohort whereas the EFe focuses on the potential impact of exposure on only 'exposed cases' in the cohort. Both measures are meaningful, but have a different focus.
6. $EFe = (ID_1 - ID_0) / ID_1$, where ID_1 and ID_0 are the incidence densities (i.e., rates) for exposed and unexposed persons in the cohort.
7. $EFe = (IDR - 1) / IDR$
8. $EF = p'(OR - 1)/[p'(OR - 1) + 1]$ and $EFe = (OR - 1) / OR$, where OR is the odds ratio and p' is the proportional of all controls that are exposed.

Q6.9
1. The etiologic fraction is $(1.4-1.2) / 1.4 = 14\%$
2. p=0.108

$$RR=(3/103)/(10/854)=2.5$$

$$EF = \frac{0.108(2.5-1)}{0.108(2.5-2)+1} = 14\%$$

3. $EFe=(2.9-1.2)/2.9=60\%$

Q6.10
1. 31.8% - prevalence of smoking = 70 million/220 million = 31.8%
2. 79.0% - The EF for lung cancer is (31.8-6.7)/21.8=79.0%.
3. 26.7% -
4. 92.2%
5. 53.3%
6. 92.2%
7. Etiologic fraction among the exposed
8. Etiologic fraction
9. Risk/rate difference
10. Etiologic fraction
11. Risk/rate difference
12. Risk/rate difference
13. Etiologic Fraction, Etiologic Fraction Among the Exposed

CHAPTER 7

IS THERE SOMETHING WRONG?
VALIDITY AND BIAS

*The primary objective of most epidemiologic research is to obtain a **valid estimate** of an **effect measure** of interest. In this chapter we illustrate three general types of **validity** problems, distinguish validity from **precision**, introduce the term **bias**, and discuss how to adjust for bias.*

Examples of Validity Problems

Validity in epidemiologic studies concerns methodologic flaws that might distort the conclusions made about an exposure-disease relationship. Several examples of validity issues are briefly described.

The validity of an epidemiologic study concerns whether or not there are imperfections in the study design, the methods of data collection, or the methods of data analysis that might distort the conclusions made about an exposure-disease relationship. If there are no such imperfections, we say that the study is **valid**. If there are imperfections, then the extent of the distortion of the results from the correct conclusions is called **bias**. Validity of a study is what we strive for; bias is what prevents us from obtaining valid results

In 1946, Berkson demonstrated that case-control studies carried out exclusively in hospital settings are subject to a type of **"selection" bias**, aptly called **Berkson's bias**. Berkson's bias arises because patients with two disease conditions or high-risk behaviors are more likely to be hospitalized than those with a single condition. Such patients will tend to be over-represented in the study population when compared to the community population. In particular, respiratory and bone diseases have been shown to be associated in hospitalized patients but not in the general population. Moreover, since cigarette smoking is strongly associated with respiratory disease, we would expect a hospital study of the relationship between cigarette smoking and bone disease to demonstrate such a relationship even if none existed in the general population.

In the 1980's and 1990's, US Air Force researchers assessed the health effects among Vietnam War veterans associated with exposure to the herbicide Agent Orange. Agent Orange contained a highly toxic trace contaminant known as TCDD. Initially, exposure to TCDD was classified according to job descriptions of the veterans selected for study. It was later determined that this produced substantial misclassification of TCDD. The validity problem here is called **information bias**. Bias could be avoided using laboratory techniques that were developed to measure TCDD from blood serum. The use of such **biologic markers** in epidemiologic research is rapidly increasing as a way to reduce misclassification and, more generally, to improve accuracy of study measurements.

As a final example, we return to the Sydney Beach Users Study described previously. A validity issue in this study concerned whether all relevant variables, other than swimming status and pollution level, were taken into account. Such variables included age, sex, duration of swimming, and additional days of swimming. The primary reason for considering these additional variables is to ensure that any observed effect of swimming on illness outcome could not be explained away by these other variables. A distortion in the results caused by failure to take into account such additional variables is called **confounding bias**.

Summary
❖ Validity: The general issue of whether or not there are imperfections in the study design, the methods of data collection, or methods of data analysis that might distort the conclusions made about an exposure-disease relationship.

❖ Bias: A measure of the extent of distortion of conclusions about an exposure-disease relationship.

❖ Validity issues are illustrated by:
  - Hospital-based case-control studies (Berkson's **selection bias**).
  - Job misclassification to assess TCDD exposure (**information bias**).
  - Control of relevant variables in the Sydney Beach Users Study (**confounding**).

Validity versus Precision

*Validity and precision concern two different sources of inaccuracy that can occur when estimating an exposure-disease relationship: **systematic error** (a validity problem) and **random error** (a precision problem). Systematic and random error can be distinguished in terms of shots at a target.*

Validity and precision are influenced by two different types of error that can occur when estimating an exposure-disease relationship. **Systematic error** affects the **validity**, and **random error**, the **precision**.

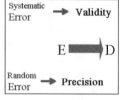

These two types of error can be distinguished by viewing an epidemiologic study as a shot at a target. The blue dot in the middle of the target symbolizes the **true measure of effect** being estimated in a population of interest. (Note: to be consistent with the CD, the use of the term "blue dot" in this text refers to the center of the target or the "bull's eye".) Each shot represents an **estimate** of the true effect obtained from one of possibly many studies in each of three populations.

For Target A, the shots are centered around the blue dot, although none of the shots actually hit it and all shots hit a different part of the target. For Target B, the shots are all far off center, but have about the same amount of scatter as the shots at

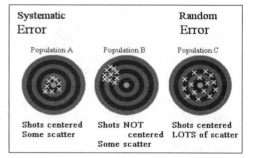

target A. For target C, the shots are centered around the blue dot, but unlike Target A, are more spread out from one another.

Systematic error is illustrated by comparing Target A with Target B. The shots at Target A are aimed at the blue dot, whereas the shots at Target B are not aimed at the blue dot, but rather centered around the red dot. (Note: to be consistent with the CD, the term "red dot" will refer to the dot above and

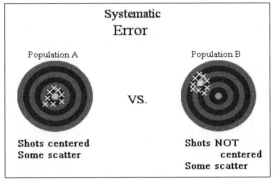

to the left of the bull's eye in Population B). The distance between the blue dot and the red dot measures the systematic error associated with Target B. In contrast, there is no systematic error associated with Target A.

Systematic error occurs when there is a difference between the true effect measure and what is actually being estimated. We say that the study is valid if there is no systematic error. Thus, validity is concerned with whether or not a study is aiming at the correct effect measure, as represented by the bull's eye. Unfortunately in epidemiologic and other research, the bull's eye is usually not known. Consequently, the amount of bias is difficult to determine and the evaluation of bias is to some extent always subjective.

All the targets illustrate random error, which occurs when there is a difference between any estimate computed from the study data and the effect measure actually being estimated. Targets A and B exhibit the same amount of random error because there is essentially the same amount of scatter of shots around the blue dot of Target A as there is around the red dot of Target B. In contrast Target C, in which shots are much more spread out, exhibits more random error than targets A or B.

Thus, the more spread out the shots, the more random error, and the less precision from any one shot. Precision therefore concerns how much individual variation there is from shot to shot, given the actual spot being aimed at. In other words, precision reflects **sampling variability**.

Problems of precision generally concern statistical inference about the parameters of the population actually being aimed at. In contrast, problems of validity concern methodologic imperfections of the study design or the analysis that may influence whether or not the correct population parameter, as represented by the blue dot in each target, is being aimed at by the study

Study Questions (Q7.1) Consider a cross-sectional study to assess the relationship between calcium intake (high versus low) in one's diet and the prevalence of arthritis of the hip in women residents of the city of Atlanta between the ages of 45 and 69. A sample of female hospital patients is selected from hospital records in 1989, and the presence or absence of arthritis as well as a measure of average calcium intake in the diet prior to enter the hospital are determined on each patient.

1. What is the target population in this study?
2. What does the center of the target (i.e., the bulls-eye) represent in epidemiologic terms?
3. What do we mean by random error associated with this study?
4. What do we mean by systematic error associated with this study?

Summary
- ❖ Validity concerns systematic error whereas precision concerns random error.
- ❖ Systematic and random error can be distinguished in terms of shots at a target.
- ❖ Systematic error: a difference between what an estimator is actually estimating and the effect measure of interest.
- ❖ Random error: a difference between any estimate computed from the study data and the effect measure actually being estimated.
- ❖ Validity does not consider statistic inference, but rather methodologic imperfections of the study design or analysis.
- ❖ Precision concerns statistical inferences about the parameter of the population actually being aimed at.

A Hierarchy of Populations

To further clarify the difference between validity and precision, we now describe a hierarchy of populations that are considered in any epidemiologic study.

We typically identify different populations when we think about the validity of an epidemiologic study. These populations may be contained within each other or they may simply overlap.

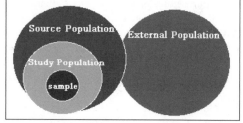

We refer to the collection of individuals from which the study data have been obtained as the **sample**. We use results from the sample to make inferences about larger populations. But what populations can we make these inferences about? What population does the sample represent?

The **study population** is the collection of individuals that our sample actually represents and is typically those individuals we can feasibly study. We may be limited to sampling from hospitals or to sampling at particular places and times. The study population is defined by what is practical, which may not be what we ideally would like.

The **source population** is the collection of individuals of restricted interest; say in a specific city, community, or occupation, who are at risk for being a case. Clearly all cases must come from the source population (if they were not at risk, they would not have become cases). The source population also is likely to include individuals who, although at risk, may not become cases. The source population has been called the **study base** or the **target population**.

We can make statistical inferences from the sample to the study population, but we would like to be able to make inferences from the sample to the source population. Unfortunately, the **study population**, the population actually represented by our sample, may not be representative of the **source population**.

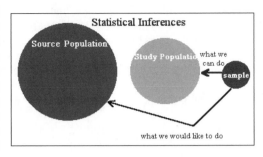

Study Questions (Q7.2) Consider an epi study carried out in New York City (NYC) to assess whether obesity is associated with hypertension in young adults. The investigators decided that it was not feasible to consider taking a sample from among all young adults in the city. It was decided that fitness centers would provide a large source of young NYC adults. A sample of subjects is taken from several randomly selected fitness centers throughout the city and their blood pressure is measured to determine hypertension status.
1. What is the source population for this study?
2. What is the study population in this study?
3. Does the sample represent the study population?
4. Does the study population represent the source population?

In a simple case every member of the study population is also in the source population -that is, we are only studying individuals who are in fact at risk. If the study population is representative of the source population and the sample is representative of the study population then there is no bias in inferring from the sample to the source population.

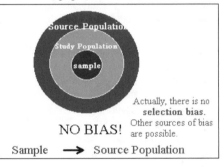

Study Questions (Q7.2) continued Recall the epi study carried out in New York City to assess whether obesity is associated with hypertension in young adults. Suppose the investigators decided that it was important to obtain a sample from all young adults within NYC. They used the 2000 census information to get a listing of all young NYC adults. A sample of subjects is taken from several randomly selected city blocks throughout the city and their blood pressure is measures to determine hypertension status.
5. What is the source population for this study?
6. What is the study population in this study?
7. Does the sample represent the study population?
8. Does the study population represent the source population?

Sometimes, however, even a sample from a study population that represents the source population can become biased. For example, in a typical cohort study, even though every member of the initial study population is also in the source population the initial sample may change in the course of the study. The initial sample may suffer from exclusions, withdrawals, non-response, or loss-to-follow-up. The final study population is then only those individuals who are willing and able to stay in such a study, a population that may not represent the initial study population or the source population as well as we might wish.

Study Questions (Q7.2) continued
9. True or False. In a cohort study, the *study* population includes persons eligible to be selected but who would have been lost to follow-up if actually followed.
10. True or False. In a cohort study, the *source* population includes persons eligible to be selected but who would have been lost to follow-up if actually followed.
11. True or False. In a case-control study, the study population may contain persons eligible to be controls who were not at risk for being a case.
12. True or False. In a cross-sectional study, the study population may contain persons who developed the health outcome but had died prior to the time at which the sample was selected.

In general, it is possible for members of the study population not even to be at risk and we may not be able to tell. We may, for example, draw our sample from a study population of persons who attend a clinic for sexually transmitted diseases. These people may or may not have an STD and may or may not be exposing themselves to STD's. For example, some of these subjects may have partners who are not infected, and thus may not be at risk themselves. If they are not at risk, they are not part of the source population, but we may not know that.

It can also happen that the study population fails to include individuals who are at risk (and thus part of the source population) either because we do not know they are at risk or because it is not practical to reach them. For example when AIDS was poorly understood, a study of gay men at risk for AIDS may have failed to include IV drug users who were also at risk.

Finally, we would often like to generalize our conclusions to a different **external population**. An external population is a population that differs from the study population but to which we nevertheless would like to generalize the results, for example, a different city, community, or occupation. In a public health setting, we are always concerned with the health of the general public even though we must study smaller subpopulations for practical reasons. For statistical conclusions that are based on a sample to generalize to an external population, the study population must itself be representative of the external population, but that is often difficult to achieve.

Study Questions (Q7.2) continued Consider an epi study carried out in New York City to assess whether obesity is associated with hypertension in young adults. Suppose it was of interest to determine whether the study results carry over to the population of the entire state of New York.

13. Considering the variety of populations described, what type of population is being considered? Explain briefly.

Summary

❖ There are a variety of populations to consider in any epi study.

❖ The **sample** is the collection of individuals from which the study data have been obtained.

❖ The **study population** is the collection of individuals that our sample actually represents and is typically those individuals we can feasibly study.

❖ The **source population** is the group of restricted interest about which the investigator wishes to assess an exposure-disease relationship.

❖ The **external population** is a group to which the study has not been restricted but to which the investigator still wishes to generalize the study results.

Internal versus External Validity

Target shooting provides an example that illustrates the difference between **internal** and **external validity**. Internal validity considers whether or not we are aiming at the center of the target. If, we are aiming at this red dot (to the left and above the bulls-eye) rather than at the bulls-eye, then our study is **not** internally valid.

Internal validity is about drawing conclusions about the source population based on information from the study population. Such inferences do not extend beyond the source population of restricted interest.

External validity concerns a different target; in particular, one at which we are not intending to shoot; whose bulls-eye we can't really see. We might imagine this external target being screened from our vision.

Suppose that this screened target is in line with the target at which we are shooting. Then, by aiming at the bulls-eye of the target we can see, we are also aiming at the bulls-eye of the external target. In this case, the results from our study population can be generalized to this external population, and thus, we have external validity. If the external target is not lined up with our target, our study does not have external validity, and the study results should not extend to this external population.

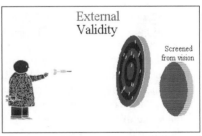

External validity is about applying our conclusions to an external population beyond the study's restricted interest. Such inferences require judgments about other findings and their connection to the study's findings, conceptualization of the disease process and related biological processes, and comparative features of the source population and the external population. External validity is therefore more subjective and less quantifiable than internal validity.

Study Questions (Q7.3) Consider an epi study carried out in New York City to assess whether obesity is associated with hypertension in young adults. Subjects are sampled from several fitness centers throughout the city and their blood pressure is measured to determine hypertension status.

1. What is required for this study to be internally valid?

Suppose it was of interest to determine whether the study results carry over to the entire State of New York.

2. Does this concern internal validity or external validity? Explain briefly.

Results from the Lipid Research Clinics Primary Prevention Trial published in 1984 (JAMA) demonstrated a significant reduction in cardiovascular mortality for white men ages 35 to 59 who were placed on a cholesterol-reducing diet and medication.

3. What question might be asked about the results of this study that concerns external validity?
4. What question(s) might be asked about the study results that concern(s) internal validity?

Summary
* Internal validity concerns whether or not we are aiming at the center of the target we know we are shooting at.
* External validity concerns a target that we are not intending to shoot at, whose bulls-eye we can't really see.
* Internal validity concerns the drawing of conclusions about the target population based on information from the study population.
* External validity concerns drawing conclusions to an external population beyond the study's restricted interest.

Quiz (Q7.4) Label each of the following statements as **True** or **False**; for questions 8-11, an additional response option is **It depends**.

1. Random error occurs whenever there is any (non-zero) difference between the value of the odds ratio in the study population and the estimated odds ratio obtained from the sample that is analyzed.   ???
2. Systematic error occurs whenever there is any (non-zero) difference between the value of the effect measure in the source population and the estimate from the sample.   ???
3. In a valid study, there is neither systematic error nor random error.   ???
4. The study population is always a subset of the source population.   ???
5. The sample is always a subset of the study population.   ???
6. The sample is always a subset of the source population.   ???
7. The estimated effect measure in the sample is always equal to the corresponding effect measure in the study population.   ???
8. Suppose the risk ratio in the source population is 3.0, whereas the risk ratio estimate in the (study) sample is 1.2. Then the study is not internally valid. ???
9. Suppose the risk ratio in the source population is 3.0, whereas the risk ratio in

the study population is 1.2. Then the study is not internally valid. **???**

10. Suppose the risk ratio in the source population is 3.0, whereas the risk ratio estimate in the study population is 3.1. Then the study is not internally valid. **???**

11. Suppose the risk ratio in the source population is 3.0, whereas the risk ratio estimate in the study population is 3.1. Then the study is not externally valid. **???**

Quantitative Definition of Bias

*A **bias** in an epidemiologic study can be defined quantitatively in terms of the **target parameter** of interest and measure of effect actually being estimated in the study population.*

A study that is not internally valid is said to have bias. Let's quantify what we mean by bias. The measure of effect in the source population is our target parameter.

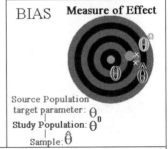

The choice of this parameter depends on the study design features, objectives of the study, and the type of bias being considered. We denote the target parameter with the Greek letter θ ("theta"). We want to estimate the value of θ in the source population.

Recalling the hierarchy of populations associated with a given study, we denote as θ^0 the measure of effect in the study population. $\hat{\theta}$ ("theta-hat") denotes the estimate of our measure of effect obtained from the sample actually analyzed. Of course, $\hat{\theta}$, θ^0 and θ may all have different values.

Any difference between $\hat{\theta}$ and θ^0 is the result of random error. Any difference between θ^0 and θ is due to systematic error.

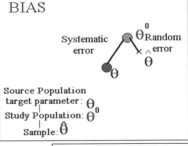

We use $\hat{\theta}$ to estimate θ. We say that $\hat{\theta}$ is a biased estimate of θ if θ^0 is not equal to θ, and we define the bias to be the difference between these two parameters:

Bias $(\hat{\theta}, \theta) = \theta^0 - \theta$

$\hat{\theta}$ is a biased estimate of θ if
$$\theta^0 - \theta \neq 0$$
meaningful difference

Thus, a bias occurs if an estimated measure of effect for the study population differs systematically from the value of the target parameter. The *not equal* sign shown below should not be strictly interpreted as any difference from zero, but rather as a meaningful difference from zero. Such a flexible interpretation of the definition is necessary because bias can rarely be quantified precisely because the target parameter is always unknown.

Study Questions (Q7.5) Consider a cohort study to evaluate whether heavy drinking during pregnancy leads to low birth weight babies. Although it is usually unknown, suppose the risk ratio in the source population (i.e., entire cohort) is 3.5. Suppose further that the study sample is representative of the source population at the start of follow-up, but that there is considerable migration out of the target population location. As a result, the risk ratio found in the final sample is 1.5.

1. For this scenario, what are the values of the target (i.e., source) population parameter and the study population parameter?
2. Is there bias in this study? Explain briefly.
3. What is the value of the bias in this study?
4. If the true effect being estimated is *high* (e.g., RR>3.5), but the study data show essentially no effect, does this indicate a bias? Explain briefly.
5. If the true effect estimated indicates *no* association, but the study data show a high association, does this indicate a bias? Explain briefly.

❖ Bias measures the extent that study results are distorted from the correct results that would have been found from a valid study.
❖ Bias occurs if an estimated measure of effect for the study population differs systematically from the value of the target parameter.
❖ Bias can rarely be quantified precisely primarily because the target parameter is always unknown.
❖ θ ("theta") is the target parameter, θ^0 is the study population parameter, and $\hat{\theta}$ is the sample estimate.
❖ $\hat{\theta}$ is a biased estimate of θ provided θ^0 is not equal to θ.
❖ Bias $(\hat{\theta}, \theta) = \theta^0 - \theta$

Relating the Target Parameter to Type of Bias

The target parameter in most epidemiologic studies is typically a measure of effect, e.g., some kind of risk ratio, odds ratio, or rate ratio, appropriate for the study design being considered. The choice of parameter depends on whether the type of bias of interest is selection bias, information bias, or confounding bias, or whether more than one of these three types of bias is of concern.

When **selection bias** is the only type of bias being considered, the target parameter is typically the value of the measure of effect of interest in the source population from which the cases are derived.

If, however, **information bias** is the only type of bias considered, then the target parameter is the measure of effect that corrects for possible misclassification or that would result from the absence of misclassification.

If there is only bias due to **confounding**, then the target parameter is the measure of effect estimated when confounding is controlled.

If more than one bias is possible, then the target parameter is the value of the measure of effect after all contributing sources of bias are corrected.

Direction of the Bias

Although the precise magnitude of bias can never really be quantified, the **direction of bias** *can often be determined. The direction of the bias concerns whether or not the target parameters is either overestimated or underestimated without specifying the magnitude of the bias.*

We have defined bias as the difference between the value of the effect measure in our target (i.e., source) population and the value of the effect measure actually being estimated in the study population. Since the target parameter is always unknown and the effect being estimated in the study population has random error, it is virtually impossible to quantify the magnitude of a bias precisely in a given epidemiologic study. Nevertheless, the investigator can often determine the direction of the bias. Such assessment usually requires subjective judgment based on the investigator's knowledge of the variables being studied and the features of the study design that are the sources of possible bias. By direction, we mean a determination of whether the target parameter is **overestimated** or **underestimated** without specifying the magnitude of the bias. If the target parameter is **overestimated**, we say that the direction of the bias is **away from the null**. If the target parameter is **underestimated**, we say that the direction of the bias is **towards the null**.

$$\mathrm{BIAS}(\hat{\theta}, \theta) = \theta^0 - \theta$$

Direction of Bias

$\theta^0 > \overset{\text{Target}}{\theta}$ Overestimated ➔ Away from the null

$\theta^0 < \theta$ Underestimated ➔ Towards the null

For example, suppose the target parameter is a risk ratio whose value is 1.5, but the risk ratio actually being estimated from our study is 4. Then the true effect has

Overestimated ➔ Away from the null

$$RR^0 = 4 > RR = 1.5 > 1$$

null value

been overestimated, since the effect from the study appears to be stronger than it really is. Both the target parameter and the study population parameter in this example are greater than the null value of 1 for a risk ratio. Thus, the bias is away from the null, since the incorrect value of 4 is further away from 1 than the correct value of 1.5.

Similarly, if the target risk ratio is less than the null value of 1, say .70 and the risk ratio being estimated is .25, the true effect is also overestimated. In this case, the true effect is

Overestimated ➔ Away from the null

$$RR^0 = 0.25 < RR = 0.70 < 1$$

More Protective   Protective

protective, since it is less than 1, and the estimated effect of .25 is even more protective than the true effect. Again, the incorrect value of .25 is further away from 1 than the correct value of .70, so the bias is away from the null.

To describe **underestimation**, or **bias towards the null**, suppose the target risk ratio is 4, but the estimated risk ratio is 1.5. Then the true effect is underestimated, since the effect from the

Underestimated ➔ Towards the null

$$1 < RR^0 = 1.5 < RR = 4$$

Study effect (1.5) appears weaker than it really is (4)

study appears to be weaker than it really is. Moreover, the incorrect value of 1.5 in this case is closer to the null value of 1 than is the correct value of 4, so the bias is

towards the null.

If the target risk ratio is 0.25 but the risk ratio being estimated is 0.70, then once again the correct value is underestimated and the bias is towards the null. In this case, the

Underestimated → Towards the null
$1 > RR^0 = 0.70 > RR = 0.25$
0.70 closer to the null than 0.25

incorrect value of 0.70 is closer to the null value of 1 than is the correct value of .25.

Suppose, however, that the target risk ratio is .50 but the risk ratio actually being estimated is 2. These two values are on opposite sides of the null value, so we cannot argue that the bias is either towards or away from the null. In this case, we call

Switchover Bias
$RR^0 = 2 > 1 > RR = 0.50$
Exposure appears to have a harmful effect when truly protective.
OR
$RR^0 = 0.7 < 1 < RR = 1.5$
Exposure appears to be protective when truly harmful.

this kind of bias a **switchover bias**. In other words, a switchover bias may occur if the exposure appears in the data to have a harmful effect on the disease when it is truly protective. Alternatively, a switchover bias can occur if the exposure appears to be protective when it is truly harmful.

Study Questions (Q7.6) Knowing the direction of the bias can be of practical importance to the investigator.

1. Suppose an investigator finds a very strong effect, say the estimated RR (in the study population) is 6, and she can also persuasively argue that any possible bias must be towards the null. Then what can be concluded about the correct (i.e., target) value of RR?
2. Suppose an investigator finds a very weak estimated RR (in the study population) of, say, 1.3, and can argue that any bias must be away from the null. Then what can be concluded about the correct value of the RR?

Summary
* The direction of the bias concerns whether or not the target parameter is either overestimated or underestimated without specifying the magnitude of the bias.
* If the target parameter is overestimated, the direction of the bias is away from the null.
* If the target parameter is underestimated, the direction of the bias is towards the null.
* A switchover bias occurs if the target parameter is on the opposite side of the null value from the parameter actually being estimated in one's study.

Quiz (Q7.7) Label each of the following statements as **True** or **False**.

1. If the estimated RR equals 2.7 in the sample and it is determined that there is a bias away from the null, then the RR in the target (i.e., source) population is greater than 2.7.   **???**
2. If the estimated RR in the sample is 1.1 and it is determined that there is bias towards the null, then there is essentially no association in the target population (as measured by RR).   **???**

3. If the estimated RR in the sample is 1.1 and it is determined that there is bias away from the null, then there is essentially no association in the target population.   **???**

4. If the estimated RR equals 0.4 in the sample and it is determined that there is a bias away from the null, then the RR in the target (i.e., source) population is less than 0.4.   **???**

5. If the estimated RR in the sample is 0.4 and it is determined that there is bias towards the null, then there is essentially no association in the target population (as measured by RR).   **???**

6. If the estimated RR in the sample is 0.98 and it is determined that there is bias away from the null, then there is essentially no association in the target population.   **???**

Fill in the Blanks; Choices <u>Away from the null</u> <u>Switchover</u>   <u>Towards the null</u>

7. If OR equals 3.6 in the target population and 1.3 in the study population, then the bias is .   **???**

8. If IDR is 0.25 in the target population and 0.95 in the study population, then the bias is   **???**

9. If the RR is 1 in the target population and 4.1 in the study population, then the bias is   **???**

10. If the RR is 0.6 in the target population and 2.1 in the study population, then the bias is   **???**

11. If the RR is 1 in the target population and 0.77 in the study population, then the bias is   **???**

12. If the RR is 4.0 in the target population and 0.9 in the study population, then the bias is   **???**

What Can be Done About Bias?

The evaluation of bias is typically subjective and involves a judgment about either the presence of the bias, the direction of the bias, or, much more rarely, the magnitude of the bias. Nevertheless, there are ways to address the problem of bias, including adjusting the sample estimate to "correct" for bias. Three general approaches are now described.

Here are three general approaches for addressing bias: 1) a priori study **design** decisions; 2) decisions during the **analysis** stage; and 3) **discussion** during the publication stage.

3 Approaches for Addressing Bias
1) a priori study design decisions
2) decisions during analysis stage
3) discussion during publication stage

When you **design** a study, you can make decisions to minimize or even avoid bias in the study's results. You can avoid **selection bias** by including or excluding eligible subjects, by choice of the source population, or by the choice of the comparison group, say the control group in a case-control study.

Study Questions (Q7.8)

1. What type of bias may be avoided by taking special care to accurately measure the exposure, disease, and control variables being studied, including using pilot studies to identify measurement problems that can be corrected in the main study?

    A. Selection bias   B. Information bias   C. Confounding bias

2. What type of bias may be avoided by making sure to measure or observe variables at the design stage that may be accounted for at the analysis stage?

    B. Selection bias   B. Information bias   C. Confounding bias

At the **analysis** stage, the investigator may be able to determine either the presence or direction of possible bias by logical reasoning about methodologic features of the study design actually used.

Study Questions (Q7.8) continued

3. In the Sydney Beach User's study, both swimming status and illness outcome were determined by subject self-report and recall. This indicates the need to assess the presence or direction of which type of bias at the analysis stage?

    A. Selection bias   B. Information bias   C. Confounding bias

4. Also, in the Sydney Beach Users study, subjects had to be excluded from the analysis if they did not complete the follow-up interview. This non-response may affect how representative the sample is. This is an example of which type of bias?

    A. Selection bias   B. Information bias   C. Confounding bias

At the **analysis** stage, bias can also be reduced or eliminated by *adjusting* a sample estimate by a guestimate of the amount of bias. Such adjustment is typically done for confounding by quantitatively accounting for the effects of confounding variables using **stratified analysis** or **mathematical modeling** methods.

> **Analysis Stage**
> **Adjustment**
> Selection/Information Bias:
>
> Limited by available information
> to measure **extent** of bias
>
> $$\hat{\theta}^c = \hat{\theta} - BÍAS$$
>
> not easy to apply
>
> θ and θ^0 always unknown
>
> θ^c - corrected estimate

Adjustment for selection bias and information bias is limited by the availability of information necessary to measure the extent of the bias. A simple formula for a "corrected" estimate involves manipulating the equation for bias by moving the target parameter to the left side of the equation. This formula is not as easy to apply as it appears. Most investigators will have to be satisfied with making a case for the direction of the bias instead. The estimated bias depends on the availability of more fundamental parameters, which are often difficult to determine. We discuss these parameters further in the chapters that follow.

The final approach to addressing bias is how you report your study. A description of the potential biases of the study is typically provided in the "Discussion" section of a publication. This discussion, particularly when it concerns possible **selection** or **information** bias, is quite subjective, but judgment is expected because of the inherent difficulty in quantifying biases. Rarely if ever does the investigator admit in the write-up that bias casts severe doubt on the study's conclusions. So, the reader must review this section with great care!

Summary – What Can be Done about Bias?

❖ The answer depends on the type of bias being considered: selection, information, or confounding.

❖ Approaches for addressing bias are: decisions in the study design stage, the analysis stage, and the publication stage.

❖ At the study design stage, steps can be taken to avoid bias.

❖ At the analysis stage, one may use logical reasoning about methodologic features of the study design actually used.

❖ Also at the analysis stage, **confounding** bias can be reduced or eliminated by quantitatively adjusting the sample estimate.

❖ A simple formula for a corrected estimate: $\theta^c = \hat{\theta} - \text{Bi}\hat{a}\text{s}$. This formula is not as easy to apply as it looks.

❖ Potential biases are described in the **Discussion** section of a publication. Beware!

Nomenclature

θ "theta", the parameter from the target population

$\hat{\theta}$ "theta-hat", the parameter estimate from the sample actually analyzed

θ^0 The parameter from the study population

RR   Risk ratio of the target population

RR^0 Risk ratio of the study population

References

Berkson J. Limitations of the application of fourfold table analysis to hospital data. Biometrics Bulletin 1946;2: 47-53.

Corbett SJ, Rubin GL, Curry GK, Kleinbaum DG. The health effects of swimming at Sydney Beaches. The Sydney Beach Users Study Advisory Group. Am J Public Health. 1993;83(12): 1701-6.

Greenberg RS, Daniels SR, Flanders WD, Eley JW, Boring JR. Medical Epidemiology (3rd Ed). Lange Medical Books, New York, 2001.

Hill H, Kleinbaum DG. Bias in Observational Studies. In Encyclopedia of Biostatistics, pp 323-329, Oxford University Press, 1999.

Horwitz RI, Feinstein AR. Alternative analytic methods for case-control studies of estrogens and endometrial cancer. N Engl J Med 1978;299(20):1089-94.

Kleinbaum DG, Kupper LL, Morgenstern H. Epidemiologic Research: Principles and Quantitative Methods. John Wiley and Sons Publishers, New York, 1982.

Perera FP, et al. Biologic markers in risk assessment for environmental carcinogens. Environ Health Persp 1991;90:247.

The Lipid Research Clinics Coronary Primary Prevention Trial results: II. The relationship of coronary heart disease to cholesterol lowering. JAMA 1984;251(2):365-74.

Warner L, Clay-Warner J, Boles J, Williamson J. Assessing condom use practices. Implications for evaluating method and user effectiveness. Sex Transm Dis 1998; 25(6):273-7.

Answers to Study Questions and Quizzes

Q7.1

1. Women residents from Atlanta between 45 and 69 years of age.
2. A measure of effect, either a prevalence ratio or a prevalence odds ratio (i.e., the blue dot or bulls eye), for the association between calcium intake and prevalence of arthritis of the hip in the target population.
3. Random error concerns whether or not the estimated odds ratio in the hospital sample (i.e., the shot at the target) differs from the odds ratio in the population of hospital patients (i.e., the red dot or the center of the actual shots) from which the sample is selected.
4. Systematic error concerns whether or not the odds ratio in the population of hospital patients being sampled (i.e., the red dot) is different from the odds ratio in the target population (i.e., the blue dot).

Q7.2

1. All young adults in New York City.
2. All young adults who attend fitness centers in New York City (NYC) and would eventually remain in the study for analysis.
3. Yes, the sample is randomly selected from the study population and is therefore representative.
4. Probably not. The group of young adults in NYC is different from the group of all young adults in NYC. Since fitness is so strongly related to health, the use of those attending fitness centers for all young adults is probably not the best choice for this study.
5. All young adults in New York City.
6. All young adults in NYC that would eventually remain in the study for analysis.
7. Yes, the sample is randomly selected from the study population (by definition of the study population) and is therefore representative of it. Nevertheless, neither the study population nor the sample may be representative of all young adults in NYC if not everyone selected into the sample participates in the study.

8. Yes, assuming that everyone selected participates (i.e., provides the required data) in the study, the study population is the same as the source population. However, if many of those sampled (e.g., a particular subgroup) do not participate, the final sample and its corresponding study population might be unrepresentative of all young adults in NYC.
9. False. Persons lost-to-follow-up are not found in the study sample, so they can't be included in the study population that is represented by the sample.
10. True. Persons lost-to-follow-up are not found in the sample, but they are still included in the source population of interest.
11. True. In the study population, controls may be specified as persons without the disease, regardless of whether they are at risk for being a case. However, the source population may only contain persons at risk for being a case.
12. False. The study population in a cross-sectional study is restricted to survivors only.
13. The population of young adults in New York State is an external population, because the study was restricted to young adults in New York City. Extrapolating the study results to New York State goes beyond considering the methodological aspects of the actual study.

Q7.3

1. The study will be internally valid provided the study population corresponding to the sample actually analyzed is not substantially distorted from the source population of young adults from fitness centers in the city. For example, if the sample eventually analyzed is a much healthier population than the source population, internal validity may be questioned.
2. External validity. The study was restricted to persons in New York City. Extrapolating the study results to New York State goes beyond considering the methodological aspects of the New York City study

3. Do the results of the study also apply to women or to men of different ages?
4. Was the study sample representative of the source population? Were the comparison groups selected properly? Did subjects consistently stick to their diet and medication regimen? Were relevant variables taken into account?

Q7.4
1. T
2. F – Systematic error occurs when there is a difference between the true effect measure and that which is actually estimated, i.e., a difference between the source and study populations.
3. F – A valid study means there is no systematic error, but there may still be random error
4. F – Not always. Ideally the study population would be equivalent to the source population. However, it may be that the study population and source population simply overlap.
5. T – The sample is always selected from the study population.
6. F – If the study population is not a subset of or equivalent to the source population, then the sample may not be a subset of (or completely contained in) the source population.
7. F – They may be different due to random error.
8. It depends – The difference may be a result of random error. If the risk ratio in the study population is meaningfully different from 3.0, then the study is not internally valid.
9. T – Any meaningful difference between the study and source population means that the study is not internally valid.
10. F – The difference between 3.0 and 3.1 would not be considered a meaningful difference.
11. It depends – We do not know about the risk ratio in the external population.

Q7.5
1. The target population parameter is 3.5. We don't know the value of the study population parameter, but it is likely to be closer to 1.5 than to 3.5 because the sample is assumed to be representative of the study population.

2. There appears to be bias in the study because the sample estimate of 1.5 is meaningfully different from the population estimate and it is reasonable to think that the final sample no longer represents the source population.
3. The bias can't be determined exactly because 1.5 is a sample estimate; however, the bias in the risk ratio is approximately $1.5 - 3.5 = -2$.
4. Yes, provided the reason for the difference is due to systematic error.
5. Yes, provided the reason for the difference is due to systematic error.

Q7.6
1. The correct RR must be even larger than 6.
2. The correct RR must indicate an even weaker, or no effect.

Q7.7
1. F – If the bias is away from the null, the RR in the source population must lie between 1 and 2.7.
2. F – If the bias is towards the null, then the RR in the source population is greater than 1.1. Since we cannot determine how much greater, we cannot conclude that these is essentially no association.
3. T – If the bias is away from the null, then the RR in the source population is between 1 and 1.1. We can thus conclude that there is essentially no association.
4. F – If the bias is away from the null, then the RR in the source population must lies between 0.4 and 1.0.
5. F – If the bias is towards the null, then the RR in the source population must be less than 0.4 and hence there is an association.
6. T – If the bias is away from the null, then the RR in the source population is between 0.98 and 1.0, which means there is essentially no association.
7. Towards the null
8. Towards the null
9. Away from the null
10. Switchover
11. Away from the null
12. Switchover

Q7.8
1. B; 2. C; 3. B; 4. A

CHAPTER 8
WERE SUBJECTS CHOSEN BADLY? SELECTION BIAS

Selection bias concerns systematic error that may arise from the manner in which subjects are selected into one's study. In his chapter we describe examples of selection bias, provide a quantitative framework for assessing selection bias, show how selection bias can occur in different types of epidemiologic study designs, and discuss how to adjust for or otherwise deal with selection bias.

Selection Bias in Different Study Designs

Selection bias is systematic error that results from the way subjects are selected into the study or because there are selective losses of subjects prior to data analysis. Selection bias can occur in any kind of epidemiologic study. In **case-control studies**, the primary source of selection bias is **the manner in which cases, controls, or both are selected** and the extent to which exposure history influences such selection. For example, selection bias was of concern in case-control studies that found an association between use of the supplement L-tryptophan and EMS (eosinophilia myalgia syndrome), an illness characterized primarily by incapacitating muscle pains, malaise, and elevated eosinophil counts. The odds ratios obtained from these studies might have overestimated the true effect.

Study Questions (Q8.1)
1. Assuming that the odds ratio relating L-tryptophan to EMS is overestimated, which of the following choices is correct?
   a. The bias is towards the null.
   b. L-tryptophan has a weaker association with EMS than actually observed.
   c. The correct odds ratio is larger than the observed odds ratio.

   Consequently, the bias would be away from the null.
   A primary criticism of these studies was that initial publicity about a suspected association may have resulted in preferential diagnosis of EMS among known users of L-tryptophan when compared with nonusers.

Study Questions (Q8.1) continued
2. Assuming preferential diagnosis of EMS from publicity about L-tryptophan, which of the following is correct? The proportion exposed among diagnosed cases selected for study is likely to be **???** the proportion exposed among all cases in the source population.
   a. larger than
   b. smaller than
   c. equal to

In cohort studies and clinical trials, the primary sources of selection bias are

loss-to-follow-up, withdrawal from the study, or **non-response**. For example, consider a clinical trial that compares the effects of a new treatment regimen with a standard regimen for a certain cancer. Suppose patients assigned to the new treatment are more likely than those on the standard to develop side effects and consequently withdraw from the study.

Study Questions (Q8.2) Clinical trial: new cancer regimen versus standard regimen. Suppose patients on new regimen are more likely to withdraw from study than those on standard.
1. Why might the withdrawal information above suggest the possibility of selection bias in this study?
2. Why won't and intention-to-treat analysis solve this problem?
3. What is the source population in this study?
4. What is the study population in this study?

In cross-sectional studies, the primary source of selection bias is what is called **selective survival**. Only survivors can be included in cross-sectional studies. If exposed cases are more likely to survive longer than unexposed cases, or vice versa, the conclusions obtained from a cross-sectional study might be different than from an appropriate cohort study.

Study Questions (Q8.2) continued Suppose we wish to assess whether there is selective survival in a cross-sectional study.
5. What is the source population?
6. What is the study population?

Summary
❖ Selection bias can occur from systematic error that results from the way subjects are selected into the study and remain for analysis.
❖ The primary reason for such bias usually differs with the type of study used.
❖ In case-control studies, the primary source of selection bias is the manner in which cases, controls, or both are selected.
❖ In cohort studies and clinical trials, the primary source of selection bias is loss to follow-up, withdrawal from the study, or non-response.
❖ In cross-sectional studies, the primary source of selection bias is what is called selective survival.

Example of Selection Bias in Case-Control Studies

In case-control studies, because the health outcome has already occurred, the selection of cases, controls, or both might be influenced by prior exposure status. In the 1970's, there was a lively published debate about selection bias in studies of whether use of estrogen as a hormone replacement leads to endometrial cancer. Early studies were case-control studies and they indicated a strong harmful effect of estrogen. The controls typically used were women with gynecological cancers other than endometrial cancer. Critics claimed that because estrogen often causes vaginal bleeding irrespective of cancer, estrogen users with endometrial cancer would be selectively screened for such cancer compared to nonusers with endometrial cancer.

Study Questions (Q8.3)
1. If the critics reasoning were correct, why would there be a selection bias problem with choosing controls to be women with gynecological cancers other than endometrial cancer?
2. If the critics reasoning were correct, would you expect the estimated odds ratio obtained from the study to be biased towards or away from the null? Explain briefly.

An alternative choice of controls was proposed; women with benign endometrial tumors, since it was postulated that such a control group would be just as likely to be selectively screened as would the cases.

Study Questions (Q8.3) continued
3. Why would estrogen users with benign endometrial tumors be more likely to be selectively screened for their tumors when compared to nonusers?
4. Assuming that estrogen users with both cancerous and benign endometrial tumors are likely to be selectively screened for their tumors when compared to non-users, what problem may still exist if the latter group is chosen as controls?

Continued research and debate, however, have indicated that selective screening of cases is not likely to contribute much bias. In fact, the proposed alternative choice of controls might actually lead to bias.

Study Questions (Q8.3) continued Researchers concluded that because nearly all women with invasive endometrial cancer will ultimately have the disease diagnosed, estrogen users will be slightly over-represented, if at all, among a series of women with endometrial cancer. Assume for the questions below that selective screening of cases does not influence the detection of endometrial cancer cases.

5. If the control group consisted of women with benign tumors in the endometrium, why would you expect to have selection bias?
6. Would the direction of the bias be towards or away from the null? Briefly explain.
7. If the control group consisted of women with gynecologic cancers other than in the endometrium, why would you not expect selection bias in the estimation of the odds ratio?

In current medical practice, the prevailing viewpoint is that taking estrogen alone is potentially harmful for endometrial cancer. Consequently, women who are recommended for hormone replacement therapy are typically given a combination of progesterone and estrogen rather than estrogen alone.

Summary
❖ Selection bias concerns a distortion of study results that occurs because of the way subjects are selected into the study.
❖ In case-control studies, the primary concern is that selection of cases, controls, or both might be influenced by prior exposure status.
❖ In the 1970's, there was a lively published debate about possible selection bias

among researchers studying whether use of estrogen, the exposure, as a hormone replacement leads to endometrial cancer.

❖ The argument supporting selection bias has not held up over time; current medical practice for hormone replacement therapy typically involves a combination of progesterone and estrogen rather than estrogen alone.

Example of Selection Bias in Cohort Studies

Selection bias can occur in cohort studies as well as in case-control studies. In prospective cohort studies, the health outcome, which has not yet occurred when exposure status is determined, cannot influence how subjects are selected into the study. However, if the health outcome is not determined for everyone initially selected for study, the study results may be biased. The primary sources of such selection bias are **loss-to-follow-up**, **withdrawal** or **non-response**. The collection of subjects that remain to be analyzed may no longer represent the source population from which the original sample was selected.

Consider this two-way table that describes the five-year follow-up for disease "D" in a certain source population. Suppose that a cohort study is carried out using a 10% random sample from this population.

Follow-up study

(Source Pop.)	E	not E	Total
D	150	50	200
not D	9850	9950	19800
Total	10000	10000	20000

$$RR = (150/10000) / (50/10000) = 3.0$$

Consider the following table of expected cell frequencies for this cohort:

10% random sample: Fill in the blanks!

(Initial Sample)	E	Not E
D	15	5
Not D	985	995
Total	1000	1000

Study Questions (Q8.4)

1. Assuming this is the sample that is analyzed, is there selection bias?

Assume that the initial cohort was obtained from the 10% sampling. However, now suppose that 20% of exposed persons are lost to follow-up but 10% of unexposed persons are

Now assume: 20% lost to follow-up 10% lost to follow-up

10% random sample plus loss-to-follow-up

	E	Not E
D	12	4.5
Not D	788	895.5
Total	800	900

lost. Also, assume that exposed persons have the same risk for disease in the final cohort as in the initial cohort and that the same is true for unexposed persons.

Study Questions (Q8.4) continued

2. Does the sample just described represent the source population or the study population?
3. What is the source population for which this sample is derived?
4. For the above assumptions, is there selection bias?

Suppose that a different pattern of loss-to follow-up results in the two-way table shown here.

10% random sample, different loss-to-follow-up:

	E	Not E
D	14	4
Not D	786	896
Total	800	900

$$\hat{RR} = 3.9$$

Study Questions (Q8.4) continued

5. Do these results indicate selection bias?
6. Do the exposed persons in the study population have the same risk for disease as in the source population?
7. Do the <u>un</u>exposed persons in the study population have the same risk for disease as in the source population?
8. Do the previous examples demonstrate that there will be selection bias in cohort studies whenever the percent lost to follow-up in the exposed group differs from the percent lost-to-follow-up in the unexposed group?

Summary

❖ The primary sources of selection bias in cohort studies are loss-to-follow-up, withdrawal, and non-response.

❖ In cohort studies, the collection of subjects that remain in the final sample that is analyzed may no longer represent the source population from which the original cohort was selected.

❖ Selection bias will occur if loss to follow-up results in risk for disease in the exposed and/or unexposed groups that are different in the final sample than in the original cohort.

Some Fine Points about Selection Bias in Cohort Studies

Reference: Hill, HA and Kleinbaum, DG, "Bias in Observational Studies", in the Encyclopedia of Biostatistics, P.A. Armitage and T Colton, eds., June 1998.

Selection bias in cohort studies may occur even with a fairly high overall response rate or with very little loss to follow-up. Consider a cohort study in which 95% of all subjects originally assembled into the cohort remain for analysis at the end of the study. That is, only 5% of subjects are lost to follow-up. If losses to follow-up are primarily found in exposed subjects who develop the disease, then despite the small amount of follow-up loss, the correct (i.e., target) risk ratio could be underestimated substantially. This is because, in the sample that is analyzed, the estimated risk for developing the disease in exposed subjects will be less than what it is in the source population, whereas the corresponding risk for unexposed subjects will accurately reflect the source population.

There may be no selection bias despite small response rates or high loss to follow-up. Suppose only 10% of all initially selected subjects agree to participate in a study, but this 10% represents a true random sample of the source population. Then the resulting risk ratio estimate will be unbiased. The key issue here is whether risks for exposed and unexposed in the sample that is analyzed are disproportionately modified because of non-response or follow-up loss from the corresponding risks in the source population from which the initial sample was selected.

We are essentially comparing two 2x2 tables here, one representing the source population and the other representing the sample:

	Source Population				**Sample for Analysis**	
	E	Not E			E	Not E
D	A	B		**D**	a	b
Not D	C	D		**Not D**	c	d
Total	N_1	N_0		**Total**	n_1	n_0

Selection bias will occur only if, when considering these tables, the risk ratio in the source population, i.e.,

$\dfrac{A/N_1}{B/N_0}$ is meaningfully different from the risk ratio in the sample, i.e., $\dfrac{a/n_1}{b/n_0}$

In the first example above (95% loss to follow-up), the argument for selection bias is essentially that the numerator a/n_1 of the risk ratio in the analyzed sample would be less than the corresponding numerator A/N_1 in the source population, whereas the corresponding denominators in these two risk ratios would be equal.

In the second example (10% non-response), the argument for no selection bias is essentially that despite the high non-response, corresponding numerators and denominators in the source population and sample are equal.

Other Examples

Here are a few more examples of studies that are likely to raise questions about selection bias.

Study Questions (Q8.5) Consider a retrospective cohort study that compares workers in a certain chemical industry to a population-based comparison group for the development of coronary heart disease (CHD).
1. In such a study, selection bias may occur because of the so-called "healthy worker effect". How might such a bias come about?

Selection bias may result from using volunteers for a study.
2. Explain the above statement in terms of study and source populations.
3. What is an alternative way to view the validity problem that arises when a study is restricted to volunteers?

In assessing long term neurologic disorders among children with febrile seizures, clinic-based studies tend to report a much higher frequency of such disorders than found in population-based studies.
4. Does the above statement indicate that clinic-based studies can result in selection bias? Explain briefly.

Summary
- ❖ Selection bias may occur because of the so-called "healthy worker effect". Workers tend to be healthier than those in the general population and may therefore have a more favorable outcome regardless of exposure status.
- ❖ Selection bias may result from using volunteers, who may have different characteristics from persons who do not volunteer.
- ❖ Clinic-based studies may lead to selection bias because patients from clinics tend to have more severe illness than persons in a population-based sample.

What Can Be Done About Selection Bias Qualitatively?

A description of quantitative formulas for correcting for selection bias, see is provided on pages 8-2 and 8-5 of the ActivEpi CD. Unfortunately the information required to apply these formulas, namely the selection ratio parameters or their ratios, is conceptually complicated, rarely available, and not easily quantified. The ideal way to address selection bias is to prevent or at least minimize such bias when designing a study rather than to attempt to correct for the bias once the data have been collected.

In case-control studies, the controls should be carefully chosen to represent the source population that produced the cases. The use of two or more control groups should also be considered.

Case-control studies using incident cases and nested case-control studies are preferable to studies that use prevalent cases or to hospital-based studies. Selection bias may also be avoided by assuring equal opportunity for disease detection among exposed and unexposed subjects.

In cohort studies, efforts should be made to achieve high response and low loss-to-follow-up.

Observational studies involving volunteers should be avoided, although clinical trials involving volunteers are possible because of randomization. Occupational cohort studies should avoid a healthy worker bias by ensuring that unexposed subjects are as healthy as exposed subjects.

At the analysis stage, it may be possible to determine the direction of the bias, even if the magnitude of the bias cannot be estimated or a numerical correction for bias is not feasible.

One approach to addressing selection bias as well as information and confounding biases is in the write-up of the study. A description of the potential biases of the study is typically provided in the "Discussion" section of a publication. This discussion, particularly when it concerns possible selection bias, is quite subjective, but such judgment is required because of the inherent difficulty in quantifying such biases.

Summary

❖ The information required to assess selection bias is conceptually complicated, rarely available, nor is easily quantifiable.

❖ At the study design stage, decisions may be made to avoid selection bias in the study's results.

❖ At the analysis stage, it may be possible to determine the direction of selection bias without being able to quantitatively correct for the bias.

❖ At the publication stage, potential biases are typically addressed qualitatively in the **Discussion** section of a paper.

The "Worst-Case Scenario" Approach

This is a practical approach for assessing the **direction** of **selection bias** that considers the most extreme changes in the estimate of effect that are realistically possible as a result of the way subjects are selected. Through such an approach it may be possible to show that the worst amount of bias possible will have a negligible effect on the conclusions of one's study.

For example, consider a cohort study involving lung-cancer-free 1000 smokers and 1000 non-smokers all over 40 years of age that are followed for 10 years. Suppose further that over the follow-up period, 200 smokers and 100 non-smokers are lost-to-follow-up. Also, suppose, that among those 800 smokers and 900 non-smokers remaining in the study, the 2x2 table relating smoking status at the start of the study to the development of lung cancer (LC) over the 10 year follow-up is shown as follows:

	Smokers	Non-smokers
LC	80	10
No LC	720	890
Total	800	900

The estimated risk ratio from these data is $(80/800)/(10/900) = 9$, which suggests a very strong relationship between smoking status and the development of lung cancer. A worst-case scenario might determine what the risk ratio estimates would be if either all 200 smokers lost-to-follow-up did not develop lung cancer and/or all 100 non-smokers lost to follow-up did develop lung. Here are comparison of estimates for "worst-case" scenarios:

Scenario	RR
1. Actual observed data	9
2. $1/10^{th}$ of 200 lost-to-follow-up smokers get LC and $1/90^{th}$ of the 100 lost-to-follow-up non-smokers get LC	9
3. $1/10^{th}$ of the 200 lost-to-follow-up smokers get LC and $2/90^{th}$ of the 100 lost-to-follow-up non-smokers get LC	8.2
4. None of the 200 lost-to-follow-up smokers get LC and $1/90^{th}$ of the 100 lost-to-follow-up non-smokers get LC	7.3
5. None of the 200 lost-to-follow-up smokers get LC and $2/90^{th}$ of the 100 lost-to-follow-up non-smokers get LC	6.6
6. None of the 200 lost-to-follow-up smokers get LC and all 100 lost-to-follow-up non-smokers get LC	0.7

Notice that scenario #6 above changes smoking from being harmful to being protective. Yet this is not a very realistic scenario. Scenario #2 is not really a "worst case" type of scenario because it assumes that those lost to follow-up have the same risk as those actually followed over the entire 10 years. The other three scenarios, i.e., #'s 3, 4, and 5, are "realistic" and of a "worst-case" type; all of these show that the risk ratio is reduced, but is still high. The difficulty with this approach, as illustrated above, concerns the extent to which the investigator can identify a "worst-case" scenario that is the most realistic among all possible scenarios.

Quiz (Q8.6)
1. Case-control studies using **???** are preferable to studies that use **???**.
2. And **???** studies are preferable to **???** studies.
3. In cohort studies, efforts should be made to achieve **???** and to avoid **???**.

Choices cases controls high response hospital-based incident cases loss-to-follow-up nested case-control prevalent cases selection bias

At the analysis stage, the extent of possible selection bias may be assessed using what are often referred to as "worst-case" analyses. Such analyses consider the most extreme changes in the estimated effect that are possible as a result of selection bias. Determine whether each of the following is **True** or **False**.

4. This approach is useful since it could demonstrate that the worst amount of bias possible will have a negligible effect on the conclusions of the study. **???**

5. This approach can rule out selection bias, but it cannot confirm selection bias. **???**

The tables below show the observed results and a 'worst-case' scenario for a clinical trial. Ten subjects receiving standard treatment and 15 subjects receiving a new treatment were lost-to-follow-up. The outcome was whether or not a subject went out of remission (D = out, not D = in) by the end of the trial. In the 'worst-case' scenario, all 10 subjects on standard treatment who were lost-to-follow-up remained in remission but all 15 subjects on the new treatment who were lost-to-follow-up went out of remission.

Observed				Worst-Case		
	Standard Rx	New Rx			Standard Rx	New Rx
D=out	32	7	D=out		a*	b*
Not D = in	100	106	Not D = in		c*	d*

6. What are the values of a*? **???**, b*? **???**, c*? **???**, d*? **???**

Choices   **106**   **110**   **121**   **22**   **32**   **42**   **90**   **91**

7. Refer to the data in the tables above. What is the risk ratio estimate based on the observed data? **???**
8. What is the risk ratio estimate based on the 'worst-case' scenario? **???**
9. In the worst-case scenario, is there selection bias? **???**
10. Does a "worst-case" assessment such as illustrated here "prove" that there is selection bias? **???**

Choices   **1.3**   **1.4**   **3.9**   **4.8**   **No**   **Yes**

References
References on Selection Bias
Berkson J. Limitations of the application of fourfold table analysis to hospital data. Biometrics Bulletin 1946;2: 47-53.
Greenberg RS, Daniels SR, Flanders WD, Eley JW, Boring JR. Medical Epidemiology (3rd Ed). Lange Medical Books, New York, 2001.
Hill H, Kleinbaum DG. Bias in Observational Studies. In Encyclopedia of Biostatistics, pp 323-329, Oxford University Press, 1999.
Horwitz RI, Feinstein AR. Alternative analytic methods for case-control studies of estrogens and endometrial cancer. N Engl J Med 1978;299(20):1089-94.
Kleinbaum DG, Kupper LL, Morgenstern H. Epidemiologic Research: Principles and Quantitative Methods. John Wiley and Sons Publishers, New York, 1982.
References on Condom Effectiveness Studies
Warner L, Clay-Warner J, Boles J, Williamson J. Assessing condom use practices. Implications for evaluating method and user effectiveness. Sex Transm Dis 1998; 25(6):273-7.
Warner DL, Hatcher RA. A meta-analysis of condom effectiveness in reducing sexually transmitted HIV. Soc Sci Med 1994;38(8):1169-70.

Answers to Study Questions and Quizzes
Q8.1
1. b
2. a; exposed cases are likely to be over-represented in the study when compared to unexposed cases.

Q8.2
1. Withdrawals from the study can distort the final sample to be analyzed as compared to the random sample obtained at the start of the trial.
2. Those who withdraw from the study have an unknown outcome and therefore cannot be analyzed.
3. A general population of patients with the specified cancer and eligible to

receive either the standard or the new treatments.

4. The (expected) sample ignoring random error that would be obtained after the withdrawals from the random sample initially selected for the trial.

5. The source population is the population cohort from which the cases would be derived if an appropriate cohort study had been carried out.

6. The study population is the expected sample obtained from the cross-sectional sample that is retained for analysis. Alternatively, the study population is the stable population from which the cross-sectional sample is obtained for study.

Q8.3

1. It is unlikely that women in this control group (e.g., with cervical or ovarian cancers) would be selectively screened for their cancer from vaginal bleeding caused by estrogen use.

2. Away from the null because of selective screening of cases but not controls. This would yield too high a proportion of estrogen users among cases but a correct estimate of the proportion of estrogen users among controls.

3. Because those who have vaginal bleeding from using estrogen will be more likely to have their benign endometrial tumor detected than those non-users with benign endometrial tumors.

4. Using benign endometrial tumors as the control group would hopefully compensate for the selective screening of cases. However, it is not clear that the extent of selective screening would be the "same" for both cases and controls.

5. Having a benign tumor in the endometrium is not readily detected without vaginal bleeding. Therefore, controls with benign endometrial tumors who use estrogen are more likely to have their tumor detected than would nonuser controls.

6. Towards the null because there would be selective screening of controls but not cases. This would yield too high a

proportion of estrogen users among controls but a correct estimate of the proportion of estrogen users among cases.

7. Because there is unlikely to be selective screening in the detection of control cases (with other gynecological cancers) when comparing estrogen users to nonusers.

Q8.4

1. No, since the risk ratio for the expected sample is 3, which equals the risk ratio in the source population.

2. Study population, because the sample just described gives the expected number of subjects obtained in the final sample.

3. The source is the population from which the initial 10% sample obtained prior to follow-up was selected. This is the population of subjects from which cases were derived.

4. There is no selection bias because the RR=3 in the study population, the same as in the source population.

5. Yes, because the estimated risk ratio in the study population of 3.9 is somewhat higher than (3) in the source population as a result of subjects being lost to follow-up.

6. No, the risk for exposed persons is 150/10,000 or .0150 in the source population and is 14/800 = .0175 in the sample.

7. No, the risk for <u>un</u>exposed persons is 50/10,000 or .0050 in the source population and 4/900 or .0044 in the sample.

8. No. There will only be selection bias if loss to follow-up results in risks for disease in the exposed and/or unexposed groups that are different in the final sample than in the original cohort.

Q8.5

1. Workers tend to be healthier than those in the general population and may therefore have a more favorable outcome regardless of exposure status.

2. Volunteers may have different characteristics from person who do not volunteer. The study population here is restricted to volunteers, whereas the

source population is population-based, e.g., a community.
3. There is lack of external validity in drawing conclusions from a source population of volunteers to an external population that is population-based.
4. Yes. Clinic-based studies may lead to spurious conclusions because patients from clinics tend to have more severe illness than persons in a population-based sample.

Q8.6
1. incident cases, prevalent cases
2. nested case-control, hospital-based
3. high response, loss-to-follow-up
4. True
5. True – Since the "worst-case" analysis can demonstrate that the worst amount of bias will have a negligible effect on the conclusions, one could rule out selection bias. However, since the "worst-case" analysis gives us the "worst possible" results, we cannot confirm selection bias. We cannot be sure that our results will be as extreme as "worst-case" results.
6. 32, 22, 110, 106
7. 3.9
8. 1.3
9. Yes
10. No - A worst-case analysis gives the "worst possible" results. Therefore, we cannot be sure that the lost-to-follow-up results that "actually" occur are as extreme as the worst-case "possible".

CHAPTER 9

ARE THE DATA CORRECT? INFORMATION BIAS

*Information bias is a systematic error in a study that arises because of incorrect information obtained on one or more variables measured in the study. The focus here is on the consequences of having inaccurate information about exposure and disease variables that are dichotomous, that is, when there is **misclassification** of exposure and disease that leads to a **bias** in the resulting **measure of effect**. We consider exposure and disease variables that are **dichotomous**. More general situations, such as several categories of exposure or disease, continuous exposure or disease, adjusting for covariates, matched data, and mathematical modeling approaches, are beyond the scope of the activities provided below.*

What is Misclassification Bias?

The two-way table to the right shows the correct classification of 16 subjects according to their true exposure and disease status. Let's see what might happen to this table and its corresponding odds ratio if some of these subjects were misclassified.

Suppose that 3 of the 6 exposed cases, shown here in the lighter shade, were actually

misdiagnosed as exposed non-cases. Suppose further that one of the two unexposed cases was also misclassified as an unexposed non-case. To complete the misclassification picture, we assume that two of the four truly exposed non-cases and two of the four truly unexposed non-cases were misclassified as cases.

The misclassified data are the data that would actually be analyzed because these data are what is observed in the study. So, what is the odds ratio for these data and how does it compare to the correct odds ratio? The odds ratio for the misclassified data is 1; the correct odds ratio is 3. Clearly, there is a bias due to misclassification. The misclassified data suggests no effect of exposure on disease, but the true effect of exposure is quite strong.

Summary
❖ If subjects are misclassified by exposure or disease status, the effect measure, e.g., the OR, may become biased
❖ Bias from misclassification can occur if the effect measure for the correctly classified data is meaningfully different from the estimated effect actually observed in the misclassified data.

❖ Subjects are misclassified if their location in one of the four cells of the correctly classified data changes to a different cell location in the (misclassified) data that is actually observed.

Misclassifying Disease Status

What are the reasons why a subject, like an exposed case, might be misclassified on exposure or disease status? In particular, why might subjects be misclassified from diseased to non-diseased or from non-diseased to diseased status? First, a subject may be incorrectly diagnosed. This can occur because of limited

Why misclassification of disease status ?
* **Incorrect Diagnosis**
Limited knowledge
Diagnostic process complex
Inadequate access to technology
Laboratory error
Disease subclinical
Detection Bias (e.g., more thorough exam if exposed)
* **Subject Self-report**
Incorrect recall
Reluctant to be truthful
* **Records Incorrectly Coded in Data-Base**

knowledge about the disease, because the diagnostic process is complex, because of inadequate access to state-of-the-art diagnostic technology, or because of a laboratory error in the measurement of biologic markers for the disease. In addition, the presence of disease may be not be detected if the disease is sub-clinical at the time of physical exam. Misdiagnosis can occur because of a detection bias if a physician gives a more thorough exam to patients who are exposed or have symptoms related to exposure.

Another source of error occurs when disease status is obtained solely by self-report of subjects rather than by physician examination. In particular, a subject may incorrectly recall illness status, such as respiratory or other infectious illness, that may have occurred at an earlier time period. A subject may be reluctant to be truthful about an illness he or she considers socially or personally unacceptable. Finally, patient records may be inaccurate or coded incorrectly in a database.

The table to the right summarizes misclassification of disease status. The columns of the table show true disease status. The rows of the table show classified disease status. We call this table a **misclassification table**.

Suppose the following numbers appear in the table:

Misclassification Table

	TRUE	
	D	Not D
D' CLASSIFIED		
Not D'		

Misclassification Table

	TRUE		
	D	Not D	
D' CLASSIFIED	6	3	9
Not D'	2	7	9
	8	10	

Study Questions (Q9.1) The following questions refer to the previous table.
1. How many truly diseased persons are misclassified?
2. How many truly non-diseased persons are correctly classified?
3. The percentage of truly diseased persons correctly classified?
4. The percentage of truly non-diseased persons correctly classified?

Summary
❖ Misclassification of disease status may occur from any of the following sources: Incorrect diagnosis, subject self-report, and coding errors
❖ A misclassification table provides a convenient summary of how disease status can be misclassified from true disease status to observed disease status.

Misclassifying Exposure Status

How can subjects be misclassified from exposed to unexposed or from unexposed to exposed? Misclassification of exposure status can occur because of imprecise measurement of exposure. This can result from a poorly constructed questionnaire or survey process that doesn't ask the right questions, or from a faulty measuring device or observation technique.

Why misclassification of exposure status?
* Imprecise measurement
* Subject's Self-report
* Interviewer bias
* Incorrect Coding of Exposure Data

Study Questions (Q9.2) A primary criticism of studies evaluating whether living near power lines increases one's risk for cancer is the quality of measurements of personal exposure to electromagnetic fields (EMFs). Which of the following "reasons" for imprecise measurement of personal EMF exposure do you think are **True** or **False**?

1. Measurements are usually made at only one time point and/or in one location of a residence.
2. Instruments for measuring EMF exposure are not available.
3. Methods for measuring distances and configuration of transmission lines near residences are poorly developed.
4. Better methods for monitoring measurements over time are needed.
5. Measuring EMF exposure from intermittent use of appliances or tools is difficult to measure.
6. Mobility patterns of individual related to EMF exposure are difficult to measure.

Exposure error may occur when exposure is determined solely from self-report by subjects, particularly when recalling prior exposure status. This is typically a problem in case-control studies, since cases may be more motivated to recall past exposures than controls. Recall error can also occur in cohort studies. For example, in the Sydney Beach Users study described in Chapter 2, subjects were asked to report their swimming status seven days after swimming may have occurred.

Subject self-report may also be incorrect because of reluctance of subjects to be truthful in reporting exposures relating to behaviors considered socially unacceptable. This problem often occurs in studies that measure food intake, sexual behavior, and illegal drug-use.

A third source of error in classifying exposure is interviewer bias. In particular, an interviewer may probe more thoroughly about exposure for cases than for controls.

Study Questions (Q9.2) continued Consider a case-control study of the effect of oral contraceptive use on the development of venous (i.e., in the vein) thrombosis (i.e., clotting). (Note: there are no questions numbered 7 to 9.)

10. Why might there be misclassification of exposure, i.e., oral contraceptive use, in such a study?
11. What you expect to be the direction of such misclassification bias?
12. How might you avoid such bias?

Finally, exposure data can be coded incorrectly in a database. The table to the right summarizes exposure status misclassifications. The columns of the table show true exposure status. The rows of the table show classified exposure status.

Misclassification Table

	TRUE	
	E	Not E
E' CLASSIFIED		
Not E'		

Study Questions (Q9.2) continued The questions are based on the table to the right.
13. How many truly exposed persons are misclassified?
14. How many truly unexposed persons are correctly classified?

Misclassification Table

	TRUE		
	E	Not E	
E' CLASSIFIED	95	10	105
Not E'	5	70	75
	100	80	

15. The percentage of truly exposed persons correctly classified?
16. The percentage of truly unexposed persons correctly classified?

Summary
❖ Misclassification of exposure status may occur from any of the following sources: Imprecise measurement, subject self-report, interviewer bias, and incorrect coding of exposure data
❖ A misclassification table provides a convenient summary of how exposure can be misclassified from true exposure to observed exposure.

Example: Misclassifying Both Exposure and Disease Status

Misclassification can sometimes occur for both exposure and disease in the same study. For example, the table to the right considers hypothetical cohort data from subjects surveyed on the beaches of Sydney, Australia

Correctly Classified Data	Swam (E)	Not Swam (Not E)	
Ill (D)	367	233	$\hat{RR} = 3.14$
not Ill (Not D)	300	1100	
Total	667	1333	

during the summer months of a recent year. The study objective was to determine if those who swam at the beach were more likely to become ill than those who did not swim.

Subjects were asked to recall one week later whether they had swum for at least a half an hour on the day they were interviewed on the beach and whether they had developed a cold, cough or flu during the subsequent week. Since both exposure and illness information were obtained by subjects' recall, it is reasonable to expect some subjects may incorrectly report either swimming or illness status or both.

Suppose of the 367 subjects who got ill and swam, only 264 reported that they got ill and swam, and 30 subjects reported that they got ill but didn't swim, 66 subjects reported that they did not get ill but swam, and 7 subjects reported that they did not get ill and did not swim.

Suppose, further, that of the 233 subjects who truly got ill but did not swim, 130 reported this correctly, but 56 reported that they got ill and swam, 14 reported that they did not get ill but swam, and 33 reported that they did not swim and did not get ill.

Continuing in this way, the table can be further revised to describe how the 300 subjects who truly did not get ill and swam were misclassified. The table can also be revised to describe the misclassification

Observed Data

	Swam'		Not Swam'	
Ill'	264	56 ¦30		130
	27	33 ..¦3		77.
not Ill'	66	14 ¦7		33
	243	297 ¦27		693

of the 1100 subjects who truly did not get ill and did not swim.

We can now separately sum up the 4 frequencies within each of the 4 cells in the table of observed data to obtain a summarized table of the observed data as shown here:

Observed Data

	Swam'	Not Swam'
Ill'	380	240
not Ill'	620	760
Total	1000	1000

Study Questions (Q9.3)

1. What is the estimated risk ratio for the observed data?
2. Why is there misclassification bias? (Hint: RR=3.14 for true data)
3. What is the direction of the bias?
4. If there is misclassification of both exposure and disease, will the bias always be towards the null?

Summary

❖ Misclassification can sometimes occur for both exposure and disease in the same study.
❖ An example of such misclassification is likely if both the exposure variable and the disease variable are determined by subject recall.
❖ When there is misclassification of both exposure and disease, the observed data results from how the cell frequencies in each of the four cells of the 2x2 table for the true data get split up into the four cells of the 2x2 table for the observed data.

Misclassification Probabilities – Sensitivity and Specificity

This misclassification table describes how a disease **D** may be misdiagnosed. Twelve subjects who were truly diseased were misclassified as non-diseased and 14 subjects who were truly not diseased were misclassified as diseased. 48 subjects who were truly diseased and 126 subjects who were truly non-diseased were correctly classified.

Misclassification of Disease Status

	TRUE		
	D	Not D	
D'	48	14	62
CLASSIFIED			
Not D'	12	126	138
	60	140	

In a perfect world, we would hope that no one was misclassified, that is, we would want our table to look like the table below. Then the proportion correctly classified as diseased would be 1 and the proportion correctly classified as non-diseased is also 1.

Perfect World	TRUE			Proportion
	D	Not D		
D'	60	0	60	$\frac{60}{60} = 1$
CLASSIFIED				
Not D'	0	140	140	$\frac{140}{140} = 1$
	60	140		

In the real world, however, these proportions are not equal to one. In our example, the proportion of truly diseased correctly classified as diseased is .80 (48/60). The proportion of truly non-diseased correctly classified as non-diseased is .90 (126/140).

$$\frac{48}{60} = .80 \rightarrow \text{Sensitivity} = \text{Prob}(\ D' |\ D\ ) \quad \text{given}$$

$$\frac{126}{140} = .90 \rightarrow \text{Specificity} = \text{Prob}(\text{not } D' |\text{not } D\ )$$

The first of these proportions is called the **sensitivity**. Generally, the sensitivity for misclassification of disease status is the probability that a subject is classified as diseased given that he or she is truly diseased.

Misclassification of Exposure Status

	TRUE	
	E	Not E
E'		
CLASSIFIED		
Not E'		

Sensitivity = Prob(E'| E) $\quad$ given
Specificity = Prob(not E'|not E)

The second of these proportions is called the **specificity**. Generally the specificity for misclassification of disease is the probability that a subject is classified as not diseased given that he or she is truly not diseased.

The ideal value for both sensitivity and specificity is 1.0 or 100%. We can also make use the misclassification table for **exposure** status to define sensitivity and specificity parameters.

Study Questions (Q9.4) Consider the numbers in the following misclassification table for exposure.

Misclassification of Exposure Status

	TRUE E	Not E	
E' CLASSIFIED	720	190	910
Not E'	180	910	1090
	900	1100	

Sensitivity = Prob(E'| E)
Specificity = Prob(not E'|not E)

1. What is the sensitivity for misclassifying exposure?
2. What is the specificity for misclassifying exposure?
3. Do your answers to the previous questions suggest that there should be some concern about misclassification bias?

Summary

❖ The underlying parameters that must be considered when assessing information bias are called **sensitivity** and **specificity**.

❖ **Sensitivity** gives the probability that a subject who is truly diseased (or exposed) will be classified as diseased (or exposed) in one's study.

❖ **Specificity** gives the probability that a subject who is truly non-diseased (or unexposed) is classified as non-diseased (or unexposed) in one's study.

❖ The ideal value for both sensitivity and specificity is 1, or 100%, which means there is no misclassification.

Nondifferential Misclassification

This table describes the true exposure and disease status for 2000 subjects in a hypothetical case-control study of the relationship between diet

True Exposure and Disease Status

Fruit/Vegetable Consumption

	Low	High	Total
CHD	600	400	1000
not CHD	300	700	1000

$\hat{OR} = \frac{600 \times 700}{400 \times 300} = 3.5$

and coronary heart disease (CHD):

The exposure variable is the amount of fruits and vegetables eaten in an average week, categorized as low or high, as recalled by the study subjects. The disease variable is the presence or absence of CHD. Suppose there is no misclassification of disease status, but that most subjects over-report their intake of fruits and vegetables because they think that diets with high amounts of fruits and vegetables are more acceptable to the investigator. In other words, there is misclassification of exposure status.

The two tables that follow describe how exposure is misclassified separately for both the CHD cases and the non-cases.

Misclassifying Exposure							
CHD cases	True Low	High	Total	CHD non-cases	True Low	High	Total
Low' Classified	480	20	500	Low' Classified	240	35	275
High'	120	380	500	High'	60	665	725
Total	600	400	1000	Total	300	700	1000

Study Questions (Q9.5)

1. What are the sensitivity and specificity for the CHD cases?
2. What are the sensitivity and specificity for the non-cases?
3. What do these two misclassification tables have in common?

This example illustrates **non-differential misclassification of exposure**. This occurs whenever the sensitivities and specificities do **not** vary with disease status. We have assumed that CHD status is not misclassified in this example. The sensitivities and specificities for misclassifying disease are all equal to 1 regardless of exposure group. Thus, in this example there is no misclassification of disease.

Study Questions (Q9.5) continued

4. Use the column total in both misclassification tables (i.e., 600, 400, 300, and 700) to determine the odds ratio for the correctly (i.e., true) classified data.

The row totals from each of the misclassification tables for exposure allow us to determine the study data that would actually be observed as a result of misclassification.

Observed (Classified) Data			
	Low	High	Total
CHD	500	500	1000
not CHD	275	725	1000

$$\hat{OR} = \frac{500 \times 725}{500 \times 275} = 2.6$$

Study Questions (Q9.5) continued

5. Why is there bias due to misclassifying exposure (Note: the correct odds ratio is 3.5)?
6. What is the direction of the bias?

This example illustrates a general rule about non-differential misclassification. Whenever there is non-differential misclassification of both exposure and disease, the bias is always towards the null, provided that there are no other variables being controlled that might also be misclassified.

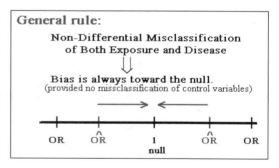

General rule:

Non-Differential Misclassification of Both Exposure and Disease

⇓

Bias is always toward the null.
(provided no misclassification of control variables)

→ ←

OR $\hat{OR}$ 1 $\hat{OR}$ OR
null

Summary

❖ **Nondifferential misclassification of disease**: the sensitivities and specificities for misclassifying disease do not differ by exposure.

❖ **Nondifferential misclassification of exposure**: the sensitivities and specificities for misclassifying exposure do not differ by disease.
❖ **Nondifferential misclassification** of **both** disease and exposure leads to a **bias towards the null**.

What Happens if a Variable <u>other</u> than Exposure or Disease Gets Misclassified?
Greenland (1980) showed that if there is non-differential misclassification of exposure and disease, but also misclassification of a covariate, then there is no guarantee that there will be a bias towards the null. However, if misclassification of exposure and disease is non-differential and a covariate that is not misclassified is controlled in the analysis (say, by stratification), then both stratum-specific and summary measures that adjust for the covariate will be biased towards the null.

Other issues about misclassification of covariates were also addressed as follows:
- Misclassification of exposure can spuriously introduce effect modification (described in Chapter 10) by a covariate.
- Misclassification of a confounder (also described in Chapter 10) can reintroduce confounding in a summary estimate that controls for confounding using misclassified data.

Differential Misclassification

This table describes the true exposure and disease status for the same 2000 subjects described in the previous section for a hypothetical case-control study of the relationship between diet and coronary heart disease:

Suppose, as before, there is no misclassification of disease status, but that subjects over-report their intake of

True Exposure and Disease Status			
Fruit/Vegetable Consumption			
	Low	High	Total
CHD	600	400	1000
not CHD	300	700	1000

$$\hat{OR} = \frac{600 \times 700}{400 \times 300} = 3.50$$

fruits and vegetables because they think that diets with high amounts of fruits and vegetables are more acceptable to the investigator. Suppose also that a CHD case, who is concerned about the reasons for his or her illness, is not as likely to over-estimate his or her intake of fruits and vegetables as is a control. Here are the two tables that describe how exposure is misclassified for both the CHD cases and controls:

Disease Status: No Misclassification
Exposure Status: Misclassification

CHD cases	True Low	High	Total
Classified Low'	580	20	600
Classified High'	20	380	400
Total	600	400	1000

CHD non-cases	True Low	High	Total
Classified Low'	240	35	275
Classified High'	60	665	725
Total	300	700	1000

Study Questions (Q9.6)
The following questions are based on the previous two tables.
1. What are the sensitivity and specificity for the CHD cases?
2. What are the sensitivity and specificity for the non-cases?
3. Is there non-differential misclassification of exposure?

This example illustrates **differential misclassification of exposure**. This occurs because the sensitivities and specificities for misclassifying exposure vary with disease status.

Differential Misclassification of Exposure		
$580 / 600 = .97$	different	$240 / 630 = .80$
Sensitivity=97%	$\longleftrightarrow$	Sensitivity=80%
$380 / 400 = .95$	same	$665 / 700 = .95$
Specificity=95%	$\longleftrightarrow$	Specificity=95%

The row totals from each of the misclassification tables for exposure allow us to determine the study data that would actually be observed as a result of misclassification:

Observed (Classified) Data			
	Low	High	Total
CHD	600	400	1000
not CHD	275	725	1000

$$\hat{OR} = \frac{600 \times 725}{400 \times 275} = 3.95$$

Study Questions (Q9.6) continued

The following questions refer to the previous table and the table with the true exposure information shown previously.

4. Is there a bias due to misclassifying exposure? (Note, the correct OR is 3.5.)
5. What is the direction of the bias, if any?

In general, when there is differential misclassification of either exposure or disease, the bias can be either **towards the null** or **away from the null** (see below for an example of bias away from the null).

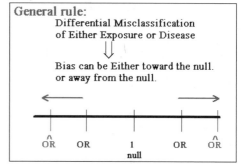

General rule:
Differential Misclassification of Either Exposure or Disease
$\Downarrow$
Bias can be Either toward the null. or away from the null.

$\hat{OR}$ OR   1 null   OR $\hat{OR}$

Summary

❖ With **differential** misclassification, either the sensitivities and specificities for misclassifying **D** differ by **E** or the sensitivities and specificities for misclassifying **E** differ by **D**.

❖ Differential misclassification of either **D** or **E** can lead to bias either towards the null or away from the null.

Quantitative Assessment of Misclassification Bias

Let's assume that we know there is a likely misclassification of exposure or disease that could bias our study results. How can we quantitatively correct for such bias to obtain an adjusted effect measure that is no longer biased?

To quantify bias, we need to adjust the cell frequencies for the observed data to obtain a two-

Observed (i.e., misclassified) Data		
	E'	Not E'
D'	a	b
Not D'	c	d

$$\hat{OR} = \frac{ad}{bc}$$

$$\hat{RR} = \frac{a/(a+c)}{b/(b+d)}$$

Corrected (i.e., adjusted) Data		
	E	Not E
D	A	B
Not D	C	D

$$\hat{OR}_{adj} = \frac{AD}{BC}$$

$$\hat{RR}_{adj} = \frac{A/(A+C)}{B/(B+D)}$$

way table of corrected cell frequencies from which we can compute a corrected effect measure. We can then compare the observed and possibly biased estimate with our corrected estimate to determine the extent of the possible bias and its direction.

Study Questions (Q9.7)   Use the information in the table below about the observed and corrected effect measures to determine whether the observed bias is towards or away from the null.

Question Number	Observed Effect	Corrected Effect	Towards the null?	Away from the null?
a.	2.2	1.7		
b.	2.5	3.8		
c.	4.0	6.1		
d.	4.1	1.2		
e.	0.5	0.9		
f.	0.8	0.9		
g.	0.3	0.2		
h.	0.7	0.1		

Suppose we have determined that whatever bias that exists results from nondifferential misclassification of exposure or disease.
1. Do we need to obtain an adjusted effect measure that corrects for such bias?
2. How can we determine whether or not misclassification is nondifferential?

Suppose we have determined that there is differential misclassification of exposure or disease.
3. Do we need to obtain an adjusted effect measure that corrects for possible misclassification bias?

   In presentations on Lesson Pages 9-3 and 9-4 of the ActivEpi CD, we give formulae for obtaining corrected estimates that consider non-differential or differential misclassification of either exposure or disease variables. Because these formulae are complex computationally, we do not provide them in the text below; the interested reader may work through the activities on 9-3 and 9-4 in the ActivEpi CD for further details.

   In any case, each of these formulae require reliable estimates of sensitivity and specificity. How can we determine the sensitivity and specificity if all we have are the observed data? One option is to take a small sample of the observed data for which true disease and exposure status is determined, so that sensitivities

Need estimates of sensitivity and specificity. How?
1. Estimate from a small sample (gold standard).
2. Determine from previous study involving same variables.
3. Make an educated guess from your clinical or other knowledge.
4. Carry out sensitivity analysis with several educated guesses to determine range of possible biases.

and specificities can be estimated (a drawback to this approach is the sample might be too small to give reliable values for sensitivity and specificity).

Another option is to determine sensitivity and specificity parameters from separate data obtained in a previous study involving the same variables. A third option is simply to make an educated guess of the sensitivity and specificity parameters from your clinical or other knowledge about the study variables. A fourth option is to carry out what is often referred to as a sensitivity analysis with several educated guesses to determine a range of possible biases.

Study Questions (Q9.7) continued Consider the following results of a sensitivity analysis for correcting for misclassification that is assumed to be nondifferential:

Observed OR	Sensitivity?	Specificity?	Corrected OR
1.5	80%	80%	3.5
1.5	80%	90%	2.5
1.5	90%	80%	2.5
1.5	90%	90%	1.8

4. Why do the observed results compared to the corresponding corrected results illustrate a bias that is towards the null?
5. Which values of sensitivity and specificity are associated with the most bias?
6. Which values of sensitivity and specificity are associated with the least bias?
7. Based on the sensitivity analysis described above, how might you decide which corrected OR is "best"?

Summary
* We can correct for misclassification bias by computing an adjusted effect measure from a two-way table whose cell frequencies are corrected from the misclassification found in observed cell frequencies.
* The correction requires accurate estimation of sensitivity and specificity parameters.
* Options for estimating sensitivity and specificity:
    o A sub-sample of the study data
    o A separate sample from another study
    o A questimate based on clinical or other theory/experience
    o A sensitivity analysis that considers several guestimates

Diagnostic Testing and Its Relationship to Misclassification

Diagnostic Test Studies

In clinical medicine, studies concerned with misclassification of disease are usually called **diagnostic test studies**. The primary goal of such a study is to evaluate the performance of a test for diagnosing a disease condition of interest. Suppose, for example, that the disease condition is deep vein thrombosis, or DVT. In a diagnostic study for DVT, the clinician targets only patients with a specific symptom, for example "acute leg swelling" and then performs both the diagnostic test, typically an ultrasound, and the gold standard procedure, typically an x-ray venogram, on these patients. Here are the results of such a diagnostic test study in the form of a misclassification table.

Using the diagnostic test, the disease classification status that is determined for a given patient is called the **test result**, and is labeled as positive "+" or negative "-" on the rows of the table. The procedure used to define true disease is called the **gold standard**, however imperfect it may be. In the misclassification table, the results from using the gold standard are labeled on the columns of the table. Typically, the gold standard is a test that is more detailed, expensive, or risky than the diagnostic test used by the physician. The gold standard might even require prolonged follow-up of the patient if the disease is expected to eventually declare itself, post-mortem examination, or a measure combining more than one strategy, sometimes in complex ways tailored to the specific disease.

Misclassification Table - Diagnostic test			
	GOLD STANDARD		
	+	-	Total
TEST RESULT +	48	14	62
-	12	126	138
Total	60	140	200

Using the information in the misclassification table, the performance of a diagnostic test can be evaluated using several important measures, including the **sensitivity**, the **specificity**, and the **prevalence**. Recall that **sensitivity** describes the test's performance in patients who truly have the disease, and is defined as the conditional probability of a positive test result given true disease, i.e.:

$P(\text{Test} + | \text{True} +)$

Study Questions (Q9.8)
1. What is the sensitivity of the test in the above table?
2. If the sensitivity had been 0.99, what could you conclude about a truly diseased patient who had a negative test result?

Specificity describes the tests performance among patients who are truly without the disease. It is defined as the conditional probability of a negative test result given the absence of disease, $P(\text{Test} - | \text{True} -)$.

Study Questions (Q9.8) continued
3. What is the specificity of the test?
4. If the specificity had been .99, what would you conclude about a truly nondiseased patient who had a positive test result?

Prevalence is calculated as the proportion of patients in the study sample who truly have the disease, $P(\text{True} +)$. If little is known about a patient, disease prevalence in a diagnostic test study is the best estimate of pre-test probability that the patient has the disease.

Study Questions (Q9.8) continued
5. What is the prevalence of true disease from these data?
6. Based on the sensitivity, specificity, and prevalence calculations above, do you think that the test is a good diagnostic tool for DVT? Explain briefly.

Although the three measures, sensitivity, specificity, and prevalence provide important summary information about the performance of the diagnostic test, a more useful measure of overall performance is called the **predictive value**. It is described in the next section.

Summary
❖ In clinical medicine, studies concerned with misclassification of disease are usually called **diagnostic test studies**.
❖ The purpose of a diagnostic test study is to evaluate test performance rather than to adjust for information bias.
❖ The procedure used to define true disease is called the **gold standard**.
❖ In a diagnostic study, the clinician targets patients with a specific symptom and then performs both the diagnostic test and the gold standard procedure on these patients.
❖ The performance of a diagnostic test can be evaluated using several important measures, including **sensitivity**, **specificity**, and **prevalence**.
❖ A more useful measure of the performance of a diagnostic test is provided by the **predictive value**.

Screening Tests

A second type of clinical study concerned with misclassification is called a **screening test**. In contrast to a diagnostic test, a screening test targets a broad population of asymptomatic subjects to identify those subjects that may require more detailed diagnostic evaluation. The subjects in a screening test have not gone to a physician for a specific complaint.

Members of the general public are typically invited to undergo screening tests of various sorts to separate them into those with higher and lower probabilities of disease. Those with higher probabilities are then urged to seek medical attention for definitive diagnosis. Those with lower probabilities receive no direct health benefit because they do not have the disease condition being screened. Also, depending on invasiveness of the screening test and/or the disease condition being targeted, persons under going screening may suffer risks as well as face some inconvenience, anxiety, personal cost, and sometimes discomfort, e.g., as with the use of a colonoscopy to screen for bowel cancer.

The Predictive Value of a Diagnostic Test

The probability of true disease status for an individual patient given the result of a diagnostic test is called the test's **predictive value**. The predictive value is particularly useful to the clinician for individual patient diagnosis because it directly estimates the probability that the patient truly does or does not have the disease depending on the results of the diagnostic test. That's what the clinician wants to know.

Study Questions (Q9.9) Suppose T+ denotes the event that a patient truly has a disease condition of interest, whereas D+ denotes the event of a positive diagnostic test result on the same patient.

1. Which of the following two probability statements describes sensitivity and which describes predictive value?
   A. $P(T+|D+)$ B. $P(D+|T+)$

The predictive value can be obtained directly from the misclassification table generated by a diagnostic test study. Because there are two possible results for a test, there are two different predictive values. The probability of actually having the disease when the test is positive is called the **positive predictive value**, and is denoted as **PV+**. The probability of actually not having the disease if the test is negative is the **negative predictive value**, and is denoted as **PV-**. Both **PV+** and **PV-** are proportions. The closer these proportions are to 1, the better the test's predictive performance.

Misclassification Table: diagnostic test study			
	TRUE DISEASE STATUS (T)		
	+	-	
DIAGNOSTIC + TEST RESULT	48	14	62
(D) -	12	126	138
	60	140	200

PV+ : P(T+ | D+) = Positive Predictive Value

PV- : P(T- | D-) = Negative Predictive Value

The positive predictive value is calculated as the number of true positive results divided by all positive results.

$$PV+ = \frac{\text{\# true positive results}}{\text{all positive results}}$$

Study Questions (Q9.9) continued
2. What is PV+ for the above table?

The positive predictive value is often referred to as the **post-test probability** of having disease. It contrasts with prevalence, which gives the average patient's **pre-test probability** of having disease.

Study Questions (Q9.9) continued
3. Based on the data in the misclassification table, what is the estimate of the average patient's probability of having DVT prior to performing an ultrasound?
4. Has the use of an ultrasound improved disease diagnosis for persons with positive ultrasound results? Explain briefly.

The **negative predictive value** is the number of true negative results divided by the total number of subjects with negative test results.

$$PV- = \frac{\text{\# true negative results}}{\text{all negative results}}$$

Study Questions (Q9.9) continued
5. What is PV- for these data?
6. Based on the data in the misclassification table, what is the estimate of the average patient's probability of not having DVT prior to performing an ultrasound?
7. Has the use of an ultrasound improved disease diagnosis for persons with negative ultrasound results? Explain briefly.

The prevalence of true disease in a diagnostic test study can greatly influence the size of the predictive values obtained. To illustrate this, we now consider a second misclassification table for a different group of patients who have presented to their clinician with pain but without swelling in their leg.

Misclassification Table: diagnostic test study

		Venogram for DVT		
		+	-	
Ultrasound	+	16	18	34
	-	4	162	166
		20	180	200

Study Questions (Q9.9) continued

8. What are the sensitivity, specificity, and prevalence in the table?
9. In the previously considered misclassification table, the sensitivity, specificity, and prevalence were 0.80, 0.90, and 0.30, respectively. How do these values compare with the corresponding values computed in the previous question?
10. What are the values of PV+ and PV- in the above table?
11. In the previously considered misclassification table, PV+ and PV- were .77 and .91, respectively, and the prevalence was .30. How do these values compare with the corresponding predicted values computed in the previous question?
12. What is the moral of this story relating predictive value to disease prevalence?

Summary

❖ The predictive value (or post-test probability) is the probability of true disease status given the result of a diagnostic test.
❖ The predictive value can be obtained directly from the misclassification table generated by a diagnostic test study.
❖ The probability of disease when the test is positive is called the positive predictive value, and is denoted as PV+
❖ The probability of disease when the test is negative is called the negative predictive value, and is denoted as PV-.
❖ PV+ = # true positives / all positive
❖ PV- = # true negatives / all negatives
❖ The closer PV+ and PV- are to 1, the better the test.
❖ The prevalence of true disease in a diagnostic test study can greatly influence the size of the predictive value.

Quiz (Q9.10) For the classification table shown on the right, determine each of the following:

		Truth		
		D	not D	
Classified	D	90	20	110
	not D	10	180	190
		100	200	300

1. What is the sensitivity? **???**
2. What is the specificity? **???**
3. What is the prevalence of the disease? **???**
4. What is the positive predictive value? **???**

Choices: <u>10%</u> <u>33.3%</u> <u>36.7%</u> <u>81.8%</u> <u>90%</u>

The sensitivity and specificity for the classification table shown on the right are still 90% as in the previous questions. For this table, answer each of the following:

Classified		Truth		
		D	not D	
	D	90	50	140
	not D	10	450	460
		100	900	600

5. What is the prevalence of the disease? **???**
6. What is the positive predictive value? **???**
7. The prevalence in this table is smaller than in the previous table; therefore, the positive predictive value is **???** than in the previous table.

Choices: 16.7%   64.3%   90%   larger   smaller

Once again, the sensitivity and specificity for the classification table shown on the right are 90%. For this table, answer each of the following:

Classified		Truth		
		D	not D	
	D	90	90	180
	not D	10	810	820
		100	900	1000

8. What is the prevalence of the disease? **???**
9. What is the positive predictive value? **???**
10. The prevalence in this table is smaller than in the previous two tables, therefore, the positive predictive value is **???** than in the previous two tables.
11. These results illustrate the fact that if the prevalence is small, the predictive value can be quite **???** even if the sensitivity and specificity parameters are quite **???**

Choices: 10%   36.7% 50%   high   larger   small   smaller

Nomenclature

Misclassification tables for disease and exposure

Misclassification table for disease:

Classified		Truth	
		D	Not D
	D′		
	Not D′		

Misclassification table for exposure:

Classified		Truth	
		E	Not E
	E′		
	Not E′		

Observed (misclassified) and corrected tables

Observed (i.e., misclassified) Data

	E′	Not E′
D′	a	b
Not D′	c	d

Corrected (i.e., adjusted) Data

	E	Not E
D	A	B
Not D	C	D

D	Truly has disease
D′	Classified as having disease
E	Truly exposed
E′	Classified as exposed
Not D	Truly does not have disease
Not D′	Classified as not having disease
Not E	Truly not exposed
Not E′	Classified as not exposed
$O\hat{R}$	Odds ratio from *observed* data = ad/bc
$O\hat{R}_{adj}$	Odds ratio from *corrected* or *adjusted* data = AD/BC
$R\hat{R}$	Risk ratio from *observed* data = [a/(a+c)]/[b/(b+d)]
$R\hat{R}_{adj}$	Risk ratio from *corrected* or *adjusted* data = [A/(A+C)]/[B/(B+D)]
Sensitivity	Of those truly with the characteristic, proportion correctly classified as having characteristic; for disease, Pr(D′|D); for exposure, Pr(E′|E)
SeD	Sensitivity of disease misclassification
SeE	Sensitivity of exposure misclassification
SpD	Specificity of disease misclassification
SpE	Specificity of exposure misclassification
Specificity	Of those truly without the characteristic, proportion correctly classified as not having the characteristic; for disease, P(not D′|not D); for exposure, P(not E′|not E).

References on Information/Misclassification Bias

Overviews

Greenberg RS, Daniels SR, Flanders WD, Eley JW, Boring JR. Medical Epidemiology (3rd Ed). Lange Medical Books, New York, 2001.

Hill H, Kleinbaum DG. Bias in Observational Studies. In Encyclopedia of Biostatistics, pp 323-329, Oxford University Press, 1999.

Kleinbaum DG, Kupper LL, Morgenstern H. Epidemiologic Research: Principles and Quantitative Methods. John Wiley and Sons Publishers, New York, 1982.

Special Issues

Barron, BA. The effects of misclassification on the estimation of relative risk. Biometrics 1977;33(2):414-8.

Copeland KT, Checkoway H, McMichael AJ and Holbrook RH. Bias due to misclassification in the estimation of relative risk. Am J Epidemiol 1977;105(5):488-95.

Dosemeci M, Wacholder S, and Lubin JH. Does nondifferential misclassification of exposure always bias a true effect toward the null value? Am J Epidemiol 1990:132(4):746-8.

Espeland MA, Hui SL. A general approach to analyzing epidemiologic data that contain misclassification errors. Biometrics 1987;43(4):1001-12.

Greenland S. The effect of misclassification in the presence of covariates. Am J Epidemiol 1980;112(4):554-69.

Greenland S, Kleinbaum DG. Correcting for misclassification in two-way tables and matched-pair studies. Int J Epidemiol 1983;12(1):93-7.

Reade-Christopher SJ, Kupper LL. Effects of exposure misclassification on regression analyses of epidemiologic follow-up study data. Biometrics 1991;47(2):535-48.

Satten GA and Kupper LL. Inferences about exposure-disease associations using probability-of-exposure information. J Am Stat Assoc 1993;88:200-8.

A Pocket Guide to Epidemiology **157**

Wynder EL. Investigator bias and interviewer bias: the problem of reporting systematic error in epidemiology. J Clin Epidemiol 1994;47(8):825-7.

Answers to Study Questions and Quizzes

Q9.1
1. 2
2. 7
3. 100 x (6/8) = 75%
4. 100 x (7/10) = 79%

Q9.2
1. False. Typically, several times and locations are used in the same residence, and a time-weighted average (TWA) is often calculated.
2. False. Good instrumentation for measuring time-weighted average has been available for some time.
3. False. A system of wire codes to measure distance and configuration has been used consistently since 1979 to rank homes crudely according to EMF intensity. However, the usefulness of this system for predicting past exposure remains an open question.
4. True
5. True
6. True
(Note: there are no questions 7 to 9)
10. Interviewer bias. Subjects known to have experienced a venous thrombosis might be probed more extensively than controls for a history of oral contraceptive use.
11. Away from the null. The proportion of exposed among controls would be less than it should have been if both cases and controls were probed to the same extent. Consequently, the odds ratio in the misclassified data would be higher than it should be.
12. Keep the interviewers blind to case-control status of the study subject.
13. 5
14. 70
15. 100 x (95/100) = 95%
16. 100 x (70/80) = 87.5%

Q9.3
1. The estimated risk ratio for the observed data is (380/1000)/(240/1000) = 1.58.
2. Because the observed risk ratio of 1.58 is meaningfully different than the true (i.e., correct) risk ratio of 3.14.

3. Towards the null, since the biased estimate of 1.58 is closer to the null value than is the correct estimate.
4. No way to tell from one example, but the answer is no, the bias might be either towards the null or away from the null.
5. The observed OR of 2.6 that results from misclassifying exposure is meaningfully different than the true odds ratio of 3.5.
6. The bias is towards the null. The biased OR estimated of 2.6 is closer to the null value of 1 than is the correct OR.

Q9.4
1. Sensitivity = 720 / 900 = .8 or 80%
2. Specificity = 910 / 1100 = .83 or 83%
3. Yes. Both sensitivity and specificity are smaller than one. However, without correcting for the bias, it is not clear that the amount of bias will be large.

Q9.5
1. Sensitivity = 480/600 = .80 or 80% and Specificity = 380/400 = .95 or 95%.
2. Sensitivity = 240/300 = .80 or 80% and Specificity = 665/700 = .95 or 95%.
3. The sensitivities for CHD cases and non-cases are equal. Also, the specificities for CHD cases and non-cases are equal. The sensitivity information indicates that 20% of both cases and non-cases with low intake of fruits and vegetables tend to over-estimate their intake. The specificity information indicates that only 5% of both cases and non-cases with high intake tend to under-estimate their intake.
4. In the correctly classified 2x2 table, a=600, b=400, c=300, and d=700, so the estimated odds ratio is ad/bc = (600 x 700) / (400 x 300) = 3.5.
5. The observed OR of 2.6 that results from misclassifying exposure is meaningfully different than the true odds ratio of 3.5.
6. The bias is towards the null. The biased OR of 2.6 is closer to the null value of 1 than the correct OR.

Q9.6

1. Sensitivity = 580/600 = .97 or 97% and Specificity = 380/400 = .95 or 95%.
2. Sensitivity = 240/300 = .80 or 80% and Specificity = 665/700 = .95 or 95%.
3. No. Although the specificities for cases and non-cases are equal (i.e., 95%), the sensitivity for the cases (97%) is quite different from the sensitivity for the non-cases (80%). This difference in sensitivities indicates that cases with low intake of fruits and vegetables are less likely to over-estimate their intake than non-cases.
4. Not much. The observed OR of 3.95 that results from misclassifying exposure is slightly higher than the true odds ratio of 3.50.
5. The bias is slightly away from the null. The biased OR of 3.95 is further away from the null value of 1 than is the correct OR of 3.5.

Q9.7

a) Away
b) Towards
c) Towards
d) Away
e) Away
f) Away
g) Towards
h) Towards

1. It depends. We know that the bias must be towards the null. If the direction of the bias is all that we are interested in, then we do not need to correct for the bias. However, if we want to determine the extent of the bias and to obtain a quantitative measure of the true effect, then we need to correct for the bias.
2. We can either reason that misclassification is nondifferential from our knowledge or experience with the exposure and disease variables of our study, or we can base our decision on reliable estimates of the sensitivity and specificity parameters.
3. It depends. The bias may be either towards the null or away from the null. We might be able to determine the direction of the bias by logical reasoning about study characteristics. Otherwise, the only way we can

determine either the extent or direction of the bias is to compare a corrected estimate with an observed estimate.

4. The biased (i.e., misclassified) observed odds ratio is closer to the null than the corrected odds ratio.
5. The greatest amount of bias is seen with the observed OR is 1.5 compared to the corrected OR of 3.5, which occurs when both the sensitivity and specificity are 80%.
6. The bias is smallest when the correct OR is 1.8, which results when both sensitivity and specificity are 90%.
7. One way to decide is to choose the corrected OR corresponding to the most realistic set of values for sensitivity and specificity. Another way is to choose the corrected OR (here, 3.5) that is most distant from the observed OR. A third alternative is to choose the corrected OR that changes least (here, 1.8) from the observed OR.

Q9.8

1. Sensitivity = 48 / 60 = 0.80.
2. The patient is very unlikely to have the disease, since the probability of getting a negative test result for a patient with the disease is .01, which is very small.
3. Specificity = 126 / 140 = 0.90
4. The patient is very likely to have the disease, because the probability of getting a positive result for a patient without the disease is .01, which is very small.
5. Prevalence of true disease = 60 / 200 = 0.30.
6. Cannot fully answer this question. Both the sensitivity and specificity are relatively high at .80 and .90, but the prevalence is only 30%. What is required is the proportion of total ultrasound positives that truly have DVT, which in this study is 48 / 62 = 0.77, which is high but not over .90 or .95.

Q9.9

1. Choice A is the predictive value and Choice B is sensitivity.
2. PV+ = 48 / 62 = 0.77
3. Based on the table, the prior probability of developing DVT is 60 / 200 = 0.30,

which is the estimated prevalence of disease among patients studied.

4. Yes, the prior probability was 0.30, whereas the (post-test) probability using an ultrasound increased to 0.77 given a positive result on the test.

5. PV- = 126 / 138 = 0.91

6. Based on the table, the prior probability of **not** developing DVT is 140 / 200 = 0.70, which is 1 minus the estimated prevalence of disease among patients studied.

7. Yes, the prior probability of not developing DVT was 0.70 whereas the (post-test) probability of not developing DVT using an ultrasound increased to 0.91 given a negative test result.

8. Sensitivity = 16 / 20 = 0.80, specificity = 162 / 180 = 0.90, prevalence = 20 / 200 = .10.

9. Corresponding sensitivity and specificity values are identical in both tables, but prevalence computed for this data is much lower at 0.10 than computed for the previous table (.30).

10. PV+ = 16 / 34 = 0.47 and PV- = 162 / 166 = 0.98.

11. PV+ has decreased from 0.77 to 0.47 and PV- has increased from 0.91 to 0.98 whereas the prevalence has dropped from 0.30 to 0.10 while sensitivity and specificity has remained the same and high.

12. If the prevalence decreases, the predictive value positive will decrease and may be quite low even if sensitivity and specificity are high. Similarly, the predictive value negative will increase and may be very high, even if the sensitivity and specificity are not very high.

Q9.10
1. 90%
2. 90%
3. 33.3%
4. 81.8%
5. 16.7%
6. 64.3%
7. smaller
8. 10%
9. 50%
10. smaller
11. small, high

CHAPTER 10

OTHER FACTORS ACCOUNTED FOR? CONFOUNDING AND INTERACTION

*Confounding is a form of bias that concerns how a measure of effect may change in value depending on whether variables other than the exposure variable are controlled in the analysis. **Interaction/effect modification**, which is different from confounding, compares estimated effects **after** other variables are controlled.*

The Concept of Confounding

Confounding is an important problem for health and medical researchers whenever they conduct studies to assess a relationship between an exposure, **E**, and some health outcome or disease of interest, **D**. Confounding is a type of bias that may occur when we fail to take into account other variables, like age, gender, or smoking status, in attempting to assess an E→D relationship.

To illustrate confounding consider the results from a hypothetical retrospective cohort study to determine the effect of exposure to a suspected toxic chemical on the development of lung cancer for workers in a chemical industry. We will call the chemical TCX. The ten-year risks for lung cancer are estimated to be 0.36 for those who were exposed to TCX and 0.17 for those who were not exposed to TCX. The estimated risk ratio is 2.1, which indicates that those exposed to TCX have twice the risk for lung cancer as those unexposed. So far, we have considered two variables, exposure to TCX, and lung cancer status, the health outcome.

Chemical Workers	TCX	no TCX	Total
LC	27	14	41
No LC	48	67	115
Total	75	81	156

Ten-year risks for LC
TCX: $27/75 = 0.36$
no TCX: $14/81 = 0.17$

$$\hat{RR} = 0.36/0.17 = 2.1$$

We haven't yet considered any other variables that might also have been measured or observed on the patients in this study. For example, we might wonder whether there were relatively more smokers among those who were exposed to TCX than those unexposed to TCX. If so, that may explain why workers exposed to TCX were found to have an increased risk of 2.1 compared to unexposed workers. Those exposed to TCX may simply have been heavier smokers and, therefore, more likely to develop lung cancer than among those not exposed to TCX, regardless of exposure to TCX. Perhaps TCX exposure is a determinant of some other form of cancer or another disease, but not necessarily lung cancer.

Suppose that we categorize our study data into two smoking history categories, non-smokers and smokers. For these tables, the estimated risk ratio is computed to be 1.0 for non-smokers and 1.3 for smokers. Notice that these two stratum-specific risk ratios suggest no association between exposure to TCX and the development of lung cancer.

Chemical Workers	TCX	no TCX	Total
LC	27	14	41
No LC	48	67	115
Total	75	81	156

$$\hat{RR} = 2.1$$

non-smokers	TCX	no TCX	Total
LC	1	2	3
No LC	24	48	72
Total	25	50	75

smokers	TCX	no TCX	Total
LC	26	12	38
No LC	24	19	43
Total	50	31	81

$\hat{RR} = 1.0$ No Association $\hat{RR} = 1.3$

When we form strata by categorizing the entire dataset according to one or more variables, like smoking history in our example here, we say that we are **controlling** for these variables, which we often refer to as **control variables**. Thus, what looks like a twofold increase in risk when we ignore smoking history, changes to no association when controlling for smoking history. This suggests that the reason why workers exposed to TCX had a twofold increase in risk compared to unexposed workers might be explained simply by noting that there were relatively more smokers among those exposed to TCX. This is an example of what we call **confounding**, and we say that smoking history is a confounder of the relationship between TCX exposure status and ten-year risk for lung-cancer. In general, confounding may be described as a distortion in a measure of association, like a risk ratio, that may arise because we fail to control for other variables, for example, smoking history, that might be risk factors for the health outcome being studied. If we fail to control the confounder we will obtain an incorrect, or biased, estimate of the measure of effect.

Summary
❖ Confounding is a distortion in a measure of effect, e.g., RR, that may arise because we fail to control for other variables, for example, smoking history, that are previously known risk factors for the health outcome being studied.
❖ If we ignore the effect of a confounder, we will obtain an incorrect, or biased, estimate of the measure of effect.

Quiz (Q10.1)

1. Confounding is a **???** in a **???** that may arise because we fail to **???** other variables that are previously known **???** for the health outcome being studied.

Choices case-control study   control for   distortion   effect modifiers eliminate   measure of effect   risk factors

A study finds that alcohol consumption is associated with lung cancer, crude OR = 3.5. Using the data below, determine whether smoking could be confounding this relationship.

2. What is the OR among smokers?   **???**
3. What is the OR among non-smokers?   **???**
4. Does the OR change when we control for smoking status?   **???**

Choices   **0.01**   **1.0**   **3.5**   **5.4**

5. Is there evidence from data shown below that smoking is a confounder of the relationship between alcohol consumption and lung cancer?   **???**

Choices   **no**   **yes**

| | Smokers | | | Non-Smokers | |
	Alcohol	No Alc		Alcohol	No Alc
Cases	560	140	Cases	40	160
Controls	240	60	Controls	160	640

Crude versus Adjusted Estimates

Confounding is assessed in epidemiologic studies by comparing the **crude estimate of effect** (e.g., $c\hat{R}R$) in which no variables are controlled, with an **adjusted estimate of effect** (e.g., $a\hat{R}R$), in which one or more variables is controlled. The adjusted estimate is typically computed by combining stratum-specific estimates into a single number.

For example, to assess confounding by smoking history in the previously described retrospective cohort study of the effects of exposure to the chemical TCX on the development of lung cancer, we can compare the crude risk ratio of 2.1 to an adjusted risk ratio that combines the risk ratios of 1.0 and 1.3 for the two smoking history categories. The method for combining these estimates into a single summary measure involves computing a weighted average of stratum-specific measures of effect; see Chapter 14 on Stratified Analysis for more details. Once we have combined these stratum specific estimates, how do we decide if there is confounding? The **data-based criterion** for confounding requires the crude estimate of effect to be different from the adjusted estimate of effect. How different must these two estimates be to conclude that there is confounding? To answer this question, the investigator must decide whether or not there is a clinically important difference.

In our retrospective cohort study the adjusted estimate would be some number between 1.0 and 1.3, which suggests a much weaker relationship than indicated by the crude estimate of 2.1. Most investigators would consider this a clinically important difference. Suppose the crude estimate had been 4.2 instead of 2.1, the difference between crude and adjusted estimates would indicate even much stronger confounding.

We can compare other crude and adjusted estimates. Suppose, for example that an estimated crude risk ratio was 4.2 and the estimated adjusted risk ratio was 3.8. Both these values indicate an association that is about equally strong, so there is no clinically important difference between crude and adjusted estimates. Similarly, if the estimated crude risk ratio is 1.2 and the estimated adjusted risk ratio is 1.3, both these values indicate about the same very weak or no association. So, here again, there is no clinically important difference between these crude and adjusted estimates.

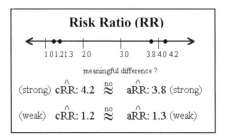

Clearly, deciding on what is clinically important requires a subjective decision by the investigators. One investigator might conclude, for example, that the difference between a 1.2 and a 1.3 is clinically important whereas another investigator might conclude otherwise. This problem may lead one to want to use a test of statistical significance to decide on whether there is a difference between the crude and adjusted estimate. However, because confounding is a validity issue, it should not be evaluated using a statistical test, but rather by looking for a meaningful difference, however imprecise.

A commonly used approach for assessing confounding is to specify, prior to looking at one's data, how much of a change in going from the crude to the adjusted estimate is required. Typically, a 10 per cent change is specified, so that if the crude risk ratio estimate is say, 4, then

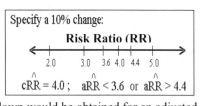

a 10% change in this estimate either up or down would be obtained for an adjusted risk ratio of either 3.6 or 4.4. Thus, if the adjusted risk ratio were found to be below 3.6 or above 4.4, we would say that confounding has occurred with at least a 10% change in the estimated association.

As another example, if a 20% change is specified and the crude risk ratio is, say, 2.5, the adjusted risk ratio would have to be either below 2 or above 3 to conclude that there is confounding.

Summary

❖ Confounding is assessed by comparing the crude estimate of effect, in which no variables are controlled, with an adjusted estimate of effect, in which one or more variables are controlled.

❖ Confounding is present if we conclude that there is a clinically important or meaningful difference between crude and adjusted estimates.

❖ We do not use statistical testing to evaluate confounding.
❖ A commonly used approach for assessing confounding is to specify, prior to looking at one's data, how much of a change in going from the crude to the adjusted estimate is required.

Quiz (Q10.2) A case-control study was conducted to study the relationship between oral contraceptive use and ovarian cancer. The crude OR was calculated as 0.77. Since age was considered a potential confounder in this study, the data were stratified into 3 age groups as shown below.

1. The OR for the 20-39 year age group is **???**
2. The OR for the 40-49 year age group is **???**
3. The OR for the 50-54 year age group is **???**
4. Do you think that this data provides some evidence that age is a confounder of the relationship between oral contraceptive use and ovarian cancer? **???**

Choices: **0.58   0.61   0.65   0.69   0.77   1.45   no   yes**

	Ages 20-39		Ages 40-49		Ages 50-54	
	OCs	No OCs	OCs	No OCs	OCs	No OCs
Case	46	12	30	30	17	44
Control	285	51	463	301	211	331

In this study described in the previous question, the crude OR was 0.77, and the adjusted OR controlling for age was 0.64.

5. If a 15% change in the crude versus adjusted OR is specified by the investigator as a meaningful difference, an adjusted OR less than **???** or greater than **???** provides evidence of confounding.
6. Is there evidence of confounding? **???**
7. Suppose the investigators determined that a 20% change was a meaningful difference. Is there evidence of confounding? **???**

Choices: **0.15   0.63   0.65   0.85   0.89   0.92   no   yes**

Quiz (Q10.3) Determine whether each of the following is **True** or **False**.
1. An adjusted estimate is a suitably chosen weighted average of the stratum specific estimates.   **???**.
2. An adjusted estimate is always less than the corresponding crude estimate.
                                                                         ???
3. Most epidemiologists prefer to give equal weight to each stratum specific estimate in case-control studies.   **???**.
4. Confounding is a validity issue and therefore, requires the use of a statistical test to determine its significance.   **???**.

Use the formula below to calculate the adjusted RR for the following examples whose stratum specific estimates are given. (Note: Although the formula below gives a weighted average, the usual formula for aRR is a more complicated "precision-based" weighted average described in Chapter 12 on Stratified Analysis.)

$$\boxed{a\hat{R}R = (w_1 \times \hat{R}R_1 + w_2 \times \hat{R}R_2)/(w_1 + w_2)}$$

5. Stratum 1: RR=1.13, w=13.1; Stratum 2: RR=1.00, w=7.7. The adjusted RR is <u>???</u>.

6. Stratum 1: RR=2.25, w=31.3; Stratum 2: RR=1.75, w=5.6. The adjusted RR is <u>???</u>

Choices:　　<u>1.06</u>　　<u>1.07</u>　　<u>1.08</u>　　<u>1.09</u>　　<u>1.98</u>　　<u>2.08</u>　　<u>2.17</u>

Criteria for Confounding

In addition to the data-based criterion for confounding, we must assess several **a priori criteria**. These are conditions to consider at the study design stage, prior to data collection, to identify variables to be measured for possible control in the data analysis.

The first a priori criterion is that a **confounder must be a risk factor for the health outcome**. This criterion ensures that a crude association between exposure and disease cannot be explained away by other variables already known to predict the disease. Such variables are called **risk factors**. For example, suppose we are studying the link between exposure to a toxic chemical and the development of lung cancer in a chemical industry. Based on the epidemiologic literature on the determinants of lung cancer, we would want to control for age and smoking status, two known risk factors. Our goal is to determine whether exposure to the chemical contributes anything over and above the effects of age and smoking on the development of lung cancer.

The second criterion is that a confounder cannot be an **intervening variable** between the exposure and the disease. A pure intervening variable (**V**) is any variable whose relationship to exposure and disease lies entirely within the causal pathway between exposure and disease.

Given a hypothetical scenario where saturated fat levels are measured to determine their effects on CHD, would we want to control for LDL levels? (Note: use of LDL in this example might

The answer: If we control for LDL level, we essentially control for the saturated fat level, and we would likely find an adjusted risk ratio or odds ratio relating saturated fat to coronary heart disease status to be close to the null value. The intervening variable here is LDL level, and we should not control for it.

$$
\begin{array}{ccc}
E & \rightarrow V \rightarrow & D \\
\text{Saturated} & & \text{Coronary} \\
\text{Fat} \rightarrow & \textbf{LDL} \rightarrow & \text{Heart} \\
& & \text{Disease}
\end{array}
$$

The third criterion is that a **confounder must be associated with the exposure in the source population being studied**. By source population we mean the underlying population cohort that gives rise to the

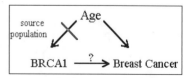

cases used in the study. Consider a study to assess whether a particular genetic factor, BRCA1, is a determinant of breast cancer. Age is a well-known risk factor for breast cancer, but is clearly not associated with the presence or absence of the gene in whatever source population is being studied.

The third a priori criterion is therefore not satisfied. Consequently, even if by some chance, age turned out to be associated with the gene in the study data, we would not control for age, even though there is data-based confounding, because age does not satisfy all a priori criteria.

All three a priori criteria plus the data-based criterion are required for a variable to be considered a true confounder.

A priori criteria
A confounder
✓ 1. must be a risk factor.
✓ 2. cannot be an intervening variable
✓ 3. must be associated with the exposure in the source population.

Data-based criterion
✓ adjusted estimate $\neq$ crude estimate

Summary
A confounder must satisfy 3 a priori criteria in addition to the data-based criterion for confounding. These are:

❖ A confounder must be a **risk factor** for the health outcome.
❖ A confounder **cannot be an intervening variable** in the causal pathway between exposure and disease.
❖ A confounder must be **related to exposure in the source population** from which the cases are derived.

Some "fine points" about risk factors
The decision regarding which variables to include in the list of risk factors is, in practice, rarely a clear-cut matter. Such is the case when only a small amount of literature is available on a given study subject. On the other hand, a large literature may be controversial in terms of which previously studied variables are truly predictive of the disease.

Also, after data collection, but prior to the primary data analysis, the list of risk factors may need to be re-evaluated to allow for the addition or deletion of variables already measured but not explicitly considered for control. Variables measured for other purposes, say in a broad study to evaluate several etiologic questions, may be added to the list of risk factors if they were previously overlooked.

Furthermore, a **surrogate** of a risk factor may have to be used when the latter is difficult to measure. For example, the number of years spent in a given job in a particular industry is often used as a surrogate measure for the actual amount of exposure to a toxic substance suspected of being an occupationally related carcinogen.

Some "fine points" about a priori criterion 3
The third a priori criterion for confounding is of particular concern in case-control studies, where the controls are usually selected into the study after the cases have already occurred. In such studies, it is possible that the study data are not representative of the source population with regard to the exposure as well as other variables.

Therefore, a variable, say C, that may be not associated with exposure in the source population may still be associated with the exposure in the actual study data. In such a case, criterion 3 says that the variable **C** cannot be considered a confounder, and should not be controlled, even if there is data-based confounding.

In cohort studies, the exposure status is determined before disease status has occurred, so that the source population is the study cohort. In such studies, a variable, **C**, that is not associated with the exposure in the study data, does not satisfy condition 3 and therefore should not be considered a confounder.

The main difficulty in assessing the third a priori criterion concerns how to determine the association of the suspected confounder, **C**, with the exposure, **E**, in the in the source population. This requires some knowledge of the epidemiologic literature about the relationship between **C** and **E** and about the source population being studied

Quiz (Q10.4) A study was conducted to assess the relationship between blood type (O-positive and O-negative) and a particular disease. Since age is often related to disease outcome, it was considered a potential confounder. Determine whether each of the a priori criteria below is satisfied.

1. A confounder must be a risk factor for the health outcome. **???**
2. A confounder cannot be an intervening variable between the exposure and the disease. **???**
3. A confounder must be associated with the exposure in the source population being studied. **???**
4. Can age be a confounder in this study? **???**

Choices: **no**   **not satisfied**   **satisfied yes**

Confounding in Different Study Designs

We have seen that the assessment of confounding requires both data-based and apriori criteria. The data-based criterion requires that the crude estimate of effect be meaningfully different from the adjusted estimate of effect. The adjusted estimate of effect is computed as a weighted average of stratum-specific estimates obtained over different categories of the potential confounder. The measure of effect used for this comparison changes with the study design but it always compares a crude estimate with an adjusted one.

We have thus far only considered follow-up studies where the measure of effect of interest is the risk ratio. For case-control studies, we compare crude and adjusted estimates of the exposure odds ratio. In cross-sectional studies, we compare crude and adjusted estimates of the prevalence odds ratio or the prevalence ratio.

Data-based Confounding
Crude vs. Adjusted
Follow-up: $c\hat{R}R$ vs. $a\hat{R}R$
Case-control: $cE\hat{O}R$ vs. $aE\hat{O}R$
Cross-sectional: $cP\hat{O}R$ vs. $aP\hat{O}R$
or
$c\hat{P}R$ vs. $a\hat{P}R$

Summary

❖ The measure of association used to assess confounding will depend on the study design.

❖ In a follow-up study, we typically compare a crude risk ratio with an adjusted risk ratio.

❖ In a case-control study, we typically compare a crude exposure odds ratio with an adjusted exposure odds ratio.

❖ In a cross-sectional study, we typically compare a crude prevalence odds ratio with an adjusted prevalence odds ratio, or we might use a prevalence ratio instead of a prevalence odds ratio.

❖ Regardless of the study design, data based confounding is assessed by comparing a crude estimated of effect with an appropriate adjusted estimate of effect.

Assessing Confounding in Case-Control Studies

These tables show results from a case-control study to assess the relationship of alcohol consumption to oral cancer. The tables describe the crude data when age is ignored and the stratified data when age has been categorized into three groups. The investigators wanted to evaluate whether there was possible confounding due to age.

Case-control Study
Alcohol consumption and oral cancer

Crude:

	Alc	no Alc
OCa	27	47
no OCa	90	443

n = 607

Stratified:

	Ages 40-49 Alc	no Alc	Ages 50-59 Alc	no Alc	Ages 60+ Alc	no Alc
OCa	4	25	12	10	11	12
no OCa	22	309	37	67	31	67

n = 360   n = 126   n = 131

From the above data, we can conclude the following:

1. The crude odds ratio relating alcohol to oral cancer is calculated by using the formula (a x d)/(b x c) which in this case equals 2.8

2. The stratum-specific odds ratio relating alcohol to oral cancer can be calculated for each strata by using the formula (a x d)/(b x c). The stratum-specific odds ratios are 2.2 for the 40 to 49 age group, 2.2 for the 50 to 59 age group and 2.0 for the 60 and higher age group.

3. There is data-based confounding because the crude odds ratio of 2.8 is meaningfully different than any weighted average of stratum-specific odds ratios, all of which are about 2.

4. There is data-based confounding because the crude odds ratio of 2.8 is meaningfully different than any weighted average of stratum-specific odds ratios, all of which are about 2.

5. Age is a confounder provided all three a priori conditions for confounding are assumed to be satisfied.

Summary

❖ As an example to assess confounding involving the exposure odds ratio, we consider a case-control study of the relationship between alcohol consumption and oral cancer.

❖ Age, a possible confounder, has been categorized into three groups.

❖ The crude estimate of 2.8 indicates a threefold excess risk whereas the adjusted estimate of 2.1 indicates a twofold excess risk for drinkers over non-drinkers.

❖ The results indicate that there is confounding due to age.

Quiz (Q10.5) These data are from a cross-sectional seroprevalence survey of HIV among prostitutes in relation to IV drug use. The crude prevalence odds ratio is 3.59.

	Black or Hispanic		White	
	IV Drug Use	No IV Drug Use	IV Drug Use	No IV Drug Use
HIV +	31	12	HIV + 16	3
HIV –	93	144	HIV – 141	124

1. What is the estimated POR among the black or Hispanic group?   **???**
2. What is the estimated POR among the whites?   **???**
3. Which table do you think should receive more weight when computing an adjusted odds ratio?   **???**

Choices: **3.25   3.59   4.00   4.31   4.69   Black or Hispanic   White**

In the study described in the previous questions, the estimated POR for the Black or Hispanic group was 4.00 and the estimated POR for the Whites was 4.69. The "precision-based" adjusted POR for this study is 4.16. Recall that the crude POR was 3.59.

4. Is there confounding? .   .   .   ..   **???**

Choices **maybe   no   yes**

Confounding versus Interaction

Another reason to control variables in an epidemiologic study is to assess for interaction. To assess interaction, we need to determine whether the estimate of the effect measure differs at different levels of the control variable. Consider the results from a case-control study to assess the potential relationship between alcohol consumption and bladder cancer. These data are stratified on race in three categories.

Case-control study								
Alcohol ➡?➡ Bladder cancer								
	White		Black		Asian		Combined	
	Alc	no Alc	Alc	no Alc	Alc	no Alc	Alc	no Alc
Case	72	41	93	54	68	33	233	128
Control	106	105	113	113	78	142	297	360
	$\widehat{OR}=1.74$		$\widehat{OR}=1.72$		$\widehat{OR}=3.75$		$c\widehat{OR}=2.21$	

The estimated odds ratios for the three race strata and the combined strata are computed to be 1.74, 1.72, 3.75, and 1.73. There is clear evidence of interaction here because the effect is strong in Asians, but less so in Whites and Blacks. It is not clear whether there is confounding, since the value of the adjusted estimate could vary between 1.72 and 3.75, depending on the weights assigned to the strata. The precision-based adjusted odds ratio is computed to be 2.16, which is not very different from the crude odds ratio of 1.73, suggesting that there is little evidence of confounding.

Confounding and interaction are different concepts. Confounding compares the estimated effects before and after control whereas interaction compares estimated effects after control. When assessing confounding and interaction in the same study, it is possible to find one with or without the other.

Consider the table shown here giving stratum specific and crude risk ratio estimates from several hypothetical data sets in which one dichotomous variable is being considered for control. For each data set in this table, do you think there is interaction or confounding? Think about your answer for a few minutes, and then continue to see the answers below.

Confounding versus Interaction					
Data Set	Stratum 1 RR	Stratum 2 RR	Crude RR	Interaction?	Confounding?
1	1.02	3.50	6.00		
2	1.02	3.50	2.00		
3	0.03	3.50	1.70		
4	1.00	1.00	4.10		
5	4.00	4.10	4.20		

Let us look at the data sets, one at a time. For dataset 1, there is clearly interaction, because the estimate for stratum 1 indicates no association but the estimate for stratum 2 indicates a reasonably strong association. There is clearly confounding, because any weighted average of the values 1.02 and 3.50 will be meaningfully different from the crude estimate of 6.0.

For data set 2, again there is clearly interaction, as in data set 1. However, it is not clear whether or not there is confounding. The value of an adjusted estimate will depend on the weights assigned to each stratum. If all the weight is given to either stratum 1 or stratum 2, then the crude estimate of 2.0 will differ considerably from the adjusted estimate, but if equal weight is given to each stratum, the adjusted estimate will be much closer to the crude estimate. Nevertheless, the use of an adjusted estimate here is not as important as the conclusion that the E→D association is different for different strata.

Dataset 3 also shows interaction, although this time the nature of the interaction is different from what we observed in datasets 1 and 2. Here, the two stratum specific estimates are on opposite sides of the null risk ratio value of 1. It appears there is a protective effect of exposure on disease in stratum 1, but a harmful effect of exposure on disease in stratum 2. In this situation, the assessment of confounding is questionable and potentially very misleading, since the important finding here is the interaction effect, especially if this strong interaction holds up after performing a statistical test for interaction.

In dataset 4, the two stratum specific estimates are identically equal to one, so there is no interaction. However, there is clear evidence of confounding, since the crude estimate of 4.0 is meaningfully different from both stratum-specific estimates.

In dataset 5, there is no interaction, because the stratum-specific estimates are both equal to 4. There is also no confounding because the crude estimate is essentially equal to both stratum specific estimates.

Data Set	Stratum 1 RR	Stratum 2 RR	Crude RR	Interaction?	Confounding?
1	1.02	3.50	6.00	yes	yes
2	1.02	3.50	2.00	yes	?
3	0.03	3.50	1.70	yes	??
4	1.00	1.00	4.10	no	yes
5	4.00 ⤾	4.10 ⤾	4.20 ⤾	no	no

Summary
❖ Confounding and interaction are different concepts.
❖ Interaction considers what happens after we control for another variable.
❖ Interaction is present if the estimate of the measure of association differs at different levels of a variable being controlled.
❖ When assessing confounding and interaction in the same study, it is possible to find one with or without the other.
❖ In the presence of strong interaction, the assessment of confounding may be irrelevant or misleading.

Quiz (Q10.6)
1. In contrast to **???** when interaction is present, the estimates of the **???** differ at various levels of the control variable.
2. When assessing confounding and interaction in the same study, it is **???** to find one without the other.

Choices **confounding**   **effect measure**   **effect modification**
not possible   **possible precision**   **variance**

For datasets 1-3 in the table below, select the best answer from the following:

    A. Confounding
    B. Interaction
    C. No confounding or interaction
    D. Calculation error (not possible)

3. Data set 1 ? **???**
4. Data set 2? **???**
5. Data set 3? **???**

	Crude OR	Stratum 1 OR	Stratum 2 OR	Adjusted OR
Dataset 1	4.0	1.0	6.0	4.0
Dataset 2	4.0	5.0	5.0	5.0
Dataset 3	4.0	4.0	4.0	3.0

Interaction versus Effect Modification

The term **effect modification** is often used interchangeably with the term **interaction**. We use effect modification from an epidemiologic point of view to emphasize that the effect of exposure on the health outcome is modified depending on the value of one or more control variables. Such control variables are called **effect modifiers** of the relationship between exposure and outcome. We use interaction from a statistical point of view to emphasize that the exposure variable and the control variable are interacting in some way within a mathematical model for determining the health outcome.

To illustrate effect modification, consider the case-control data to assess the relationship between alcohol consumption and bladder cancer. The data showed clear evidence of interaction, since the estimated effect was much stronger in Asians than in either Blacks or Whites. This evidence suggests that race is an effect modifier of the relationship between alcohol consumption and bladder cancer. Such a conclusion is supported by the epidemiologic literature, which indicates that alcohol is metabolized in Asians differently than in other racial groupings.

	White		Black		Asian		Combined	
	Alc	no Alc	Alc	no Alc	Alc	no Alc	Alc	no Alc
Case	72	41	93	54	68	33	233	128
Control	106	105	113	113	78	142	297	360

$$\hat{OR} = 1.74 \qquad \hat{OR} = 1.72 \qquad \hat{OR} = 3.75 \qquad c\hat{OR} = 2.21$$

The assessment of interaction or effect modification is typically supported using the results of statistical testing. Recall that confounding does not involve significance testing because it is a validity issue. Nevertheless, statistical testing of interaction is considered appropriate in epidemiologic studies because effect modification concerns understanding the underlying causal mechanisms involved in the E→D relationship, which is not considered a validity issue. One such test for stratified data that has been incorporated into available computer software, is called the **Breslow-Day test**

Summary
* ❖ Effect modification and interaction are often used interchangeably.
* ❖ If there is effect modification, then the control variable or variables involved are called effect modifiers.
* ❖ The assessment of effect modification is typically supported by statistical testing for significant interaction.
* ❖ One popular statistical test for interaction is called the **Breslow-Day** test.

Is There Really a Difference between Effect Modification and Interaction?
Although the terms effect modification and interaction are often used interchangeably, there is some controversy in the epidemiologic literature about the precise definitions of effect modification and interaction (see Kleinbaum et al., Epidemiologic Research: Principles and Quantitative Methods, Chapter 19, John Wiley and Sons, 1982).

One distinction frequently made is that effect modification describes a non-quantitative clinical or biological attribute of a population, whereas interaction is typically quantitative and data-specific, and in particular, depends on the scale on which the "interacting" variables are measured. Nevertheless, this conceptual distinction is often overlooked in the applied research studies.

Why Do Epidemiologists Statistically Test for Interaction but not for Confounding?

We have previously pointed out that the assessment of confounding should not involve statistical testing, essentially because **confounding is a validity issue** involving systematic rather than random error. Moreover, if there is a meaningful difference between estimated crude and adjusted effects, then a decision has to be made as to which of these estimates to report; consequently, the adjusted effect must be used, without consideration of a statistical test, because it controls for the variables (i.e., risk factors) designated for adjustment.

Furthermore, it is not obvious, even if we wanted to statistically test for confounding, exactly how to properly perform a test for confounding. What is typically done, though incorrect, is to test whether the potential confounder, e.g., age, is significantly associated with the health outcome, possibly also controlling for exposure status. Such a test does not really assess confounding, since it concerns random error (i.e., variability) rather than whether or not the crude and adjusted estimates are different in the data!

As to whether or not one should do a statistical test for assessing interaction/effect modification, the answer is not as clear-cut. If we consider interaction as a data-based manifestation of a population-based phenomenon (i.e., effect modification), then a statistical test can be justified to account for the random error associated with a data-based result. Moreover, in contrast, to the assessment of confounding, there are several 'legitimate' approaches to testing for interaction, one of which is the Breslow-Day test for stratified data (described in Chapter 14) and another is a test for the significance of product terms in a logistic model.

Furthermore, it may be argued that the assessment of interaction/effect modification isn't a validity issue, but rather concerns the conceptual understanding/explanation of the relationships among variables designated for control. The latter argument, in this author's opinion, is a little too esoteric to accept at face value. In fact, a counter argument can be made that the presence of interaction/effect modification implies that the most "valid" estimates are obtained by stratifying on effect modifiers, provided that one can determine which variables are the "true" effect modifiers.

As in many issues like this one that arise in the undertaking of epidemiologic research, the best answer is probably, "it depends!" That is, it depends on the researcher's point of view whether or not a statistical test for interaction/effect modification is appropriate. Nevertheless, this author tends to weigh in with the opinion that effect modification is a population phenomenon that can be assessed using 'legitimate' statistical testing of a data-based measure of interaction.

Effect Modification – An Example

In the early 1990's, investigators of the Rotterdam Study screened 8,000 elderly men and women for the presence of Alzheimer's disease. One of the research questions was whether the presence of atherosclerosis increased the risk of this disease. In a cross-sectional study, the investigators found that patients with high levels of atherosclerosis had a three times increased risk of having Alzheimer's disease compared to participants with only very little atherosclerosis. These results were suggestive of a link between cardiovascular disease and neurodegenerative disease.

The investigators knew from previous research that one of the genes involved in lipid metabolism influences the risk of Alzheimer's disease. For this gene, there are two alternative forms, allele A and allele B. Each person's genetic make-up consists of two of these alleles. Persons with at least one B-allele have a higher risk of Alzheimer's disease than persons with two A-alleles.

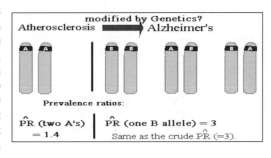

The investigators hypothesized that a person's genetic make-up might modify the association they found between atherosclerosis and Alzheimer's disease. Therefore, they divided the study population into a group of participants who had at least one B-allele, and a group of participants with two A-alleles. They found the following results: Among those with at least one B allele, the prevalence of Alzheimer's disease for those with high levels of atherosclerosis was three times the prevalence of those with low levels. This result is the same as the crude. However, among those with two A-alleles, the prevalence for those with high levels of atherosclerosis was only 1.4 times the prevalence of those with low levels.

These results provide an example of effect modification. Genetic make-up is the effect modifier. The investigators showed that the extent of atherosclerosis is associated with Alzheimer's disease, but only in those whose genetic make-up predisposes them to the development of this disease.

Study Questions (Q10.7)

Prevalence of Alzheimer's Disease	
High ATH, 1 B-allele: 13.3% Low ATH, 1 B-allele: 4.4%	$\hat{PR} = 3.0$
High ATH, 2 A-alleles: 4.8% Low ATH, 2 A-alleles: 3.4%	$\hat{PR} = 1.4$

The prevalence of Alzheimer's and the prevalence ratios for each gene group are listed above. Answer the following assuming the group with low ATH and two A-alleles is the reference.

1. What is the prevalence ratio comparing those with high ATH and two A-alleles to the reference group?
2. What is the prevalence ratio comparing those with low ATH and at least one B-allele to the reference group?
3. What is the prevalence ratio comparing those with both high ATH and at least one B-allele to the reference group?
4. What is the difference between the three prevalence ratios you just calculated and the two listed above?

Quiz (Q10.8)   True or False

1. The term effect modification emphasizes that the effect of exposure on the health outcome is modified depending on the value of one or more control variables.
    ???
2. Evidence for effect modification is present when the stratum-specific measures of association are approximately the same.   **???**
3. This assessment can be supported by a statistical test known as the Breslow-Day test.   **???**

A measles vaccine may be highly effective in preventing disease if given after a child is 15 months of age, but less effective if given before 15 months.
4. This example illustrates **???**, where the exposure is **???**, the outcome is **???**, and the effect modifier is **???**.

Choices: **age at vaccination**   **confounding**   **effect modification**
        measles   **measles vaccine**

Nomenclature

aEÔR	Estimate of the adjusted exposure odds ratio
aPÔR	Estimate of the adjusted prevalence odds ratio
aP̂R	Estimate of the prevalence ratio
aR̂R	Estimate of an adjusted risk ratio
C	Confounding variable
cEÔR	Estimate of the crude exposure odds ratio
cPÔR	Estimate of the prevalence odds ratio
cP̂R	Estimate of the prevalence ratio
cR̂R	Estimate of the crude risk ratio
D	Disease
E	Exposure
V	Intervening variable
w or w_i	Weight; with a subscript i, denotes the weight for a stratum

References

Hofman A, Ott A, Breteler MM, Bots ML, Slooter AJ, van Harksamp F, van Duijn CN, Van Broeckhoven C, Grobbee DE. Atherosclerosis, apolipoprotein E, and prevalence of dementia and Alzheimer's disease in the Rotterdam Study. Lancet 1997;349 (9046):151-4.

Greenland S, Morgenstern H. Confounding in health research. Annu Rev Public Health 2001;22:189-212.

Kleinbaum DG, Kupper LL, Morgenstern H. Epidemiologic Research: Principles and Quantitative Methods. John Wiley and Sons Publishers, New York, 1982.

Miettinen O. Confounding and effect modification. Am J Epidemiol 1974;100(5):350-3.

Mundt KA, Shy CM. Interaction: An epidemiological perspective for risk assessment. In: Fan AM, Chang LW (eds.). Toxicology and risk assessment: Principles, methods, and applications. Marcel Dekker, Inc., New York, NY, p.p. 329-351, 1996

Whittemore AS. Collapsibility of multidimensional contingency tables. J R Stat Soc B 1978;40:328-40.

Answers to Study Questions and Quizzes

Q10.1
1. distortion, measure of association, control for, risk factors
2. 1.0
3. 1.0
4. yes
5. yes – The data-based assessment of confounding is made by determining whether the crude estimate of the measure of association is meaningfully different from an adjusted measure of association.

Q10.2
1. 0.69
2. 0.65
3. 0.61
4. yes – The data-based assessment of confounding is made by determining whether the crude estimate of the measure of association is meaningfully different from an adjusted measure of association.
5. 0.65, 0.89 – To determine whether there is a meaningful difference in the crude and adjusted estimates based on a specified percent change required between the crude and adjusted estimates, multiply the crude estimate by the specified percent change, and then add and subtract that value to the crude estimated. If the interval obtained contains the adjusted estimate, then there is no meaningful difference.
6. yes
7. no

Q10.3
1. True
2. False – The adjusted estimate can be greater or less than the corresponding crude estimate.
3. False – Most epidemiologists prefer to give unequal weight to each stratum specific estimate. Weights are usually determined based on sample size or precision.
4. False – Since confounding is a validity issue, it should not be evaluated by statistical testing, but by looking for a meaningful difference in the crude and adjusted estimates.
5. 1.08
6. 2.17

Q10.4
1. satisfied
2. satisfied
3. not satisfied – Age cannot possibly be associated with blood type.
4. no – Age cannot possibly be associated with blood type.

Q10.5
1. 4.00
2. 4.69
3. Black or Hispanic – You might think that the table for the white group should receive more weight since it has a slightly larger sample size, however, the table for the Black or Hispanic group is actually more balanced. See Chapter 14 for a more complete explanation on balanced data.
4. maybe – It depends on whether the investigator considers the difference between 3.59 and 4.16 a meaningful difference.

Q10.6
1. confounding, effect measure
2. possible
3. B
4. A
5. D – Data set 3: Recall that the adjusted estimate is a weighted average of the two stratum specific estimates and therefore, must lie between them.

Q10.7
1. 4.8% / 3.4% = 1.4
2. 4.4% / 3.4% = 1.3
3. 13.3% / 3.4% = 3.9
4. The two PRs above are the stratum-specific PRs for each of the two gene groups. The three calculated here use one group as a reference and compare the other three to that group. In this example, having low ATH and 2 A-alleles is the reference group compared to those having either one or both of the risk factors (high ATH, 1 B-allele). To

see how these 3 PRs can be used to define two different types of interaction, see the first asterisk on the ActivEpi CD lesson page (10-4) or the box labeled **Two Types of Interaction - Additive and Multiplicative.**

Q10.8

1. True
2. False – Evidence for effect modification is present when the stratum-specific measures of association are different.
3. True
4. effect modification, measles vaccine, measles, age at vaccination

CHAPTER 11

CONFOUNDING CAN BE CONFOUNDING - SEVERAL RISK FACTORS

*This chapter considers how the assessment of **confounding** gets somewhat more complicated when controlling for more than one risk factor. In particular, when several **risk factors** are being controlled, we may find that considering all risk factors simultaneously may not lead to the same conclusion as when considering risk factors separately. We have previously (Chapter 10) argued that the assessment of confounding is not appropriate for variables that are **effect modifiers** of the exposure-disease relationship under study. Consequently, throughout this chapter, our discussion of confounding will assume that **none** of the variables being considered for control are effect modifiers (i.e., there is no interaction between exposure and any variable being controlled).*

Assessing Confounding in the Presence of Interaction

We have restricted our discussion of confounding involving several variables to the situation where **none** of the variables considered for control are effect modifiers of the exposure-disease relationship under study. This restriction has been made primarily for pedagogical reasons, since it is easier to discuss the confounding among several variables when there is no effect modification.

Nevertheless, **it is often quite appropriate to consider confounding even when interaction is present**. For example, if we are only controlling for one variable, say gender, and we find that the odds ratio for males is 1.3 whereas the odds ratio for females is 3.6 and the crude odds ratio is 10.1, then both confounding and interaction are present and each may be addressed. A similar situation may present itself when two or more variables are being controlled.

Moreover, when several variables are being controlled and there is interaction of, say, only one of these variables with the exposure variable, then the remaining variables considered for control may be assessed as potential confounders. For example, if in a cohort study of risk factors for coronary heart disease (CHD), it was determined that cholesterol level (CHL) was the only effect modifier of the exposure variable (say, physical activity level) among risk factors that included age, smoking status, gender and blood pressure, then these latter variables may still be assessed for possible confounding.

In the latter situation, one method for carrying out confounding assessment involves **stratifying on the effect modifier** (CHL) and assessing confounding involving the other variables separately within different categories of CHL.

Another approach is to use a **mathematical model** (e.g., using logistic regression) that contains all risk factors considered as main effects and also contains a product term of exposure with cholesterol. Those risk factors other than CHL can then be assessed for confounding provided the main effect of cholesterol, the exposure variable, and the product of exposure with CHL remains in the model throughout the assessment.

Two Important Principles

We have thus far considered only the control of a single confounder in an epidemiologic study. But usually several risk factors are identified and measured for possible control. Recall the a priori criteria for confounding. When several factors meet these criteria, how do we determine which to control for in the analysis?

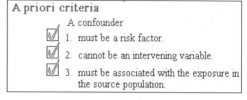

Suppose age and race are two risk factors identified and measured for possible control in a case-control study to assess an exposure disease relationship. It is possible that the adjusted odds ratio, which simultaneously controls for both age and race to give different results from those obtained by controlling for each variable separately.

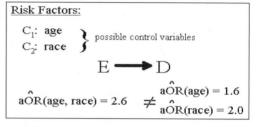

If the odds ratio that controls for all potential risk factors is our standard, then should we **always** control for **all** risk factors? Not necessarily. It is possible that only a subset of these factors needs to be controlled to obtain valid results.

Suppose these results were obtained from our case-control study:

$$a\hat{O}R(\text{age, race}) = 2.6 \qquad a\hat{O}R(\text{age}) = 2.6$$
$$\downarrow \qquad\qquad a\hat{O}R(\text{race}) = 2.0$$
$$\text{the standard}$$

Here, the odds ratio controlling for age alone is equivalent to the odds ratio controlling for both age and race. In this case, we would not lose anything with regards to validity by selecting only age for control.

These examples illustrate two fundamental principles about the control of confounding when several risk factors have been identified and measured. First, the joint (or simultaneous) control of two or more variables may give different results from those obtained by controlling for each variable separately. The adjusted estimate (denoted here as a theta hat, $\hat{\theta}$) that simultaneously controls for all risk factors under consideration should be the standard on which all conclusions about confounding and the identification of specific confounders must be based.

Second, not all the variables in a given list of risk factors may need to be controlled; it is possible that different subsets of such variables can correct for confounding. We will discuss these two principles in the activities that follow.

Confounding With Several Covariates
Two Fundamental Principles

1. Joint (i.e., simultaneous) control of two or more variables may give different results from controlling for each variable separately.

$$\hat{a\theta}\,(C_1, C_2, \ldots, C_p) \rightarrow \text{standard}$$

2. Not all the variables in a given list of risk factors may need to be controlled; it is possible that different subsets of such variables can correct for confounding.

Note: θ denotes any effect measure of interest.

Study Questions (Q11.1) Suppose age, race, gender, and smoking status are the only risk factors considered for control in assessing an exposure-disease relationship.

1. Describe the adjusted estimate that should be the standard on which all conclusions about confounding and the identification of specific confounders be based.
2. If one fails to consider all potential confounders simultaneously, what might be some of the problems to arise?
3. If the gold standard adjusted estimate controls for all risk factors, is it possible that a subset of such risk factors may also control for confounding?
4. Why might the use of such a subset of variables be advantageous over the use of the adjusted estimate that controls for all potential confounders?

Summary

❖ There are two fundamental principles about the control of confounding when two or more risk factors have been identified and measured for possible control.

   1. The joint or simultaneous control of two or more variables can give different results from those obtained by controlling for each variable separately.
   2. Not all variables in a given list of risk factors may need to be controlled.

❖ Moreover, depending on the relationships among these risk factors, it is possible that confounding can be corrected by using different subsets of risk factors on the list.

Joint Versus Marginal Confounding

We defined **data-based confounding** involving a single potential confounder to mean that there is a meaningful difference between the estimated crude effect (which completely ignores a potential confounder) and the **estimated adjusted**

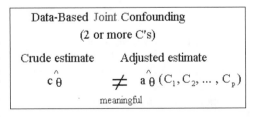

Data-Based Joint Confounding
(2 or more C's)

Crude estimate   Adjusted estimate

$$\hat{c\theta} \neq \hat{a\theta}\,(C_1, C_2, \ldots, C_p)$$

meaningful

effect (which controls for a potential confounder). We now define **data-based joint confounding** in the presence of 2 or more potential confounders. This occurs when there is a meaningful difference between the estimated crude effect and the estimated adjusted effect, which simultaneously controls for all the potential confounding.

Study Questions (Q11.2) Suppose a follow-up study was conducted to evaluate an E→D relationship. Age and smoking status were determined as possible control variables. Suppose further that:

aRR(age, smoking) =	2.4
aRR(age) =	1.7
aRR(smoking) =	1.9
cRR =	1.5

1. Is this evidence of joint confounding? Why or why not?

Suppose for a different follow-up study of the same E→D relationship that once again age and smoking status were possible control variables. Suppose further that:

aRR(age, smoking) =	1.4
aRR(age) =	2.4
aRR(smoking) =	2.4
cRR =	1.5

2. Is this evidence of joint confounding? Why or why not?

In contrast, we define **data-based marginal confounding** to mean that there is a meaningful difference between the estimated crude effect and the estimated adjusted effect that controls for only one of several potential confounders.

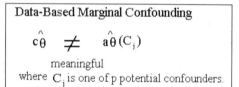

Study Questions (Q11.2) continued Suppose a follow-up study was conducted to evaluate an E→D relationship. Age and smoking status were determined as possible control variables. Suppose that:

aRR(age, smoking) =	2.4
cRR =	1.5

3. Is there evidence of marginal confounding? Why or why not?
4. If the aRR(age) = 1.4, does this provide evidence of marginal confounding?
5. Does this mean that we should not control for age as a confounder?

Joint confounding is the primary criterion for determining the presence of data-based confounding when all are eligible for control. Nevertheless, data-based marginal confounding can help determine whether **some** potential confounders **need not** be controlled.

Study Questions (Q11.2) continued

6. In the follow-up study described in the previous study question, the:

aRR(age, smoking) =	2.4
aRR(age) =	1.5
aRR(smoking) =	2.4
cRR =	1.5

Does this mean that we do not have to control for age?
7. What problem might there be in practice that could prevent the estimate of the effect that controls for all risk factors (e.g., C_1, C_2, ..., C_k)?
8. What should we do if there are too many potential confounders in our list and we are unable to determine the appropriate adjusted estimate?
9. What if the choice of such a subset becomes difficult?

Summary

❖ **Data-based joint confounding** occurs when there is a meaningful difference between the estimated crude effect and the estimated adjusted effect that simultaneously controls for *all* the potential confounders.

❖ **Data-based marginal confounding** occurs when there is a meaningful difference between the estimated crude effect and the estimated adjusted effect, which controls for only *one* of the several potential confounders.

❖ Our conclusions regarding confounding should be based on joint confounding whenever possible.

Quiz (Q11.3) Suppose **F** and **G** are two distinct risk factors for some disease with dichotomous levels F_1, F_0, and G_1, G_0, respectively. The estimated risk ratios describing the association between the disease and some exposure are listed below for various combinations of levels of **F** and **G**. Assume that the risk ratio estimates are of high precision (i.e., are based on large sample sizes).

$\hat{RR}(F_1 G_1) = 3.0$	$\hat{RR}(F_1) = 1.0$	$c\hat{RR} = 1.0$
$\hat{RR}(F_1 G_0) = 3.0$	$\hat{RR}(F_0) = 1.0$	
$\hat{RR}(F_0 G_1) = 0.3$	$\hat{RR}(G_1) = 1.0$	
$\hat{RR}(F_0 G_0) = 3.0$	$\hat{RR}(G_0) = 1.0$	

Determine whether the following statements are **True** or **False**.

1. There is evidence of interaction in the data.   ???
2. There is evidence of confounding in the data.   ???
3. At level G_0, there is no confounding due to factor **F**.   ???
4. At level F_1, there is no interaction due to factor **G**.   ???
5. At level F_0, there is no interaction and no confounding due to factor **G** .???
6. At level G_0, there is confounding but no interaction due to factor **F**   ???
7. It is not necessary to control for either **F** or **G** (or both) in order to understand the relationship between D and E.   ???.

Variable Selection and Control of Confounding

The adjusted estimate that controls for all potential risk factors is the standard on which conclusions about confounding should be based. However, if an adjusted, estimate that controls for only a subset of risk factors is equivalent to this standard, we may then choose such a subset for control.

$$\hat{a\theta}(C_1, C_2 \ldots, C_p) \rightarrow \text{standard}$$
$$=$$
$$\hat{a\theta}(C_1, C_2)$$
$$\hat{a\theta}(C_2, C_3, C_7) \quad \text{Maybe this subset is 'best'}$$
$$\hat{a\theta}(C_3)$$

Consider a case-control study in which three risk factors, **F**, **G**, and **H** are being considered for control. The crude odds ratio differs from the adjusted odds ratio that controls for all three factors. Because the crude and adjusted estimates differ, we have evidence of data-based joint confounding in these data.

> **Case-control study**
>
> F, G, and H eligible for control
>
> $c\hat{O}R = 3.1$
> $\neq$
> $a\hat{O}R(F,G,H) = 1.6 \text{ (standard)}$
>
> Joint Confounding

Suppose now that controlling for any two of these factors provides the same results as controlling for all three. **F**, **G**, and **H** do not **all** need to be controlled simultaneously. Controlling for any two of the three risk factors will provide the same results as the standard.

We may also wish to consider marginal confounding to see if any single variable is an appropriate subgroup. These results indicate that there is no marginal confounding because each of these results differs from the standard estimate, not one of these variables alone would be an appropriate subgroup for control.

> **Case-control study**
>
> F, G, and H eligible for control
>
> $c\hat{O}R = 3.1$
> $\neq$
> $a\hat{O}R(F,G,H) = 1.6 \text{ (standard)}$
> $\hat{a\theta}(F,G) = 1.6$
> $\hat{a\theta}(F,H) = 1.6$ Do not need to control for all 3!
> $\hat{a\theta}(G,H) = 1.6$

> Case-control study
>
> F, G, and H eligible for control
>
> $c\hat{O}R = 3.1$ Marginal   NO!
> $\neq$ Confounding?
> $a\hat{O}R(F,G,H) = 1.6 \text{ (standard)}$
> $a\hat{O}R(F) = 3.0$
> $a\hat{O}R(G) = 2.7$
> $a\hat{O}R(H) = 3.2$

Study Questions (Q11.4)

$a\hat{O}R(F,G,H) = 1.6$ (standard)	
$a\hat{O}R(F,G) = 1.6$	$a\hat{O}R(F) = 3.0$
$a\hat{O}R(F,H) = 1.6$	$a\hat{O}R(G) = 2.7$
$a\hat{O}R(G,H) = 1.6$	$a\hat{O}R(H) = 3.2$

1. What might be the advantage to controlling for only two of these risk factors rather than all three even though it is the standard?
2. How might you determine which two variables to controls?
3. Why can't we control for **F**, **G**, or **H** separately?

Assume that F, G, H, I, and J are the only risk factors in a case-control study. Suppose further that:

$$cOR \neq aOR(F, G, H, I, J)$$

but

$$aOR(F, G, H, I) = aOR(G, J) = aOR(I) = aOR(F, G, H) = aOR(F, G, H, I, J)$$

and that

$$aOR(\text{any other subset of risk factors}) \neq aOR(F, G, H, I, J)$$

Determine whether each of the following is a proper subset of confounders that controls for (joint) confounding in this study by answering **Yes** or **No**:

4. {G, J}?
5. {I}?
6. {G, H, I}?
7. {F, G, H}?

Summary

❖ When two or more risk factors are considered for control, we can select an appropriate subset of confounders for control.
❖ When the results from controlling for various subsets of risk factors are equivalent to the joint control of all risk factors, we can select any one of which provides valid and precise results.

Confounding: Validity versus Precision

The fully adjusted estimate that controls for all factors simultaneously is the standard on which all decisions should be based. Why then would we want to go through the process of seeking out candidate subsets of confounders? If we cannot improve on the validity of the effect measure, why not just use the fully adjusted estimate?

$a\hat{\theta} (C_1, C_2, C_3, \cdots, C_k)$ → Standard
controls all risk factors simultaneously

$a\hat{\theta} (C_1, C_2)$

$a\hat{\theta} (C_2, C_3, C_7)$

$a\hat{\theta} (C_3)$ } **Why bother?**

The precision of the estimate may justify such an effort. Controlling for a smaller number of variables may yield a more precise estimate of effect. The identification of the subset of confounders giving the most precise estimate is important enough to make such examination worthwhile. Consider the following exercise to illustrate this point.

Study Questions (Q11.5) A clinical trial was conducted to determine the effectiveness of a particular treatment on the survival of stage 3 cancer patients. The following variables were considered in the analysis:

RX = exposure **AGE** = age at trial entry
SERH = serum hemoglobin level **TSZ** = size of primary tumor
INSG = combined index that measures tumor stage and grade.

1. The cRR = 6.28 and the aRR(AGE, SERH, TSZ, INSG) = 8.24. Does this provide evidence of joint confounding in the study? (Assume all quantities above are estimates.)

We calculated the aRR for all possible subsets of the four potential confounders. Excluding the crude results and the gold standard, there are 14 possible subsets of these 4 confounders.

2. What criteria may we use to reduce the number of candidate subsets?

Below are the results from the gold standard and the 4 candidate subsets whose aRR is within 10% of the gold standard:

Covariates	aRR	95% CI	CI Width
INSG, AGE, SEHR, TSZ	8.24	(3.59, 18.91)	15.32
AGE, SERH, TSZ	8.26	(3.64, 18.75)	15.11
INSG, AGE	7.63	(3.75, 15.56)	11.81
INSG, SERH	7.63	(3.64, 15.97)	12.33
SERH	8.25	(4.06, 16.76)	12.70

3. The most valid estimate results from controlling which covariates?
4. The most precise estimate results from controlling which covariates?
5. Which covariates do you think are most appropriate to control?

This exercise has illustrated that we need to consider both validity and precision when assessing an exposure-disease relationship. Getting a valid estimate of effect is most important. Nevertheless, you must also consider the trade-off between controlling for enough risk factors to maintain validity and the possible loss in precision from the control of too many variables.

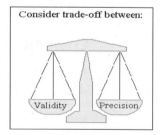

Consider trade-off between:

Validity Precision

Summary
❖ The reason for seeking candidate subsets of all potential confounders is the possibility of improving the precision of the estimated effect.
❖ Controlling for fewer variables may (or may not) lead to a more precise estimate of effect.

❖ When controlling for several potential confounders, you should consider the possible trade-offs between:
  o Controlling for enough risk factors to maintain validity *versus*
  o Possible loss in precision from the control of too many variables.

Quiz (Q11.6) Suppose that variables **F**, **G**, and **H** have been measured in a certain study and that only **F** and **G** are considered to be risk factors for some disease (D). Suppose that it is of interest to describe the relationship between this disease and some study factor (E), and that there is no interaction of any kind present in the data. Finally, suppose that the following relationships hold among various odds ratios computed from the data:

$$
\begin{array}{ll}
c\hat{O}R \neq a\hat{O}R\,(F) & a\hat{O}R\,(F,G) = a\hat{O}R\,(F) \\
c\hat{O}R = a\hat{O}R\,(G) & a\hat{O}R\,(F,G) \neq a\hat{O}R\,(G) \\
c\hat{O}R = a\hat{O}R\,(H) & a\hat{O}R\,(F,H) = a\hat{O}R\,(H) \\
c\hat{O}R = a\hat{O}R\,(F,G,H) & a\hat{O}R\,(F,G,H) = a\hat{O}R\,(G,H) \\
c\hat{O}R \neq a\hat{O}R\,(F,G) &
\end{array}
$$

Determine whether the following statements are **True** or **False**.
1. There is confounding in the data. ???
2. Variable **F** needs to be controlled to avoid confounding. ???
3. Variable **G** needs to be controlled to avoid confounding. ???
4. Variable **H** needs to be controlled to avoid confounding. ???
5. Both variables **F** and **G** do not need to be controlled simultaneously in order to avoid confounding. ???

A ten-year follow-up study was conducted to determine if someone experiencing food allergies is at increased risk of coronary heart disease. The following covariates were considered in the analysis: **AGE** = age at enrollment, **BMI** = body mass index, and **SMK** = smoking status. The results for the standard and all possible subsets are listed below. The crude risk ratio = 1.02.

	Covariates	aRR	95%CI	
1.	AGE, BMI, SMK	4.10	(1.7, 8.8)	(standard)
2.	AGE, BMI	2.70	(1.6, 7.8)	
3.	AGE, SMK	4.12	(1.4, 9.5)	
4.	BMI, SMK	2.50	(1.8, 6.2)	
5.	AGE	4.01	(1.6, 8.7)	
6.	BMI	2.50	(1.4, 7.5)	
7.	SMK	4.16	(1.5, 8.6)	

6. Is there evidence of confounding? ???.
7. Besides the standard, which are candidate subgroups for control? ???, ???, ???.
8. Which of the candidate subgroups corresponds to the most valid estimate (including the standard)? ???.
9. Is there more than one candidate subgroup that is the most precise? ???.
10. Which estimate should be used? ???.

Choices **#2** **#3** **#4** **#5** **#6** **#7** **no** **yes**

Nomenclature

$\hat{\theta}$	Estimated measure of effect
aOR	Adjusted odds ratio
aRR	Adjusted risk ratio
C_i	Confounding variable
CI	Confidence interval
cOR	Crude odds ratio
cRR	Crude risk ratio
D	Disease
E	Exposure

Reference

Kleinbaum DG, Kupper LL, Morgenstern H. Epidemiologic Research: Principles and Quantitative Methods. John Wiley and Sons Publishers, New York, 1982 (Chapter 14).

Answers to Study Questions and Quizzes

Q11.1

1. The adjusted estimate that simultaneously controls for all 4 risk factors under consideration.
2. Confounding might not be controlled if there is not a subset of potential confounders that yields (essentially) the same adjusted estimate as obtained when all confounders are controlled.
3. Yes, provided the subset yields essentially the same adjusted estimate as the gold standard.
4. Adjusting for a smaller number of variables may increase precision. Also, such a subset provides a more parsimonious description of the exposure-disease relationship.

Q11.2

1. Yes, the cRR of 1.5 differs from the aRR(age, smoking) of 2.4 that controls for both potential confounders.
2. No, the cRR of 1.5 is essentially equal to the aRR(age, smoking) of 1.4 that controls for both potential confounders.
3. No, the cRR of 1.5 differs from the aRR(age, smoking) of 2.4, which controls for all potential confounders. This is evidence of joint confounding.
4. No, since the cRR of 1.5 is approximately equal to the aRR(age) of 1.4, there is no evidence of marginal confounding due to age.

5. Not necessarily. Our conclusions regarding confounding should be based on the joint control of all risk factors.
6. Yes. Controlling for smoking alone gives us the same result as controlling for both risk factors. We might still wish to evaluate the precision of the estimates before making a final conclusion.
7. There may be so many risk factors in our list relative to the amount of data available that the adjusted estimate cannot be estimated with any precision at all.
8. Then we may be forced to make decisions by using a subset of this large initial set of risk factors.
9. The use of marginal confounding may be the only alternative.

Q11.3

1. True – There is interaction because the risk ratio estimated in one stratum (F_0G_1) is 0.3, which is quite different from the stratum-specific risk ratios of 3.0 in the other strata.
2. True – The presence of strong interaction may preclude the assessment of confounding. Also, the value of an adjusted estimate may vary depending on the weights chosen for the different strata.
3. False – The RR for F_1 and F_0 at level G_0 are both 3.0. These differ from the overall RR at level G_0 of 1.0.

Therefore, at level G_0, there is confounding due to factor F.
4. True
5. False – There is interaction and possibly confounding. At level F_0, the RR for G_1 and G_0 are very different, and both are very different from the overall risk ratio at level F_0.
6. True
7. False – Both confounding and interaction are present and each should be addressed.

Q11.4
1. Controlling for fewer variables will likely increase the precision of the results.
2. The two that provide the most precise adjusted estimate.
3. Controlling for any of these three factors alone yields different results than controlling for all three, which is the standard on which our conclusions should be based.
4. Yes
5. Yes
6. No
7. Yes

Q11.5
1. Yes, the cRR differs from the aRR controlling for all potential confounders, which is the gold standard.
2. We may choose to only consider those results within 10% of the gold standard. In this case, that would be 8.24 ± 0.82 which is a range of values between 7.42 and 9.06.
3. Controlling for all the covariates provides the most valid estimate. It is the gold standard.
4. Controlling for both INSG and AGE provides the narrowest confidence interval and hence is the most precise.

5. Debatable: Controlling for SERH alone yields an almost identical aRR as the gold standard, increases precision, and is the stingiest subset. Controlling for INSG and AGE provides a slightly larger increase in precision (than controlling for SERH only) and its aRR is within 10% of the standard. Consider the trade-off between parsimony and political/scientific implications of not controlling for all risk factors, and more precision from controlling for fewer risk factors.

Q11.6
1. True
2. True
3. False – Variable G does not need to be controlled since aOR(F,G)=aOR(F). In other words, controlling for F alone yields the same results as the gold standard, controlling for both F and G.
4. False – Variable H is not a risk factor in this study, and therefore should not be considered a confounding.
5. True
6. Yes – The cRR of 1.02 differs from the standard RR of 4.10 that controls for all potential confounders.
7. #3, #5, #7
8. #1 – The most valid estimate controls for all risk factors measured.
9. Yes – Candidate subgroups 1 and 7 are equally precise.
10. #1 – The gold standard is the most valid estimate; has the same precision as obtained for candidate 7. No precision is gained by dropping any risk factors so it can be argued the gold standard is the 'political' choice for it controls for all considered risk factors. Controlling only for SMK is the best choice for it gives the smallest, most precise subset of variables.

CHAPTER 12

SIMPLE ANALYSES-
2×2 TABLES ARE NOT THAT SIMPLE

*This chapter discusses methods for carrying out **statistical inference** procedures for epidemiologic data given in a simple two-way table. We call such procedures **simple analyses** because we are restricting the discussion here to dichotomous disease and exposure variables only and we are ignoring the typical analysis situation that considers the control of **other** variables when studying the effect of an exposure on disease.*

WHAT IS SIMPLE ANALYSIS?

When analyzing the crude data that describes the relationship between a dichotomous exposure and dichotomous disease variable, we typically want to make statistical inferences about this relationship. That is, we would like to determine whether the measure of effect being estimated is statistically significant and we would like to obtain an interval estimate that considers the sample variability of the measure of effect.

The tables shown here have been described in previous chapters to illustrate data from three different studies, a cohort study to assess whether quitting smoking after a heart attack will reduce one's risk for dying, a case-control study to determine the source of an outbreak of diarrhea at a resort

Heart Attack Patients	Smoke	Quit	Total
Death	27	14	41
Survival	48	67	115
Total	75	81	156

COHORT

Quit Smoking ➡ Mortality

$\hat{RR} = 2.1$

Resort Study	Raw Hamburger Ate	Did not Eat	Total
Cases	17	20	37
Controls	7	26	33
Total	24	46	70

CASE-CONTROL

Source ➡ Diarrhea

$\hat{OR} = 3.2$

Cholestrol Study	Cholestrol Level Borderline High	Normal
Deaths	26	14
P–Years	36,581	60,239

PERSON-TIME COHORT

Cholesterol ➡ Mortality

$\hat{IDR} = 3.5$

in Haiti, and a person-time cohort study to assess the relationship between serum cholesterol level and mortality.

In each study, a measure of effect was computed to estimate the extent of the relationship between the exposure variable and the health outcome variable. In the quit smoking cohort study, the effect measure was a risk ratio and its estimate was 2.1. In the outbreak study, the effect measure was an odds ratio and its estimate was 3.2. And in the cholesterol mortality study, the effect measure was a rate ratio, also called an incidence density ratio, and its estimate was 3.5.

We have discussed how to interpret each of these estimates in terms of the exposure disease-relationship being studied. All three estimates, even though dealing with different study types and different study questions, are similar in that they are all larger than the **null value of one**, and they all indicate that there is a moderately large effect from exposure. Nevertheless, we must be careful to realize that each of these three estimates is based on sample data. If a different sample had been drawn, any of these estimates might have resulted in a different value, maybe a lot larger, maybe closer to the null value of one. That is, there is always **random error** associated with any sample estimate.

We call these estimates **point estimates** because they each represent a single number or point from the possibly wide range of numbers that might have been obtained if different samples had been drawn. So, we might wonder, given the inherent variability in a point estimate, how can we draw conclusions about the **population parameters** being estimated?

For example, in the first cohort study, what can we say about the **population risk ratio** based on the **estimated risk ratio**? Or, in the case-control study, what can we conclude about the **population odds ratio** based on the **estimated odds ratio**? In the person-time study what can we conclude about the **population rate ratio** based on the **estimated rate ratio**? In answering these questions, we typically have one of two objectives. We may want to determine whether we have evidence from the sample that the population risk ratio, odds ratio or rate ratio being estimated is different from the null value of one. For this objective, we use **hypothesis testing**. Or, we may want to determine the precision of our point estimate by accounting for its **sampling variability**. For this objective, we use **interval estimation**.

The methods used to achieve these objectives comprise the general subject matter of **statistical inference**. When our attention is focused on the relatively simple situation involving only one dichotomous exposure variable and one dichotomous disease variable, as illustrated by these three studies, we call these methods **simple analyses**.

<u>Summary</u>
- ❖ Estimates of measures of effect such as RR, OR, and IDR are **point estimates**, since each estimate represents a single number that may vary from sample to sample.
- ❖ **Statistical inference** involves drawing conclusions about the value of a measure of effect in a population, based on its estimate obtained from a sample.
- ❖ The two types of **statistical inference** procedures are **hypothesis testing** and **interval estimation**.

STATISTICAL INFERENCES – A REVIEW

The activities in this section review fundamental concepts and methods of statistics. Our primary focus concerns how to draw conclusions about populations based on data obtained in a sample. We assume that you already have some previous exposure to basic statistical concepts, including the distinction between a <u>sample</u> and a <u>population</u>, a sample <u>statistic</u> and a population <u>parameter</u>, some important distributions like the <u>normal</u>, <u>binomial</u>, <u>Student's t</u>, and <u>chi square</u> distributions. We also assume that you have some previous exposure to *the concepts underlying statistical tests of hypothesis and confidence intervals, which are the two types of statistical inferences possible. Our focus here will be to review statistical inference concepts in the context of the statistical questions that apply to the analysis of a 2 x 2 table, which is the kind of data we are considering in a simple analysis. You may wish to skip this entire review section and proceed to the next section, Cohort Studies, on page 12-4. We begin by using data from a famous "incident" to distinguish between the two types of statistical inference procedures: hypothesis (significance) testing and confidence interval estimation. See if you can guess what "incident" we illustrate.*

Statistical Inference Overview

Here are some data from an incident in which a group of persons were at risk of dying. From these data, we can find the proportions who died for men and women, separately. We can see that 79.7% of the men died, but only 25.6% of the women died.

AN INCIDENT
Persons at Risk

	Men	Women	Total
Died	1329	109	1438
Lived	338	316	654
Total	1667	425	2092

	.797	.256	Meaningfully
	79.7 %	25.6 %	different !

Clearly these two percentages are meaningfully different since the men had a much higher risk for dying than the women. But can we also claim that there is a difference in the risk for dying among men and women in the population from which these samples came? In other words, is the difference in the risks for men and women **statistically significant**?

If we wish to draw conclusions about a population from data collected from a sample, we must consider the methods of **statistical inference**. In particular, we must view the two proportions or percentages as estimates obtained from a sample. Let's focus on the two sample proportions, which we denote $\hat{p}_M$ and $\hat{p}_W$. The corresponding population proportions are denoted p_M and p_W, without "hats".

Statistical inference draws conclusions about a population parameter based on information obtained from a sample statistic. So, what is the population parameter considered for these data and what is its corresponding sample statistic?

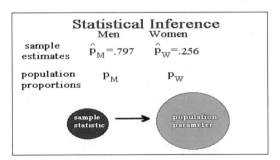

Since our focus here is to **compare** the proportions for males and females, one logical choice for our parameter of interest is the difference between the two population proportions. The corresponding sample statistic is the difference between the two estimated proportions.

Statistical Inference

	Men	Women	
sample statistic	$\hat{p}_M$	– $\hat{p}_W$	= .541
population parameter	p_M	– p_W	

Study Questions (Q12.1)
1. What other (epidemiologic) parameters could also be considered as alternatives to the difference in the two proportions?

Hypothesis testing can be used here to determine whether the difference in the two proportions is statistically significant. This is one of the two types of statistical inference questions we may ask. Our hypothesis in this case, usually stated as what we want to disprove, is that the true difference in the two population proportions is zero. This is called the **null hypothesis**. In hypothesis testing, we seek evidence from the sample to disprove the null hypothesis in favor of the **alternative hypothesis** that there is a difference in the population proportions.

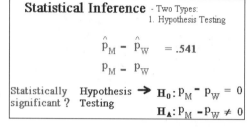

Statistical Inference - Two Types:
1. Hypothesis Testing

$$\hat{p}_M - \hat{p}_W = .541$$

$$p_M - p_W$$

Statistically significant ? | Hypothesis Testing → $H_0 : p_M - p_W = 0$
$H_A : p_M - p_W \neq 0$

Study Questions (Q12.1) continued
2. If the parameter of interest is the risk ratio (RR), how would you state the null hypothesis?
3. If the parameter of interest is the odds ratio (OR), how would you state the null hypothesis?

We can use **interval estimation** to determine the precision of our point estimate. Here, our goal is to use our sample information to compute two numbers, say, **L** and **U**, that define a confidence interval for the difference between the two population proportions. Using a confidence interval, we can predict with a certain amount of confidence, say 95%, that the limits, **L** and **U**, bound the true value of the parameter. For our data, it turns out, that the lower and upper limits for the difference in the two proportions are .407 and .675, respectively.

$$L = .407 < p_M - p_W < U = .675$$
$$\hat{p}_M - \hat{p}_W = .541$$

It may appear from these two numbers that an interval estimate is less precise than a point estimate. The opposite is actually true. The range of values specified by the interval estimate actually takes into account the unreliability or variance of the point estimate. It is therefore more precise, since it uses more information to describe the point estimate.

In general, interval estimation and hypothesis testing can be contrasted by their different approaches to answering questions. A test of hypothesis arrives at an answer by looking for rare or unlikely sample results. In contrast, interval estimation arrives at its answer by looking at the most likely results, that is, those values that we are confident lie close to the parameter under investigation.

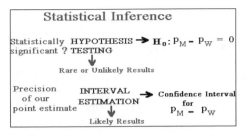

Summary

❖ **Statistical inference** concerns drawing conclusions about a population parameter based on information obtained from a sample statistic.

❖ The two types of statistical inference are **hypothesis testing** and **interval estimation**.

❖ When we test a hypothesis, we typically want to disprove a null hypothesis.

❖ When doing interval estimation, we want to obtain a confidence interval that provides upper and lower limits that we can be, say 95%, confident covers the population parameter of interest.

❖ A test of hypothesis looks for rare or unlikely results from our sample, where a confidence interval looks for likely results.

The Incident

The story of the Titanic is well known. The largest ship that had ever been built up to that time, she left Southampton, England on her maiden voyage to New York on Wednesday, April 10, 1912, carrying many of the rich and famous of England and the United States, but also many of more modest means. Because the Titanic was so large and so modern, many thought that she could not sink.

After a stop at Cherbourg France, where she took on many 3rd class passengers seeking new lives in the New World, and a brief stop off Queenstown, Ireland, she set out across the Atlantic. At 11:40 on the evening of April 14th, the Titanic struck an iceberg and, by 2:15 the next morning, sank.

Of 2,201 passengers and crew, only 710 survived. Some facts can be gleamed about the passengers, about who survived and who did not. One underlining question of interest in any disaster of this sort is did everyone have an equal chance of surviving? Or, stated in statistics terms, was the probability of surviving independent of other factors.

Hypothesis Testing

We illustrate how to carry out a statistical test of hypothesis to compare survival of men and women passengers on the Titanic. We want to assess whether the difference in sample proportions for men and

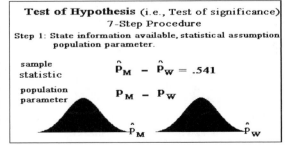

women is statistically significant.

A **test of hypotheses**, also called a **test of significance**, can be described as a seven-step procedure. In **step one** we state the information available, the statistical assumptions, and the population parameter being considered. In our example, the information includes the numbers of men and women passengers and the sample proportions. We need to assume that the data represents a sample from a larger population and that each sample proportion is approximately normally distributed. The **population parameter** of interest is the difference between the two population proportions being estimated ($P_M - P_W$). The corresponding **sample statistic** is the difference between the two estimated proportions ($\hat{P}_M - \hat{P}_W$).

In **step 2**, we specify the **null** and **alternative hypotheses**. A hypothesis is a claim about a value of a population parameter. The hypothesis that we plan to test is commonly called the null hypothesis. This is often the accepted state of knowledge that we want to question. The null hypothesis in our example is that the difference in the two population proportions is zero. H_0 is essentially treated like the defendant in a trial. It is assumed true, or innocent, until the evidence from the data makes it highly unlikely to have occurred by chance. Our testing goal here is to see if we have evidence to disprove this null hypothesis. The alternative hypothesis, typically called H_A, gives the values the parameter may take if the null is false. In our example, the alternative hypothesis is that the difference in population proportions is not equal to zero. This is called a **two-sided alternative** because it states that we are interested in values both above and below the null. The alternative hypothesis would be called **one-sided** if, before looking at our data, we were interested in determining only whether men were at greater risk for dying than women. To avoid biasing one's analysis, both the null and alternative hypothesis should be made without looking at the study data and be based only on the a priori objectives of the study.

Step 2: Specify the null and alternative hypotheses.
H_0: $P_M - P_W = 0$
H_A: $P_M - P_W \neq 0$ Two-sided APRIORI
$P_M - P_W > 0$ One-sided

In **step 3**, we specify the **significance level, alpha**. We will set the significance level for our example at .05 or 5 percent. This means that in carrying out our procedure, we are willing to take a 5 percent risk of rejecting the null hypothesis even if it is actually true. Equivalently, the significance level tells us how rare or unlikely our study results have to be under the null hypothesis in order for us to reject the null hypothesis in favor of the alternative hypothesis. An alpha of 5 percent means that, if the null hypothesis is actually true, we will have a 5% chance of rejecting it.

Step 3: Specify the significance level α.
$\alpha = .05$ (i.e., 5%)
Even if H_0 true, 5% risk of rejecting H_0
How unlikely must our study results be (under H_0) in order to reject H_0.

Summary of first 3 steps.

❖ A statistical test of hypothesis can be described as a seven-step procedure. The first three steps are:

Step 1: State the information available, the statistical assumptions, and the population parameter being considered.

Step 2: Specify the null and alternative hypotheses.
Step 3: Specify the significance level alpha (α).

In **step 4** of our hypothesis testing procedure, we must select the **test statistic** to use, and we must state its **sampling distribution** under the assumption that the null hypothesis is true. Because the parameter of interest is the difference between two proportions, the test statistic T is given by the difference in the two sample proportions divided by the estimated standard error of this sample difference under the null hypothesis. The denominator here is computed using an expression involving the pooled estimate, $\hat{p}$, of the common proportion for both groups that would result under the null hypothesis.

Step 4: Select the test statistic and state its sampling distribution under H_0.

$$T = \frac{\hat{p}_M - \hat{p}_W}{\sqrt{\hat{p}(1-\hat{p})(\frac{1}{n_M} + \frac{1}{n_W})}} \qquad \hat{p} = \frac{n_M \hat{p}_M + n_W \hat{p}_W}{n_M + n_W}$$

Study Question (Q12.2) The pooled estimate of the common proportion for two groups is a weighted average of the two sample proportions, where the weights are the sample sizes used to compute each proportion. The sample size proportions and their corresponding sample sizes are .7972 and 1667, respectively for men, and .256 and 425 for women.

1. Compute the pooled estimate from the above information. (You will need a calculator to obtain your answer.)

The sampling distribution of this test statistic is approximately the standard normal distribution, with zero mean and unit standard deviation, under the null hypothesis.

In **step 5**, we formulate the decision rule that partitions the possible outcomes of the test statistic into acceptance and rejection regions. Because our test statistic has approximately the standard normal or Z distribution under the null hypothesis, the acceptance and rejection regions will be specified as intervals along the Z-axis under the curve of this distribution. In particular, because our alternative hypothesis is two-tailed and since our significance level is .05, these two regions turn out to be as shown here by the red and green lines. (Note: the red lines are in the tail areas < -1.96 and > 1.96; the green line between −1.96 and 1.96.) The area under the standard normal curve above the interval described as the acceptance region is .95 .The area under the curve in each tail of the distribution identified as rejection regions is .025. The sum of these two areas is .05, which is our chosen significance level. The -1.96 on the left side under the curve is the 2.5 percentage point of the standard normal distribution, and the 1.96 on the right side under the curve is the 97.5 percentage point.

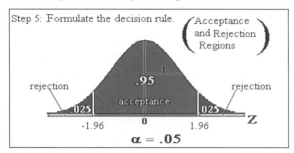

Our decision rule can now be described as follows. If the value of the **test statistic T** computed from our data falls into the rejection region, we reject the null hypothesis in favor of the alternative hypothesis. However, if the observed study value falls into the acceptance region, we do not reject the null hypothesis.

Step 6 of our process simply requires us to compute the value of the test statistic T from the observed data. We will call the computed value **T*** to distinguish it from the test statistic T. Here again are the sample results:

Step 6: Compute the test statistic T from the data

$$T = \frac{\hat{p}_M - \hat{p}_W}{\sqrt{\hat{p}(1-\hat{p})(\frac{1}{n_M} + \frac{1}{n_W})}} \qquad \hat{p} = \frac{n_M \hat{p}_M + n_W \hat{p}_W}{n_M + n_W}$$

Computed T = T*
$\hat{p} = .6874$ (men and women combined)
$\hat{p}_M = .7972 \; n_M = 1667$ (men)
$\hat{p}_W = .2565 \; n_W = 425$ (women)

Substituting the sample information into the formula for T, our computed value T* turns out to be 21.46.

$$T^* = \frac{.7972 \; .2565}{\sqrt{.6874 \, (1 - .6874) \, (\frac{1}{1667} + \frac{1}{425})}}$$

$$= 12.00$$

Finally, in **Step 7**, we use our computed test statistic to draw conclusions about our test of significance. In this example, the computed test statistic falls into the extreme right tail of the rejection region because it is much larger than 1.96.

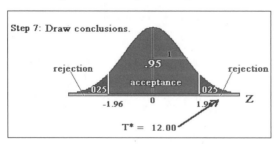

Consequently, we reject the null hypothesis and conclude that we have a statistically significant difference between the two proportions at the .05 significance level. We therefore conclude that of all those that could have been aboard the Titanic, men were more likely to die than women.

<u>Summary</u>
❖ A statistical test of hypothesis can be described as a seven-step procedure. The first three steps are:
Step 1: State the information available, statistical assumptions, and the population parameter being considered.
Step 2: Specify the null and alternative hypotheses.
Step 3: Specify the significance level alpha (α).
Step 4: Select the test statistic and state its sampling distribution under the null hypothesis.
Step 5: Formulate the decision rule in terms of rejection and acceptance regions under the null hypothesis.
Step 6: Compute the test statistic using the observed data.
Step 7: Draw conclusions, i.e., reject or do not reject the null hypothesis at the alpha significance level.

Hypothesis Testing – The P-value

We have found that the difference in the sample proportions of the men and women who died on the Titanic was statistically significant at the 0.05 significance level. In particular, the computed value of the test statistic fell into the extreme right tail of the rejection region. This tells us that if the null hypothesis were true, the observed results had less than a 5% chance of occurring. That is, the results were quite unlikely under the null hypothesis.

We may wonder, then, exactly how unlikely, or how rare, were the observed results under the null hypothesis? Were they also less than 1% likely, or less than 0.1% likely, or even rarer? The answer to these questions is given by the **P-value**. The P-value gives the probability of obtaining the value of the test statistic we have computed or a more extreme value if the null hypothesis is true.

Let's assume, as in our example, that the test statistic has the standard normal distribution under the null hypothesis. To obtain the P-value, we must determine an area under this curve. Here, we show four different areas that correspond to where the computed value T* falls under the curve and to whether the alternative hypothesis is one-sided or two-sided.

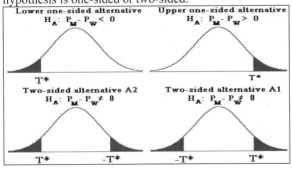

If the alternative hypothesis is an upper one-sided hypothesis, then the P-value is the area under the curve to the right of T* (upper right distribution in the above figure). If the alternative hypothesis is a lower one-sided hypothesis, then the P-value is the area under the curve to the left of T* (upper left distribution in the above figure). If the alternative hypothesis is two-sided and T* falls in the right tail under the curve, then the P-value is the sum of the areas under the curve to the right of T* and to the left of -T*. If the alternative hypothesis is two-sided and T* falls in the left tail under the curve, then the P-value is the sum of the areas under the curve to the left of T* and to the right of -T*. The P-value gives the area under the curve that shows the probability of the study results under the null hypothesis.

Study Questions (Q12.3)
1. Which of the four scenarios above correspond to the P-value for our Titanic example? (Hint: T* = 12, H_A is two-sided.)
2. To obtain the P-value for a 2-sided H_A, why is it not necessary to compute 2 areas under the normal curve?

Now, let's see how rare our computed test statistic is under the null hypothesis. The computed test statistic is 12.0, so we need to find the area under the normal curve to the right of the value 12.0, and to the left of -12.0. One way to determine this area is to use a table of the percentage points of the standard normal or Z distribution. In one such table, as illustrated in the figure that follows this paragraph, the highest percentage point is 3.8, corresponding to the 99.99 percentage point. Although we can't find the area to the right of 12.0 under the normal curve exactly, we can say this area is less than .0001, clearly a very small value.

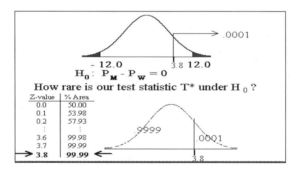

How rare is our test statistic T* under H_0?

Z-value	% Area
0.0	50.00
0.1	53.98
0.2	57.93
⋮	⋮
3.6	99.98
3.7	99.99
→ 3.8	99.99 ⟵

Study Questions (Q12.3) continued
3. If our alternative hypothesis had been one-tailed, what would be our P-value?
4. Since our alternative hypothesis was actually two-tailed, what is our P-value?
5. Based on your answer to question 2, has a rare event occurred under the null hypothesis?
6. Based on the P-value here, what should you conclude about whether or not the test of hypothesis is significant?

P-values are often used as an alternative way to draw conclusions about a test of hypothesis rather than specifying a fixed significance level in advance of computing the test statistic. If the P-value is small enough, so that a rare event has occurred, then we reject the null hypothesis. If the P-value is not small, then we would not reject the null hypothesis.

So, how small must the P-value be for our results to be considered rare? The answer here essentially depends on the alpha (α) significance level we wish to use. A conventional choice for alpha is 0.05, although a frequent alternative choice is 0.01. Thus if the P-value is <0.05 or <0.01, then the test results are typically considered rare enough to reject the null hypothesis in favor of the alternative hypothesis.

Study Questions (Q12.3) continued If your significance level was .05, what conclusions would you draw about the null hypothesis for the following P-values?
7. a) P > .01?   b) P = .023?
8. c) P < .001?   d) P = .54?   e) P = .0002?

If your significance level was .001, what conclusions would you draw about H_0 for the following P-values?
9. a) P > .01?   b) P = .023?
10. c) P < .001?   d) .01 < P = .05?   e) P = .0002?

Summary
- The P-value describes how unlikely, or how rare, are the observed results of one's study under the null hypothesis.
- For one-tailed alternative hypotheses, the P-value is determined by the area in the tail of the distribution, beyond the computed test statistics (i.e., to the right or left), under the null hypothesis.
- For two-tail alternative hypotheses, the P-value is twice the area in the tail of the distribution, beyond the computed test statistic, under the null hypothesis.
- The P-value is often used as an alternative way to draw conclusions about a null hypothesis rather than specifying a significance level prior to computing the test statistics.
- If the P-value is considered small by the investigators, say, less than .05, .01, we reject the null hypothesis in favor of the alternative hypothesis.
- If the P-value is not considered small, usually greater than .10, we do not reject the null hypothesis.

Z-scores and Relative Frequencies – The Normal Density Function

Most statistics texts include a table that lets you relate z-scores and relative frequencies in a **normal density**. The tables always give this information for the **Standard Normal Density**, so that the x-axis of the density is marked out in z-scores. The normal density tool we have been working with provides the same information more easily. For example, to find the relative frequency of values with z-scores below -1.5, just drag the left flag to the z-score value -1.5 and read the relative frequency in the lower left box, 0.067.

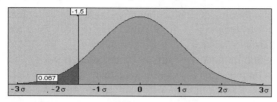

Summary

❖ The Standard Normal Density curve, for which tables are usually given in statistics textbooks, relates z-scores and relative frequencies.

❖ The Normal Density tool (lesson page 12-2 of the ActivEpi CD ROM) provides the same information and gives you some practice exercises.

Quiz (Q12.4) Fill in the Blanks.

1. We use **???** to assess whether the population parameter is different from the null value.
2. When determining the precision of a point-estimate, **???** accounts for sampling variability.
3. **???** looks for rare or unlikely results.
4. By looking at the most likely results, **???** finds those values that we are confident lie close to the population parameter.

Choices: **hypothesis testing   interval estimation**

5. The **???** gives the risk we are willing to take for rejecting the null hypothesis when the null hypothesis is false.
6. The **???** can be either upper-one-sided, lower one-sided or two-sided.
7. If the computed value of the test statistic falls into the **???**, we reject the **???** and conclude that the results are **???** significant.

Choices **acceptance region   alternative hypothesis   meaningfully
null hypothesis   rejection region   significance levels   statistically**

8. The **???** describes how rare or how unlikely are the observed results of one's study under the **???**.
9. If the P-value satisfies the inequality P>.30, we should **???** the null hypothesis.
10. If the P-value satisfies the inequality P<.005, we should reject the null hypothesis at the **???**. significance level, but not at the **???** level.

Choices **.001   .01   P-value   alternative hypothesis   not reject
null hypothesis   reject   significance level**

Confidence Intervals Review

*A **confidence interval (CI)** provides two numbers **L** and **U** between which the population parameter lies with a specified level of confidence. Here we describe how to compute a large-sample 95% CI for the difference in two proportions.*

Confidence Interval for Comparing Two Proportions

We now show how to calculate a confidence interval for the difference in two proportions using the Titanic data. Our goal is to use our sample information to compute two numbers, **L** and **U**, about which we can claim with a certain amount of confidence, say 95%, that they surround the true value of the parameter. Here is the formula for this 95 percent confidence interval:

CONFIDENCE INTERVAL for $P_M - P_W$

The data: $\hat{p}_M = .797$ $\hat{p}_W = .256$

$n_M = 1667$ $n_W = 425$

The goal: $L < P_M - P_W < U$

e.g., 95% Confidence

$$(\hat{p}_M - \hat{p}_W) \pm 1.96 \sqrt{\frac{\hat{p}_M(1 - \hat{p}_M)}{n_M} + \frac{\hat{p}_W(1 - \hat{p}_W)}{n_W}}$$

The standard error of the difference is the square root of the sum of the variances of the proportions, where each variance is of the form $(\hat{p})(1-\hat{p})$ / (sample size). The value 1.96 is the 97.5 percent point of the standard normal distribution. This percent point is chosen because the area between -1.96 and +1.96 under the normal curve is .95, corresponding to the 95% confidence level we specified. The normal distribution is used here because the difference in the two sample proportions has approximately the normal distribution if the sample sizes in both groups are reasonably large, which they are for these data. This is why the confidence interval formula described here is often referred to as a **large-sample** confidence interval.

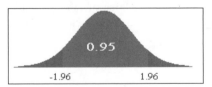

-1.96   1.96

Study Question (Q12.5)
1. Why is the standard error formula used here different from the standard error formula used when testing the null hypothesis of no difference in the two proportions?

S.E. for testing: $\sqrt{\hat{p}(1-\hat{p})(\frac{1}{n_M} + \frac{1}{n_W})}$

We can calculate the confidence interval for our data by substituting into the formula the values for $\hat{p}_M$, $\hat{p}_W$, n_M, and n_W:

$$
\begin{array}{l}
\textbf{CONFIDENCE INTERVAL for } P_M - P_W \\[4pt]
\text{The data: } \hat{p}_M = .797 \quad \hat{p}_W = .256 \\[4pt]
\qquad\qquad n_M = 1667 \quad n_W = 425
\end{array}
$$

$$
(\hat{p}_M - \hat{p}_W) \pm
$$
$$
1.96 \sqrt{\dfrac{.797(1 - .797)}{1667} + \dfrac{.256(1 - .256)}{425}}
$$

The standard error turns out to be .0234. The lower and upper limits of the 95% interval are then .495 and .587, respectively. Thus, the 95 percent confidence interval for the difference in proportions of men and women who died on the Titanic is given by the range of values between .495 and .587.

$$
(\hat{p}_M - \hat{p}_W) \pm (1.96)\ (.0234)
$$
$$
.495 < P_M - P_W < .587
$$

Summary
- ❖ A **confidence interval (CI)** provides two numbers **L** and **U** between which the population parameter lies with a specified level of confidence.
- ❖ A large-sample 95% CI for the difference in two proportions is given by the difference ± 1.96 times the estimated standard error of the estimated difference.
- ❖ The estimated standard error is given by the square root of the sum of the estimated variances of each proportion.

Interpretation of a Confidence Interval

How do we interpret this confidence interval? A proper interpretation requires that we consider what might happen if we were able to repeat the study, in this example, the sailing and sinking of the Titanic, several times. If we computed 95 percent confidence intervals for the data resulting from each repeat, then we would expect that about 95 percent of these confidence intervals would cover the true population difference in proportions.

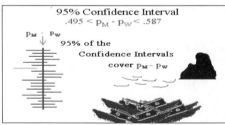

This is equivalent to saying that there is a probability of .95 that the interval between .495 and .587 includes the true population difference in proportions.

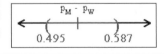

The true difference might actually lie outside this interval, but there is only a 5% chance of this happening.

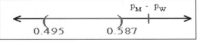

The probability statement that describes the confidence interval, which has the population parameter, $P_M - P_W$, without any hats, at its center, suggests that this parameter is a random variable. This is not so. The parameter $P_M - P_W$ does not vary at all; it has a single fixed population value. The random elements of the interval are the limits 0.495 and .587, which are computed from the sample data and will vary from sample to sample.

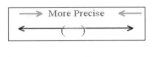

$$\text{Pr } (0.495 < P_M - P_W < 0.587) = 0.95$$

Random   Fixed   Random

In general, a confidence interval is a measure of the precision of an estimate of some parameter of interest, which for our example, is the difference between two population proportions. The narrower the width of the confidence interval, the more precise the estimate.

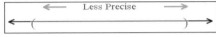

In contrast, the wider the width is, the less precise the estimate will be.

The extreme case of no precision at all would occur for difference measures (e.g., risk difference and incidence rate difference) where the confidence interval goes from minus infinity to infinity; for ratio measures (e.g., odds ratio, risk ratio, and incidence density ratio), it would be a confidence interval from zero to infinity; and for proportions, it would be a confidence interval from zero to 1.

Study Questions (Q12.6)
1. For a confidence interval that goes from minus infinity to infinity, how much confidence do we have that the true parameter is being covered by the interval?
2. If 90%, 95%, and 99% confidence intervals were obtained for the difference between two proportions based on the same data, which confidence interval would be the widest, and which would be the narrowest?
3. Suppose two different datasets yielded 95% confidence intervals for the difference between two proportions. Which dataset (A or B below) gives the more precise estimate?
   Dataset A: $.49 < p1 - p2 < .58$
   Dataset B: $.40 < p1 - p2 < .52$

Summary
* A 95% CI can be interpreted using the probability statement $P(L < $ the parameter $ < U) = .95$
* If a CI is computed for several repeats of the same study, we would expect about 95% of the CI's to cover the true population parameter.
* The random elements of a confidence interval are the limits L and U.
* It is incorrect to assume that the parameter in the middle of a confidence interval statement is a random variable.
* The larger the confidence level chosen, the wider will be the confidence interval.

A Debate: Does the Titanic data represent a population or a sample?

Our example, as previously indicated, describes the survival data for all men and women passengers on the Titanic, the "unsinkable" ocean liner that struck an iceberg and sank in 1912. Since these data consider all men and women passengers, it can be argued that the proportions being compared are actually population proportions, so that it is not appropriate to carry out either a statistical test of significance or to compute a confidence interval with these data.   Nevertheless, a counter-argument is that the 1667 men and 425 women passengers represent a sample of men and women who were eligible to be chosen for the Titanic's journey, whereas the population difference in proportions refers to the proportions of all those eligible for the trip.

These two arguments are debatable, and from our point of view, there is no clear-cut reason to conclude that either argument is correct. In fact, similar debates often occur when analyzing data from an epidemiologic outbreak investigation. For example, when seeking the source of an outbreak of diarrhea from a picnic lunch, statistical tests are often carried out on data that represent everyone who attended the picnic. Such tests are justifiable only if the data being analyzed is considered a sample rather than a population.

Quiz (Q12.7) Fill in the blanks.
1. A large-sample 95% confidence interval for the difference in two proportions adds and subtracts from the estimated difference in the two proportions 1.96 times the **???** of the estimated difference.
2. The confidence interval example shown below does not contain the null value for the **???** of the two proportions.
3. The **???** within a confidence interval has a single fixed value and does vary at all.

**Choices   confidence level difference   estimated mean
estimated standard error estimated variance   population parameter ratio**

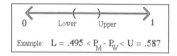

Example: $L = .495 < P_M - P_W < U = .587$

4. The **???** of a confidence interval may vary from sample to sample.
5. For a **???** confidence interval, the probability is 0.95 that the interval between the upper and lower bounds includes the true population parameter.
6. The true population parameter might actually lie outside this interval, but there is only a **???** chance of this happening.

Choices: 5% 95% 97.5% confidence level population parameter upper limit

COHORT STUDIES INVOLVING RISK RATIOS

Hypothesis Testing for Simple Analysis in Cohort Studies

We return to the data from a cohort study to assess whether quitting smoking after a heart attack will reduce one's risk for dying. The effect measure in this study was a risk ratio and its estimate was 2.1. What can we say about the population risk ratio based on the estimated risk ratio obtained from the sample?

Heart Attack Patients	Smoke	Quit	Total
Death	27	14	41
Survival	48	67	115
Total	75	81	156

COHORT

Smoking ➝ Mortality

$\hat{RR} = 2.1 \xrightarrow{?} RR$

We wish to know if we have evidence from the sample that the risk ratio is statistically different from the null value. That is, we wish to perform a **test of hypothesis** to see if the risk ratio is significantly different from 1.   The null hypothesis being tested is that the population risk ratio is 1. The logical alternative hypothesis here is that the risk ratio is >1, since prior to looking at the data the investigators were interested in whether continuing smoking was more likely than quitting smoking to affect mortality.

TEST OF HYPOTHESIS H_0 : RR = 1
$\qquad\qquad\qquad\quad H_A$: RR > 1

Because the risk ratio is the ratio of cumulative incidences for the exposed group (CI_1), divided by cumulative incidences for the unexposed group (CI_0), we can equivalently state the null hypothesis in terms of the difference in population cumulative incidences as shown here:

$$H_0: RR = \frac{CI_1}{CI_0} = 1$$
$$H_0: P_1 - P_0 = 0$$
$$H_0: ROR = 1$$

Equivalent

Because the risk ratio equals one if and only if the risk odds ratio equals one, we can also equivalently state the null hypothesis in terms of the risk odds ratio. Because cumulative incidence is a proportion, the cumulative incidence version of the null hypothesis implies that our test about the risk ratio is equivalent to testing a hypothesis about the difference between two proportions: $H_0: p_1 - p_0 = 0$.

The test statistic is the difference in the two estimated cumulative incidences divided by the estimated standard error of this difference, under the null hypothesis that the risk ratio is one. Because the sample

$$T = \frac{\hat{P}_1 - \hat{P}_0}{\sqrt{\hat{p}(1-\hat{p})\left(\frac{1}{n_1}+\frac{1}{n_0}\right)}}$$ where $P_1 = CI_1$, $P_0 = CI_0$
p = pooled CI

sizes in both groups are reasonably large, this test statistic has approximately a standard normal distribution under the null hypothesis.

The computed value of the test statistic is obtained by substituting the estimated cumulative incidences and corresponding sample sizes into the test statistic formula as shown here. The resulting value is 2.65.

$$T^* = \frac{(27/75) - (14/81)}{\sqrt{\frac{41}{156}\left(1-\frac{41}{156}\right)\left(\frac{1}{75}+\frac{1}{81}\right)}} = 2.65$$

The P-value for this test is then obtained by finding the area in the right tail of the standard normal distribution above the computed value of 2.65. The exact P-value turns out to be .0040. Because the P-value of .0040 is well below the conventional significance level of .05, we reject the null hypothesis and conclude that the risk ratio is significantly greater than the null value of one. In other words, we have found that among heart attack patients who smoke, continuing smokers have a significantly higher risk for dying than smokers who quit after their heart attack.

Summary

❖ When testing the hypothesis about a risk ratio (RR) in a cumulative-incidence cohort study, the null hypothesis can be equivalently stated as either RR = 1, $CI_1 - CI_2 = 0$, or ROR = 1, where CI_1 and CI_2 are the cumulative incidences for the exposed and unexposed groups, respectively.

❖ The alternative hypothesis can be stated in terms of the RR either as RR $\neq$ 1, RR > 1, or RR < 1 depending on whether the alternative is two-sided, upper one-sided, or lower one-sided, respectively.
❖ To test the null hypothesis that RR = 1, the test statistic is the same as that used to compare the difference between two proportions.
❖ Assuming large samples, the test statistic has approximately the N(0,1) distribution under H_0.

Chi Square Version of the Large-sample Test

The large-sample test for a risk ratio can be carried out using either the **normal distribution** or the **chi square distribution**. The reason for this equivalence is that if a standard normal variable Z is squared, then Z square has a chi square distribution on 1 degree of freedom.

More specifically, for our mortality study of heart attack patients, here is the test statistic that we previously described, it follows a standard normal distribution under the null hypothesis that the risk ratio equals 1. The square of this statistic is shown next to its corresponding chi square distribution:

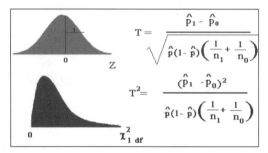

$$T = \frac{\hat{p}_1 - \hat{p}_0}{\sqrt{\hat{p}(1-\hat{p})\left(\frac{1}{n_1}+\frac{1}{n_0}\right)}}$$

$$T^2 = \frac{(\hat{p}_1 - \hat{p}_0)^2}{\hat{p}(1-\hat{p})\left(\frac{1}{n_1}+\frac{1}{n_0}\right)}$$

With a little algebra, we can rewrite the statistic in terms of the cell frequencies a, b, c and d of the general 2 by 2 table that summarizes the exposure disease information in a cohort study that estimates cumulative incidence.

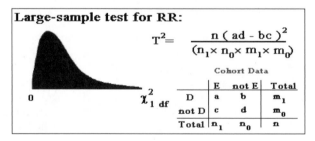

Large-sample test for RR:

$$T^2 = \frac{n\,(ad-bc)^2}{(n_1 \times n_0 \times m_1 \times m_0)}$$

Cohort Data

	E	not E	Total
D	a	b	m_1
not D	c	d	m_0
Total	n_1	n_0	n

For the mortality study of heart attack patients, the values of the cell frequencies are shown following this paragraph. Substituting these values into the chi square statistic formula, we obtain the value 7.04. This value is the square of the computed test statistic we found earlier ($2.65^2 \approx 7.04$)

$$\frac{156\ [(27)(67)-(48)(14)]^2}{(75)\ (81)\ (41)\ (115)}$$

$$= 7.04$$

Mortality Study

	E	not E	Total
D	27	14	41
not D	48	67	115
Total	75	81	156

Is the chi square version of our test significant? The normal distribution version was significant at the .01 significance level, so the chi square version had better be significant.

But in comparing these two versions of the test, we need to address a small problem. A chi-square statistic, being the square of a Z statistic, can never be negative, but a standard normal statistic can either be positive or negative. Large values of a chi square statistic that might indicate a significant result could occur from either large positive values or large negative values of the normal statistic. In other words, if we use a chi square statistic to determine significance, we are automatically performing a test of a **two-sided** alternative hypothesis even though we are only looking for large values in the right tail of the distribution.

Study Questions (Q12.8) The .99 and .995 percentage points of the chi square distribution with 1 df are given by the values 6.635 and 7.789, respectively.
1. Does the computed chi square value of 7.04 fall in the upper 1 percent of the chi square distribution?
2. Does the computed chi square value of 7.04 fall in the upper .5 percent of the chi square distribution?
3. Would a test of a two-sided alternative for RR be significant at the .01 significance level? (Note: The computed test statistic is 7.04.)
4. Would a test of a two-sided alternative for RR be significant at the .005 significance level?

So, if our chi square statistic allows us to assess a two-sided alternative hypothesis about the risk ratio, how can we assess a one-sided alternative? One way is simply to carry out the normal distribution version of the test as previously illustrated. The other way is to divide the area in the right tail of the chi square curve in half.

Study Questions (Q12.8) continued

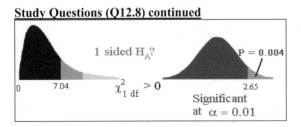

5. Using the above results, would a test of an upper one-sided alternative RR > 1 be significant at the .01 significance level?
6. Would a test of an upper one-sided alternative RR > 1 be significant at the .005 significance level?

Summary
❖ An alternative but equivalent way to test for the significance of a risk ratio is to use a chi square test.
❖ The square of a standard normal variable has the chi square distribution with one degree of freedom.
❖ We can directly compute the chi square statistic using a formula involving the cell frequencies of a 2 x 2 table for cohort data that allows for estimation of risk.
❖ When we use a chi square statistic to determine significance, we are actually performing a test of a two-sided alternative hypothesis.
❖ We can assess a one-sided alternative either using the normal distribution version of the test or by using the chi square distribution to compute a P-value.

The P-value for a One-Sided Chi Square Test

We now describe how to compute a P-value when using a chi square test involving a one-sided alternative hypothesis about a risk ratio. We will illustrate this computation once again using data from the mortality study on smoking behavior of heart attack patients. To determine the P-value, we must first compute the area shaded as pink (lighter shaded in the right tail of the distribution) under the chi-square distribution above the value of the computed chi-square statistic 7.04. This area actually gives the P-value for a 2-sided alternative hypothesis. In fact, it is equivalent to the combined area in the two tails of the corresponding normal distribution defined by the computed value of 2.65.

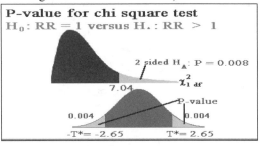

For the upper one-sided alternative that the population risk ratio is greater than 1, we previously found the P-value to be the area only in the right tail of the normal curve above 2.65. This right tail area is but one-half of the corresponding area in the right tail of the chi-square curve above 7.04. Consequently, the area in the right tail of the chi square curve gives twice the P-value for a one-tailed alternative. Therefore, this area must be divided by 2 in order to get a one-sided P-value.

$$P = \frac{.008}{2} = .004$$

Study Questions (Q12.9)
1. Suppose the alternative hypothesis in our example above was a **lower** one-sided alternative and the computed value of the chi square statistic is 7.04, corresponding to a computed Z statistic of +2.65. What is the corresponding P-value?

2. Based on your answer to the previous question, what would you conclude about the null hypothesis that the RR equals 1?
3. Suppose the alternative hypothesis was a **lower** one-sided alternative and the computed value of the chi square statistic is 7.04, but this time corresponding to a computer Z statistic of −2.65. What is the corresponding P-value?
4. Based on your answer to the previous question, what would you conclude about the null hypothesis that the RR equals 1?

Summary
❖ When using a chi square test of a two-sided alternative hypothesis about a risk ratio, the P-value is obtained as the area under the chi square curve to the right of the computed test statistic.
❖ If the alternative hypothesis is one-sided, e.g., RR > 1, then the P-value is one-half the area in the right tail of the chi square curve.

Testing When Sample Sizes Are Small

This table displays hypothetical results from a five-month randomized clinical trial comparing a new anti-viral drug for shingles with the standard anti-viral drug "Valtrex". Only 13 patients were involved in the trial, which was a pilot study for a larger clinical trial. The estimated risk ratio from these data is 3.2, which indicates that, in the sample of 13 patients, the new drug was 3.2 times more successful than the standard drug.

Pilot Clinical Trial for Shingles Patients			
	Drug		
	New	Standard	Total
Success	4	2	6
Failure	1	6	7
Total	5	8	13

new drug: $4/5 = 0.80$
standard drug: $2/8 = 0.25$ $\implies \hat{RR} = 3.2$

Is this risk ratio significantly different from the null value of one? We are considering a small sample size here, so a large-sample test of hypothesis is not appropriate. (Note: How large is large is somewhat debatable here, but it is typically required that the sample size for a proportion must be large enough (e.g., >25) for the sample to be normally distributed.) However, there is a statistical test for sparse data, called **Fisher's Exact Test**, that we can use here. Fisher's Exact Test is appropriate for a 2x2 table relating a dichotomous exposure variable and a dichotomous disease variable. To use Fisher's exact test, we must assume that the values on the margins of the tables are fixed values prior to the start of the study. If we make this 'fixed marginals assumption', we can see that once we identify the number in anyone cell in the table, say the exposed cases or **a** cell, the numbers in the other three cells can be determined by using only the frequencies on the marginals.

Study Questions (Q12.10)
1. Determine the formulas for calculating the values for **b**, **c**, and **d** in terms of **a** and the fixed marginal values.

General Layout	E	not E	Total
D	4		6
not D			7
Total	5	8	13

2. Calculate the values in the other cells of the table above knowing only the marginal values and the value in one cell.

To test our hypothesis about the risk ratio, we need only consider the outcome for one of the four cells of the table. For example, we would like to know what values we might get in the **a** cell that would be unlikely to occur under the null hypothesis that the risk ratio, or for that matter the risk odds ratio, equals 1. In particular, we would like to determine whether the value obtained in the **a** cell for our study, which turned out to be 4, is a rare enough event under the null hypothesis for us to reject the null hypothesis and conclude that the observed risk ratio is statistically significant. We can answer this question by computing the P-value for our test.

Study Questions (Q12.10) continued

General Layout	E	not E	Total
D	5		6
not D			7
Total	5	8	13

3. Suppose the **a** cell value was 5 instead of 4, assuming the marginals are fixed. What would be the corresponding revised values for **b**, **c**, and **d**?
4. What would be the risk ratio for the revised table?
5. Is the revised risk ratio further away from the null risk ratio than the risk ratio of 3.2 actually observed?
6. Are there any other possible values for the **a** cell that would also be further away from the null risk ratio than 3.2?
7. Based on the previous questions, why would we want to compute the probability of getting an **a** cell value of 4 or 5 under the null hypothesis?

To compute the P-value for Fisher's Exact test, we need to determine the probability distribution of the **a** cell frequency under the null hypothesis. Assuming fixed-marginals, this distribution is called the **hypergeometric distribution**. The formulae for the hypergeometric distribution and the corresponding P-value for Fisher's Exact Test are described in an asterisk on Lesson Page 12-4 (cohort studies) and 12-6 (case-control studies) of the **ActivEpi CD ROM**.

Study Questions (Q12.10) continued Using the hypergeometric distribution, the (Fisher's Exact Test) one-sided P-value for the study described in this section is $P(a = 4 \text{ or } 5 | Rr=1) = P(a=4|RR=1) + P(a=5|RR=1) = .0816 + .0046 = .0863$.

8. What are your conclusions about the null hypothesis that RR = 1?

Summary

❖ Fisher's Exact Test provides a test of significance for a risk ratio or an odds ratio when the data are sparse.

❖ To use Fisher's exact test, we must assume that the values on the margins of a 2x2 table are fixed values prior to the start of the study.

❖ The marginal frequencies of a 2x2 table provide no information concerning the strength of the association.

❖ To compute the P-value for Fisher's Exact test, we need to determine the probability distribution of the **a** cell frequency under the null hypothesis.

❖ Assuming fixed-marginals, the **a** cell has the **hypergeometric distribution**.

❖ Computer programs, including a DataDesk program for ActivEpi, are available to calculate the P-value for this test.

COHORT STUDIES INVOLVING RISK RATIOS
(continued)

Large-sample version of Fisher's Exact Test - The Mantel-Haenszel Test

Let's consider again the mortality study data on smoking behavior of heart attack patients. For these data, we have previously described a large-sample chi square statistic for testing the null hypothesis that the risk ratio is 1.

Heart Attack Patients	Smoke	Quit	Total
Death	27	14	41
Survival	48	67	115
Total	75	81	156

$$\chi^2 = \frac{n(ad - bc)^2}{(n_1 \times n_0 \times m_1 \times m_0)}$$

$$H_0 : RR = 1$$

Because the mortality data involves a large-sample, we do not need to use Fisher's Exact Test for these data. Nevertheless, we could still compute the Fisher's Exact test statistic. To compute Fisher's Exact test, we assume that the frequencies on the margins of

Fisher's Exact Test

compute $P(a \geq 27 | H_0)$

$P(27|RR=1) + P(28|RR=1) + P(29|RR=1) +$
$P(30|RR=1) + P(31|RR=1) + P(32|RR=1) +$
$P(33|RR=1) + P(34|RR=1) + P(35|RR=1) +$
$P(36|RR=1) + P(37|RR=1) + P(38|RR=1) +$
$P(39|RR=1) + P(40|RR=1) + P(41|RR=1)$

the table are fixed and then we compute the probability under the null hypothesis of getting an **a** cell value at least as large as the value of 27 that was actually obtained. We would therefore compute and sum 15 probability values, from a= 27 to a= 41 to obtain the P-value for Fisher's Exact Test.

Although such a calculation can be accomplished with an appropriate computer program, a more convenient large-sample approximation to Fisher's Exact Test is often used instead when the cell frequencies in the two by two table are moderately large. This large-sample approach is called the **Mantel-Haenszel** (**MH**) test for simple analysis. The Mantel-Haenszel statistic is shown below. This statistic has an approximate chi square distribution with one degree of freedom under the null hypothesis that the risk ratio is 1. Consequently, the P-value for a one-sided alternative using this

Mantel-Haenszel test (MH)

$$\chi^2(MH) = \frac{(n-1)(ad - bc)^2}{(n_1 \times n_0 \times m_1 \times m_0)}$$

approx. $\chi^2_{1\,df}$

under $H_0 : RR=1$

statistic is obtained in the usual way by finding the area under the chi-square distribution above the computed test statistic and then dividing this area by 2.

If we compare the large-sample chi square statistic for Fisher's exact test with the large-sample chi square statistic previously described for comparing two proportions, we see that these two test statistics are remarkably similar. In fact, they differ only in that the statistic for approximating Fisher Exact Test contains n-1 in the numerator but the earlier large-sample version contains n in the numerator. When n is large, using either n or n-l in the numerator will have little effect on the computed chi square statistic.

Mantel-Haenszel test (MH)
$$\chi^2(MH) = \frac{(n-1)(ad - bc)^2}{(n_1 \times n_0 \times m_1 \times m_0)}$$
$$\chi^2 = \frac{n(ad - bc)^2}{(n_1 \times n_0 \times m_1 \times m_0)}$$

In our mortality data example, for instance, the value of the chi square approximation to Fisher's exact test is equal to 6.99. The large-sample chi square statistic for comparing two proportions was previously shown to be 7.04. Clearly, the two chi square statistics are very close, although not exactly equal. The corresponding one-sided P-values are .0040 and .0041, respectively, essentially equal.

Heart Attack Patients	Smoke	Quit	Total
Death	27	14	41
Survival	48	67	115
Total	75	81	156

Mantel-Haenszel test (MH)

$$\chi^2(MH) = \frac{(n-1)(ad - bc)^2}{(n_1 \times n_0 \times m_1 \times m_0)} = \frac{(156-1)(27 \times 67 - 14 \times 48)^2}{(75 \times 81 \times 41 \times 115)}$$
$$= 6.99 \ (P = .0040)$$

$$\chi^2 = \frac{n(ad - bc)^2}{(n_1 \times n_0 \times m_1 \times m_0)} = \frac{(156)(27 \times 67 - 14 \times 48)^2}{(75 \times 81 \times 41 \times 115)}$$
$$= 7.04 \ (P = .0041)$$

*Note: in the box above one-sided p-values are provided.

This example illustrates that in large-samples, these two chi square versions are essentially equivalent and will lead to the same conclusions about significance.

Study Questions (Q12.11)

	Drug		
	New	Standard	Total
Success	4	2	6
Failure	1	6	7
Total	5	8	13

For the above data, we previously showed that the one-sided P-value for Fisher's Exact test is .0863. The MH statistic computed from these data turns out to be 3.46.

1. The P-value for a two-sided MH test is .0630. What is the P-value for a one-sided Mantel-Haenszel test?
2. Why is the P-value for the Mantel-Haenszel test different from the P-value for Fisher's Exact test?

3. The computed value for the large-sample chi square statistic for comparing two proportions is 3.75. Why is this latter value different from the computed Mantel-Haenszel test statistic of 3.46?

Summary

❖ A large-sample approximation to Fisher's Exact test is given by the Mantel-Haenszel (MH) chi-square statistic for simple analysis.

❖ The MH statistic is given by the formula:

$$\chi^2 = \frac{(n-1)(ad-bc)^2}{n_1 n_0 m_1 m_0}$$

❖ The MH chi square statistic contains n-1 in the numerator whereas the large-sample chi square version for comparing two proportions contains n in the numerator.

❖ In large-samples, either of these two chi square versions are essentially equivalent and will lead to the same conclusions about significance.

Large-Sample Confidence Interval for a Risk Ratio

We once again use the data from the mortality study on smoking behaviors of heart attack patients, this time to describe how to obtain a large-sample confidence interval for a risk ratio.

Heart Attack Patients	Smoke	Quit	Total
Death	27	14	41
Survival	48	67	115
Total	75	81	156

A risk ratio is a ratio of two proportions, each of which is a measure of cumulative incidence. If we were interested in the **difference** rather than the **ratio** between two cumulative incidences, the large sample confidence interval would be given by the commonly used confidence interval formula for two proportions shown here:

Large-sample confidence interval for $p_1 - p_2$

$$(\hat{p}_1 - \hat{p}_2) \pm 1.96 \sqrt{\frac{\hat{p}_1(1-\hat{p}_1)}{n_1} + \frac{\hat{p}_2(1-\hat{p}_2)}{n_2}}$$

This formula says that we must add and subtract from the difference in the two estimated proportions 1.96 times the estimated standard error of this difference. The corresponding 95 percent confidence interval formula for a risk ratio is slightly more complicated. In contrast to the risk difference formula, the risk ratio formula looks like as shown to the right:

Large sample confidence interval for RR $(= \frac{p_1}{p_2})$?

$$\widehat{RR} \exp\left[\pm 1.96 \sqrt{\frac{1-\hat{CI}_1}{n_1 \hat{CI}_1} + \frac{1-\hat{CI}_0}{n_0 \hat{CI}_0}}\right]$$

Note: $\exp[a] = e^a$

An equivalent version of the risk ratio formula, which helps explain where this formula comes from, is shown here:

$$e^{\ln(\hat{RR}) \pm 1.96\sqrt{\hat{Var}\{\ln(\hat{RR})\}}}$$

The confidence interval for a risk ratio is obtained by exponentiating a large sample confidence interval for the natural log of the risk ratio. The formula used for the estimated variance of the log of the risk ratio is actually an approximate, not an exact formula.

$$\frac{1-\hat{CI}_1}{n_1\hat{CI}_1} + \frac{1-\hat{CI}_0}{n_0\hat{CI}_0} \approx \hat{Var}\{\ln(\hat{RR})\}$$

There are two reasons why the formula for the risk ratio is more complicated than for the risk difference. First, the estimated difference in two proportions is approximately normally distributed, but the estimated ratio of two proportions is highly skewed. In contrast, the log of the risk ratio is more closely normally distributed.

Second, the variance of a ratio of two proportions is complicated mathematically and is not equal to the ratio of the variances of each proportion. However, since the log of a ratio is the difference in logs, approximating the variance of a difference is much easier.

We now apply the risk ratio formula to the mortality study data set. Substituting the values for the estimated risk ratio, the cumulative incidences in each group, and the sample sizes, we obtain the lower and upper confidence limits shown here:

Heart Attack Patients	Smoke	Quit	Total
Death	27	14	41
Survival	48	67	115
Total	75	81	156

$$2.08\exp\left[\pm 1.96\sqrt{\frac{1-27/75}{75*27/75} + \frac{1-14/81}{81*14/81}}\right]$$

$$1.185 < RR < 3.661$$

Study Question (Q12.12)
1. Interpret the above results.

Summary
- ❖ The confidence interval formula for a ratio of two proportions is more mathematically complicated than the formula for a difference in two proportions.
- ❖ The 95% risk ratio formula multiplies the estimated risk ratio by the exponential of plus or minus the quantity 1.96 times the square root of the variance of the log of the estimated risk ratio.
- ❖ This risk ratio formula is obtained by exponentiating a large sample confidence interval for the natural log of the risk ratio.
- ❖ The estimated ratio of two proportions is highly skewed whereas the log of the risk ratio is more closely normally distributed.
- ❖ The variance of the log of a risk ratio is mathematically easier to derive than is the variance of the risk ratio of itself, although an approximation is still required.

Quiz (12.13)

For the cohort study data shown below, the estimated probability of death among continuing smokers (CS) is 0.303, and the estimated probability of death among smokers who quit (OS) is 0.256.

Heart Attack Patients	Smoke	Quit	Total
Death	277	243	520
Survival	638	705	1343
Total	915	948	1863

$$T = \frac{\hat{P}_{CS} - \hat{P}_{OS}}{\sqrt{\hat{P}(1-\hat{P})\left(\frac{1}{n_{CS}} + \frac{1}{n_{OS}}\right)}}$$

1. What is the estimated probability of death among the entire sample: **???**.
2. Based on the computed probability values, use a calculator or computer to compute the value of the test statistic T for testing the null hypothesis that the RR equals 1. Your answer is T* = **???**.

Choices 0.279   0.475   0.491   0.533   0.721   2.20   2.23   2.27   2.31   2.36

3. Find the P-value for based on the computed T statistic (2.23) and assuming an upper-one-sided alternative hypothesis. Your answer is: P-value = **???**.
4. Based on the P-value, you should reject the null hypothesis that RR=1 at the **???** significance level but not at the **???** significance level.

Choices   0.003 0.013 0.021 0.120 1%   5%

The computed Z statistic for testing RR = 1 for these data is 2.23.

5. Using the computed Z statistic, what is the value of the Mantel-Haenszel chi-square statistic for these data? MH CHISQ = **???**.

6. What is the P-value for a two-sided test of the null hypothesis that RR=1? (You may wish to use the chi square distribution tool located on lesson page 16-2 of the ActivEpi CD-ROM.) P-value =**???**.

7. Fisher's exact test is not necessary here because the sample size for this study is **???**.

Choices: 0.006 0.013 0.026 0.120 0.240 4.970 4.973 large small

---

Calculating Sample Size for Clinical Trials and Cohort Studies

When a research proposal for testing an etiologic hypothesis is submitted for funding, it is typically required that the proposal demonstrate that the number of subjects to be studied is "large enough" to reject the null hypothesis if the null hypothesis is not true. This issue concerns the **sample size** advocated for the proposed study. The proposer typically will prepare a section of his/her proposal that describes the sample size calculations and resulting decisions about sample size requirements.

Since most epidemiologic studies, even if considering a single dichotomous exposure variable, involve accounting for several (**control**) variables in the analysis, the methodology for determining sample size can be very complicated. As a result, many software programs have been developed to incorporate such multivariate complexities, e.g., **Egret SIZ**, **PASS**, and **Power and Precision** (a web-based package). The use of such programs is likely the most mathematically rigorous and computationally accurate way to carry out the necessary sample size deliberations.

Nevertheless, there are basic principles from which all sophisticated software derive, and such principles are conveniently portrayed in the context of a 2x2 table that considers the simple (i.e., crude) analysis of the primary exposure-disease relationship under study. Moreover, the use of sample size formulae for a simple analysis is often a convenient and non-black-box approach for providing a reasonable as well as understandable argument about sample size requirements for a given study. A description of such formulae now follows.

All formulae for sample size requirements for hypothesis testing consider the two types of error that can be made from a statistical test of hypothesis. A **Type I error** occurs if the statistical test (incorrectly) rejects a true null hypothesis, and a **Type II error** occurs if the test (incorrectly) does not reject a false null hypothesis. The probability of making a Type I error is usually called α, the **significance level of the test**. The probability of making a Type II error is usually called β, and **1-β** is called the **power of the test**. All sample size formulae that concern hypothesis testing are aimed at determining that sample size for a given study that will achieve desired (small) values of α and β and that will detect a specific departure from the null hypothesis, often denoted as Δ. Consequently, the investigator needs to specify values for α, β, and Δ into an appropriate formula to determine the required sample size.

For clinical trials and cohort studies, the sample size formula for detecting a risk ratio (RR) that differs from the null value of 1 by at least Δ, i.e. ($\Delta = RR - 1$) is given by the formula:

$$n = \frac{(Z_{1-\alpha/2} + Z_{1-\beta})^2 \, \overline{p}\overline{q}(r+1)}{[p_2(RR-1)]^2 \, r}$$

where

$Z_{1-\alpha/2}$ = the $100(1 - \alpha/2)$ percent point of the N(0,1) distribution

$Z_{1-\beta}$ = the $100(1 - \beta)$ percent point of the N(0,1) distribution

p_2 = expected risk for unexposed subjects

$\overline{p}$ = $p_2(RR + 1) / 2$

$\overline{q} = 1 - \overline{p}$

r = ratio of unexposed to exposed subjects

(Note: if the sample sizes are to be equal in the exposed and unexposed groups, then r = 1. When **r** does not equal 1, the above formula provides the sample size for the exposed group; to get the sample size for the unexposed group, use **n x r**.)

To illustrate the calculation of **n**, suppose α = .05, β = .20, **RR** = 2, p_2 = .04, and r = 3. Then:

$$\overline{p} = (.04)(2 + 1) / 2 = .06$$

and substituting these values into the formula for **n** yields:

$$n = \frac{(1.96 + 0.8416)^2 (.06)(.94)(3+1)}{[(.04)(2-1)]^2 \, 3} = 368.9$$

Thus, the **sample size (n)** needed to detect a risk ratio **(RR)** of 2 at an α of .05 and a β of .20, when the expected risk for exposed (p_2) is .04 and the ratio of unexposed to exposed subjects (**r**) is 3, is 369 exposed subjects and 368.9 x 3 = 1,107 unexposed subjects. The above sample size formula can also be used to determine the sample size for estimating a prevalence ratio (i.e., **PR**) in a cross-sectional study; simply substitute **PR** for **RR** in the formula.

CASE-CONTROL STUDIES AND CROSS-SECTIONAL STUDIES

Below we provide summaries of techniques for carrying out the analysis of a 2 x 2 table in case-control and cross-sectional studies. In case-control studies, the measure of effect of interest is the exposure odds ratio (i.e., EOR), and in cross-sectional studies, the measure of effect of interest is either the prevalence odds ratio (i.e., POR) or the prevalence ratio (i.e., PR).

Large sample Z tests and Mantel-Haenszel chi square tests for the EOR, POR, and PR use identical computational formula as used for tests about risk ratios (i.e., RR). Large sample confidence intervals for these parameters require different formulae for different parameters. Formulae for such tests and confidence intervals are provided at the end of this chapter.

For more details on large sample tests for EOR, POR, and PR, as well as Fisher's Exact Test for small samples and sample size calculation, see lesson page 12-6 in the ActivEpi CD ROM.

Summary- Large Sample Tests

❖ When testing the hypothesis about an odds ratio (OR) in a case-control study, the null hypothesis can be equivalently stated as either EOR = 1 **or** $p_1 - p_2 = 0$, where p_1 and p_2 are estimated exposure probabilities for cases and non-cases.

❖ The alternative hypothesis can be stated in terms of the EOR either as EOR ≠ 1, EOR > 1, or EOR < 1, depending on whether the alternative is two-sided, upper one-sided, or lower one-sided, respectively.

❖ One version of the test statistic is a large-sample N(0,1) statistic used to compare two proportions.

❖ An alternative version is a large-sample chi square statistic, which is the square of the N(0,1) statistic.

❖ A Mantel-Haenszel large-sample chi square statistic can alternatively be used for the chi square test.

Summary- Fishers Exact Test

❖ Fisher's exact test provides a test of significance for an odds ratio as well as a risk ratio with the data are sparse.

❖ To use Fisher's exact test, we must assume that the values on the margins of a 2x2 table are fixed values prior to the start of the study.

❖ To compute the P-value for Fisher's exact test, we need to determine the probability distribution of the a cell frequency under the null hypothesis.

❖ Assuming fixed-marginals, the a cell has the hypergeometric distribution.

❖ Computer programs, including DataDesk for ActivEpi, are available to calculate the P-value for this test.

Summary- Large Sample Confidence Intervals

❖ The formula for a 95% confidence interval for an odds ratio formula multiplies the estimated odds ratio by the exponential of plus or minus the quantity 1.96 times the square root of the variance of the log of the estimated odds ratio.

❖ The odds ratio formula is obtained by exponentiating a large sample confidence interval for the natural log of the odds ratio.

❖ The variance of the log of an odds ratio is approximately equal to the sum of the inverses of the four cell frequencies in the 2x2 table layout.

COHORT STUDIES INVOLVING RATE RATIOS USING PERSON-TIME INFORMATION

In cohort studies that use person-time information, the measure of effect of interest is the rate ratio (i.e., incidence density ratio, IDR). Formulae for large sample tests and confidence intervals for the IDR are provided at the end of this chapter. **For more details, see lesson page 12-7 in the ActivEpi CD ROM.**

Summary- Large Sample Tests
❖ When testing the hypothesis about a rate ratio in a person-time cohort study, the null hypothesis can be equivalently stated as either IDR = 1 or IR1 – IR0 = 0.
❖ IDR denotes the rate ratio (i.e., incidence density ratio) and IR1 and IR0 are the incidence rates for the exposed and unexposed groups.
❖ The alternative hypothesis can be stated in terms of the IDR ≠ 1, IDR > 1, or IDR < 1 depending on whether the alternative is two-sided, upper one-sided, or lower one-sided, respectively.
❖ One version of the test statistic is a large sample $N(0,1)$ or Z statistic used to compare two incidence rates.
❖ An alternative version is a large-sample chi square statistic, which is the square of the Z statistic.

Summary- Large Sample Confidence Interval
❖ The 95% CI formula for a rate ratio multiplies the estimate rate ratio by the exponential of plus or minus the quantity 1.96 times the square root of the variance of the log of the estimated rate ratio.
❖ This rate ratio formula is obtained by exponentiating a large sample confidence interval for the natural log of the rate ratio.
❖ The variance of the log of a rate ratio is approximately equal to the sum of the inverses of the exposed and unexposed cases.

Nomenclature

Table setup for cohort, case-control, and prevalence studies:

	Exposed	Not Exposed	Total
Disease/cases	a	b	n_1
No Disease/controls	c	d	n_0
Total	m_1	m_0	n

Table setup for cohort data with person-time information:

	Exposed	Not Exposed	Total
Disease (New cases)	I_1	I_0	I
Total disease-free person-time	PT_1	PT_0	PT

χ^2_{MH}	Mantel-Haenszel chi square
CID	Cumulative incidence difference or risk difference, $CI_1 - CI_0$; same as risk difference (RD)
$\hat{ID}$	Incidence density (or "rate") in the population (I/PT)
$\hat{ID}_0$	Incidence density (or "rate") in the not exposed (I_0/PT_0)
$\hat{ID}_1$	Incidence density (or "rate") in the exposed (I_1/PT_1)
IDD	Incidence density difference or rate difference, $ID_1 - ID_0$
IDR	Incidence density ratio or rate ratio: ID_1 / ID_0; same as Incidence Rate Ratio (IRR)
MH	Mantel-Haenszel

Formulae

Statistical Tests

T statistic for the difference between two sample proportions

$$T = \frac{\hat{p}_1 - \hat{p}_0}{\sqrt{\hat{p}(1-\hat{p})\left(\frac{1}{n_1} + \frac{1}{n_0}\right)}} \qquad where \qquad \hat{p} = \frac{n_1 \hat{p}_1 + n_0 \hat{p}_0}{n_1 + n_0}$$

Chi square statistic for a 2x2 table

$$\chi^2 = \frac{n(ad - bc)^2}{n_1 n_0 m_1 m_0}$$

Mantel-Haenszel chi square statistic for a 2x2 table

$$\chi^2_{MH} = \frac{(n-1)(ad - bc)^2}{n_1 n_0 m_1 m_0}$$

T statistic for the difference between two sample rates

$$T = \frac{I_1 - Ip_0}{\sqrt{Ip_0(1 - p_0)}} \qquad where \qquad p_0 = \frac{PT_1}{PT}$$

Chi square statistic for comparing two rates

$$\chi^2 = \frac{(I_1 PT_0 - I_0 PT_1)^2}{IPT_1 PT_0}$$

Confidence intervals

Large sample 95% confidence interval for the difference between two proportions (cumulative or risk difference)

$$\hat{p}_1 - \hat{p}_0 \pm 1.96 \sqrt{\frac{\hat{p}_1(1-\hat{p}_1)}{n_1} + \frac{\hat{p}_0(1-\hat{p}_0)}{n_0}}$$

Large sample 95% confidence interval for the risk ratio (ratio of two proportions)

$$\hat{RR} \ \exp\left[\pm 1.96 \sqrt{\frac{1-\hat{CI}_1}{n_1 \hat{CI}_1} + \frac{1-\hat{CI}_0}{n_0 \hat{CI}_0}} \right]$$

Large sample 95% confidence interval for the odds ratio

$$\hat{OR} \ \exp\left[\pm 1.96 \sqrt{\frac{1}{a} + \frac{1}{b} + \frac{1}{c} + \frac{1}{d}} \right]$$

Large sample 95% confidence interval for the incidence density ratio

$$\hat{IDR} \ \exp\left[\pm 1.96 \sqrt{\frac{1}{I_1} + \frac{1}{I_0}} \right]$$

Large sample 95% confidence interval for the incidence density difference

$$\hat{IDD} \pm 1.96 \sqrt{\frac{I_1}{PT_1^2} + \frac{I_0}{PT_0^2}}$$

References

Basic Statistics References

There are a great many beginning texts that cover the fundamental concepts and methods of statistics and/or biostatistics. (Note: biostatistics concerns applications of statistics to the biological and health sciences.) Consequently, it is not our intention here to provide an exhaustive list of all such texts, but rather to suggest a few references that this author has used and/or recommends. Among these, we first suggest that you consider Velleman's ActivStats CD ROM text, which has the same format has ActivEpi. Suggested references include:

Kleinbaum DG, Kupper LL, Muller KA, Nizam A Applied Regression Analysis and Other Multivariable Methods, 3rd Edition. Duxbury Press, 1998. (Chapter 3 provides a compact review of basic statistics concepts and methods.)

Moore D. The Active Practice of Statistics. WH Freeman Publishers, 1997 (This book is designed specifically to go with ActivStats and matches it closely.)

Remington RD and Schork MA. Statistics with Applications to the Biological and Health Sciences. Prentice Hall Publishers, 1970.

Velleman P. ActivStats - A Multimedia Statistics Resource (CDROM), Addison-Wesley Publishers, 1998.

Weiss N. Introductory Statistics, 6th Edition. Addison-Wesley Publishing Company, Boston, 2002.

References on Simple Analysis

Fleiss JL. Confidence Intervals for the odds ratio in case-control studies: the state of the art. J Chronic Dis 1979;32(1-2):69-77.

Goodman SN. Toward evidence-based medical statistics. 1: The P value fallacy. Ann Intern Med 1999;130(12):995-1004.

Goodman SN. Toward evidence-based medical statistics. 2: The Bayes factor. Ann Intern Med 1999;130(2):1005-13.

Kleinbaum DG, Kupper LL, Morgenstern H. Epidemiologic Research: Principles and Quantitative Methods, Chapter 15 , John Wiley and Sons, 1982.

Miettinen O. Estimability and estimation in case-referent studies. Am J Epidemiol 1976;103(2):226-235.

Mantel N, Haenszel W. Statistical aspects of the analysis of data from retrospective studies of disease. J Natl Cancer Inst 1959;22(4):719-48.

Thomas DG. Exact confidence limits for an odds ratio in a 2x2 table. Appl Stat 1971;20:105-10.

Answers to Study Questions and Quizzes

Q12.1

1. RR, the ratio or two proportions, or OR, the ratio of two odds, each of the form $p/(1-p)$.
2. The usual null hypothesis for a risk ratio is RR $= 1$, where 1 is the null value of the risk ratio.
3. The usual null hypothesis for an odds ratio is OR $= 1$, where 1 is the null value of the odds ratio.

Q12.2

1. The pooled estimate of the common proportion is given by $\{(.7972 \times 1667) + (.2565 \times 425)\} / \{1667 + 425\} = .6874$.

Q12.3

1. The 2-sided alternative A1, in the lower right corner.
2. Because the normal curve is symmetric, the left and right tails have equal areas. Thus, compute one tail's area and then multiply by two.
3. For an upper one-sided alternative, the P-value is the area under the normal curve to the right of T*=12.0. From the table, we find P<.0001. Thus, if the null hypothesis were true and our alternative hypothesis had been one-tailed, our results had less than a .01% chance of occurring.
4. The P-value is twice the area beyond the value of 12.0 under the curve, so P < 0.0002. This is because a computed T* less than –12.0 in the left tail of the normal distribution would also

represent a worse value under the null hypothesis than the T* = 12.0 that was actually observed. Thus, if the null hypothesis were true and our alternative hypothesis had been two-tailed, our results had less than a .02% chance of occurring.

5. Yes, the P-value, which represents the chance that our results would occur if the null hypothesis were true, is extremely small.
6. Conclude that the test is significant, i.e., reject the null hypothesis and conclude that the proportions for men and women are significantly different.
7. a) P > .01: Do not reject H_0. b) P = .023: Reject H_0.
8. c) P < .001: Reject H_0. d) P = .54: Do not reject H_0. e) P = .0002: Reject H_0.
9. a) P > .01: Do not reject H_0. b) P = .023: Do no reject H_0.
10. c) P < .001: Reject H_0. d) .01 < P < .05: Do not reject H_0. e) P = .0002: Reject H_0.

Q12.4

1. hypothesis testing
2. interval estimation
3. hypothesis testing
4. interval estimation
5. significance level
6. alternative hypothesis
7. rejection region, null hypothesis, statistically
8. P-value, null hypothesis
9. not reject

10. .01, .001

Q12.5
1. The standard error used here does not assume that the null hypothesis is true. Thus, the variance for each proportion must be computed separately using its sample proportion value.

Q12.6
1. 100% confidence.
2. The 99% confidence interval would be the widest and the 90% confidence interval would be the narrowest.
3. Dataset A gives the more precise estimate because it's confidence interval is narrower than that for Dataset B.

Q12.7
1. estimated standard error
2. difference
3. population parameter
4. upper limit
5. 95%
6. 5%

Q12.8
1. Yes, because 7.04 is larger than 6.635, which is the .99 percent point of the chi square distribution with 1 df.
2. No, because 7.04 is less than 7.879, which is the .995 percent point of the chi square distribution with 1 df.
3. Yes, because the P-value for a two-sided test is the area above 7.04, which is less than the area above 6.635, which is .01.
4. No, because the P-value is the area above 7.04, which is greater than the area above 7.879, which is .005.
5. Yes, because the upper one-sided test using the normal curve was significant at the 1 percent level.
6. Yes, the one-tailed P-value using the normal distribution was .0040, which is less than .005.

Q12.9
1. The correct P-value is the area under the normal curve below +2.65, which is 1 minus the area above 2.65, which is calculated to be 1 - .004 = .996. The value of .996 can equivalently be obtained from the chi square curve by taking one half of .008 and subtracting from 1, i.e., 1 – (.008 / 2) = .996. It would be incorrect, therefore, to take

one-half of the area of .008 under the chi-square curve nor would it be correct to take one-half of 1 minus .008.
2. Do not reject the null hypothesis because the P-value is very high.
3. The correct P-value is the area under the normal curve below –2.65, which is .004. This can also be obtained by taking half of the area above the chi square value of 7.04, which is .008/2 = .004.
4. Reject the null hypothesis because the P-value is very small, and much smaller than .05 and .01.

Q12.10
1. $b = m_1 - a; c = n_1 - a; d = m_0 - n_1 + a$
2. $b = 2; c = 1; d = 6$
3. $b = 1; c = 0; d = 7$
4. $RR = (5/5) / (1/8) = 8$
5. Yes
6. No. An **a** cell value greater than 5 is not possible because the assumed fixed column marginal of 5 would then be exceeded.
7. $P(a=4 \text{ or } 5|RR=1) = P(a=4|RR=1) + P(a=5|RR=1)$. This tells us how rare our observed results are under the null hypothesis. It is the P-value for testing this hypothesis.
8. Since P is greater than .05, we fail to reject at the .05 significance level for the null hypothesis that the RR = 1.

Q12.11
1. The one-sided p-value is .0630 / 2 = .0315
2. The large-sample assumption does not hold.
3. The sample size n = 13 is not large, so that the difference between n = 13 and n – 1 = 12 has a stronger effect on the calculation of each test statistic.

Q12.12
1. This confidence interval has a 9% probability of covering the true risk ratio that compares *continuing smokers* to *smokers who quit*. Even though the confidence interval contains the null value of 1, it is wide enough to suggest that the true risk ratio might be either close to one or as large as 3.6. In other words, the point estimate of 2.1 is somewhat imprecise, and the true effect

of quitting smoking after a heart attack
may be either very weak or very strong.

Q12.13

1. $520/1863 = 0.279$
2. 2.23: $T^* = (.303 - .256) / [\text{sqrt}\{.279 * (1-.279) * [(1/915) + (1/948)]\}] = 2.23$
3. .013
4. 5%, 1%
5. 4.970: MH chi square $= (1862 * 2.23^2)/1863 = 4.970$
6. 0.026
7. large

CHAPTER 13

CONTROL- WHAT IT'S ALL ABOUT

*In previous chapters, we have discussed and illustrated several important concepts concerning the **control** of additional (**extraneous**) variables when assessing a relationship between an exposure variable and a health-outcome variable. In this chapter, we briefly review these concepts and then provide an overview of several options for the process of control that are available at both the design and analysis stages of a study.*

What do we Mean by Control?

Suppose we are studying whether there is a link between exposure to a toxic chemical and the development of lung cancer in a chemical industry. To answer this question properly, we would want to isolate the effect of the chemical from the possible influence of other variables, particularly age and smoking status, two known risk factors for lung cancer. That is, our goal is to determine whether or not exposure to the chemical contributes anything over and above the effects of age and smoking to the development of lung cancer.

Variables such as age and smoking in this example are often referred to as **control variables**. When we assess the influence of such control variables on the $E \rightarrow D$ relationship, we say we are **controlling for extraneous variables**. By extraneous, we simply mean that we are considering variables other than E and D that are not of primary interest but nevertheless could influence our conclusions about the $E \rightarrow D$ relationship.

In general, we typically carry out a simple analysis of an exposure-disease relationship as the starting point for more complicated analyses that we will likely have to undertake. A simple analysis allows us to see the **crude association** between exposure and disease and therefore allows us to make some preliminary insights about the exposure-disease relationship. Unfortunately, a simple analysis by definition ignores the influence that variables other than the exposure may have on the disease. If there are other variables already known to predict the disease, then the conclusions suggested by a simple analysis may have to be altered when such risk factors are taken into account.

Consequently, when we control for extraneous variables, we assess the effect of the exposure E on the disease D at different combinations of values of the variables we are controlling. When appropriate, we evaluate the overall $E \rightarrow D$ relationship by combining the information over the various combinations of control values.

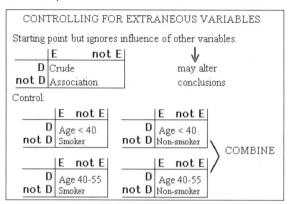

Study Questions (Q13.1) Consider a case-control study to assess whether a certain toxic chemical (**E**) is associated with the development of lung cancer (**D**) in a chemical industry. Suppose we wish to consider the control of age and smoking status. Assume that we categorize age into three groups: below 40, 40-55, and over 55. We also categorize smoking as "ever smoked" versus "never smoked".

1. How many combinations are there of the categories of age and smoking?

Two kinds of pooled analyses with these data are:
- Pool 2x2 tables of these combinations into one overall "pooled" table and compute an odds ratio for this pooled table, and
- Compute an odds ratio for each 2x2 table corresponding to each combination and then average these separate odds ratios in some way.

2. Which of these two analyses controls for age and smoking?

Several questions arise when considering the control of extraneous variables. Why do we want to control in the first place? That is, what do we accomplish by control? What are the different options that are available for carrying out control? Which option for control should we choose in our study? Which of the variables being considered should actually be controlled? What should we do if we have so many variables to control that we run out of data? These questions will be considered in the activities to follow.

Questions about Control:
Why control?
What are the options for control?
Which option should we choose?
Which variables should actually be controlled?
What if we run out of data?

Summary
- ❖ When assessing an E→D relationship, we determine whether **E** contributes anything over and above the effects of other known predictors (i.e., **control variables**) of **D**.
- ❖ When we assess the influence of control variables, we say we are **controlling for extraneous variables**.
- ❖ A simple analysis ignores the control of extraneous variables.

❖ Controlling assesses the **E→D** relationship at combinations of values of the control variables.
❖ When appropriate, controlling assesses the **overall E→D** relationship after taking into account control variables.

Reasons for Control

The typical epidemiologic research question assesses the relationship between one or more health outcome variables, **D**, and one or more exposure variables, **E**, taking into account the effects of other variables, **C**, already known to predict the outcome.

D = health outcome variables
E = exposure variables
C = control variables

When there is only one **D** and one **E**, and there are several control variables, the typical research question can be expressed as shown here, where the arrow indicates that the variable **E** and the **C** variables on the left are to be evaluated as predictors of the outcome **D**, on the right.

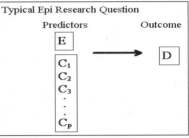

Why are the **C** variables here? That is, what are the reasons why we want to control for the **C**'s? One reason for control is to ensure that whatever effect we may find of the exposure variable cannot be explained away by variables already known to have an effect on the health outcome. In other words, we want to make sure we have accounted for the possible confounding of the **E→D** relationship due to the influence of known risk factors for the health outcome.

A second reason for control is to ensure that we remove any variability in the estimate of the E→D effect contributed by other known predictors. We might gain **precision** in our effect estimate, for example, a narrow confidence interval, as a result of controlling. In some situations there may be a loss of precision when controlling for confounders.

A third reason for control is to allow us to assess whether the effect of the exposure may vary depending on the characteristics of other predictors. For example, there may be a strong effect of exposure for smokers but no effect of exposures for non-smokers. This issue concerns **interaction**, or **effect modification**.

These are the primary three reasons for controlling: 1) to control for confounding; 2) to increase precision; and 3) to account for the possibility of **effect modification**.

1. Confounding
2. Precision
3. Effect Modification

All three reasons are important, but there is nevertheless an ordering of when they should be considered in the course of an analysis.

Ordering for Analysis ?
1. Effect Modification
2. Confounding (validity)
3. Precision (random error)

The possibility of **effect modification** should be considered first, because if there is an effect modification, then a single adjusted estimate that controls for confounding may mask the fact that the **E→D** relationship differs for different categories of a control variable.

Once effect modification is addressed or found to be absent, **confounding** should be considered, particularly in terms of those control variables **not** found to be effect modifiers. Confounding should be assessed prior to precision because confounding concerns the **validity** of an estimate. **Precision** only concerns **random error**. We would rather have a valid estimate than a narrow confidence interval around a biased estimate.

Study Questions (Q13.2) Consider again a case-control study to assess whether a certain toxic chemical (**E**) is associated with the development of lung cancer (**D**) in a chemical industry, where we wish to control for age and smoking status. Also, assume that we categorize age into three groups: below 40, 40-55, and >55 years of age; and we categorize smoking as "ever smoked" versus "never smoked."

1. True of False. We can assess confounding of either age or smoking by determining whether the **E**→**D** relationship differs within different categories of either age or smoking or both combined.
2. True or False. A more precise estimate of the odds ratio (OR) for the **E**→**D** association will be obtained if we control for both age and smoking status.

Suppose that when controlling for both age and smoking status, the OR for the **E**→**D** association is 3.5, but when ignoring both age and smoking status, the corresponding crude OR is 1.3.

3. Does this indicate confounding, precision, or interaction?

Suppose that when controlling for age and smoking status, the adjusted OR is 3.5, as above, with a 95% confidence interval ranging from 2.7 to 4.5, but that the crude OR of 1.3 has a 95% confidence interval from 1.1 to 1.5.

4. Which of these to OR's is more appropriate?

Suppose in addition to the above information, you learned that the estimated OR relating **E** to **D** is 5.7 for smokers but only 1.4 for non-smokers?

5. Would you want to control for confounding of both age and smoking?

Summary
❖ The typical epi research question assesses the relationship of one or more **E** variables to one or more **D** variables controlling for several **C** variables.
❖ The three reasons to control are confounding, precision, and effect modification.
❖ The possibility of effect modification should be considered first, followed by confounding, and then precision.

Options for Control

Design Options

Suppose you wish to assess the possible association of personality type and coronary heart disease. You decide to carry out a cohort study to compare the CHD risk for a group of subjects with Type A personality pattern with the corresponding risk for Type B subjects. You plan to follow both groups for the same duration, say 5 years.

Your exposure variable, **E**, is therefore dichotomous. You recognize that age, gender, ethnicity, blood pressure, smoking status, and cholesterol level are important CHD risk factors that you need to observe or measure for control in your study. You also recognize that there are other factors such as genetic factors, daily stress level, physical activity level, social class, religious beliefs, that you might also like to consider but you don't have the resources to measure.

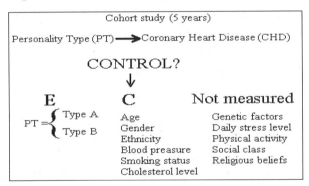

How do you carry out your study to control for any or all of the variables we have just mentioned? That is, what are your options for control? Some of your options need to be carried out at the study design stage **prior** to data collection. Other options are carried out **during the analysis stage** after the data has been obtained. It is possible to choose more than one option in the same study.

Design Options - prior to data collection
Analysis Options - after data collection

We first focus on the **design options**. One design option is **randomization**. You might wish to randomly assign an initial disease-free individual to either Type A or Type B personality type. If you could randomize, then the variables you want to control for, even those you don't actually measure, might be distributed similarly for both exposure groups. However, this option is unavailable here. You can't force people to be one personality type or another; they are what they are.

A second design option is called **restriction**. This means specifying a narrow range of values for one or more of the control variables. For example, you might decide to restrict the study to African-Americans, to women, to persons older than 50, or to all three, but not to restrict any of the other variables on your list.

Study Questions (Q13.3)
1. What is a drawback to limiting the study to women only?
2. Other than generalizing to other age groups, what is another drawback to limiting the age range to persons over 50?

A third design option is **matching**. Matching imposes a "partial restriction" on the control variable being matched. For example, if we match on smoking status using what is called **pair matching**, our cohort would consist of pairs of subjects, where each pair would have a Type A subject and Type B subject who are either both smokers or both non-smokers. Smoking status would therefore not be restricted to either all smokers or all non-smokers. What would be restricted, however, is the smoking status distribution, which would be the same for both Type A and Type B groups. Matching is often not practical in cohort studies such as the study described here, so it is rarely used in cohort studies. Rather it is most often used in case-control studies or in clinical trials.

Study Questions (Q13.3) continued Suppose you carry out a case-control study to compare CHD risks for Type A with Type B subjects. You decide to pair-match on both smoking status (ever versus never) and gender. Your cases are CHD patients identified from a cardiovascular disease registry and your controls are disease-free non-CHD subjects that are community-based.

3. What is the smoking status and gender of a control subject who is matched with a male non-smoking case?
4. If there are 110 cases in the study, what is the total number of study subjects? (Assume pair matching, as described above.)
5. Is there any restriction on the smoking status or gender of the cases?
6. Is there any restriction on the smoking status or gender of the controls?

Summary
Three design options for controlling extraneous variables are:
- ❖ **Randomization** – randomly allocating subjects to comparison groups
- ❖ **Restriction** – specifying a narrow range of possible values of a control variable.
- ❖ **Matching** – a partial restriction of the distribution of the comparison group.

Analysis Options

What control options are available at the analysis stage of a study? We'll continue the illustration of a 5-year cohort study to assess the possible association of personality type and coronary heart disease. Once the data are collected, the most direct and logical analysis option is a **stratified analysis**.

In our cohort study, if we have not used either restriction or matching at the design stage, **stratification** can be done by categorizing all control variables and forming combinations of categories called **strata**. For example, we might categorize age in three groups, say under 50, 50-60, and 60 and over; ethnicity into non-whites verses whites; diastolic blood pressure into below 95 and 95 or higher; and HDL level at or below 35 versus above 35. Because there are 6 variables being categorized into 3 categories for age and 2 categories for the other 5 variables, the total number of category combinations is 3 times 2^5, or 96 strata.

Control: AGE, GENDER, ETHNIC, DBP, SMK, HDL

Categorize all control variables   Combine categories
AGE - Under 50, 50 - 60, Over 60   **6 Variables**
ETHNIC - Non-white, White
DBP - Below 95, 95 and higher $3 \times 2^5 = 96$ **(Strata)**
HDL - At or below 35, Above 35
GENDER - Male, Female
SMK - Yes, No

An example of a stratum is subjects over 60, female, non-white, with a diastolic blood pressure greater than 95, a smoker, and with HDL level below 35. For each stratum we form the 2x2 table that relates exposure, here personality type, to the disease, here, CHD status.

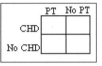

A stratified analysis is then carried out by making decisions about the **E-D** relationship for individual strata and if appropriate, combining the information over all strata to provide an overall adjusted estimate that controls for all variables together.

| | Stratum 1 | Stratum 2 | ··· | Stratum k |

Make decisions about individual strata

Obtain overall adjusted estimate (if appropriate)

<u>**Study Questions (Q13.4)**</u>
1. When would it not be appropriate to compute an overall adjusted estimate that combines the information over all strata?
2. How would you assess the E→D relationship within any given stratum?
3. For the cohort study illustrated here, what is the biggest obstacle in carrying out stratum-specific analyses?
4. How might you carry out stratified analyses that avoid dealing with a large number of strata containing zero cells?
5. What would be an advantage and a disadvantage of doing several stratified analyses one variable at a time?

A major problem with doing stratified analysis when there are many variables to control is that you quickly run out of subjects. **An alternative option that gets around this problem is to use a mathematical *model*.** A mathematical model is a mathematical expression or formula that describes how an outcome variable, like CHD status in our example, can be predicted from other variables, which in our example are the exposure variable and the control variables we have measured or observed. In other words, we have a variable to be **predicted**, often referred to as the **dependent variable** and typically denoted **Y**, and **predictors**, often called

independent variables and typically denoted with **X**'s.

Mathematical Model

Formula that describes how an outcome variable can be predicted from other variables

$$Y \;=\; f(X_1, X_2, X_3, ..., X_p)$$

(dependent variable) (independent variables)

f denotes "formula"

When modeling is used, we do not have to split up the data into strata. Instead, we obtain a formula to predict the dependent variable from the independent variables. We can also use the formula to obtain estimates of effect measures such as risk ratios or odds ratios. But modeling has difficulties of its own. These include the choice of the model form to use, the variables to be included in the initial and final model, and the assumptions required for making statistical inferences.

Difficulties:
Choice of model form to use
Variables to be included
Assumptions for inferences

For dichotomous dependent variables like CHD in our example, the most popular mathematical model is called the **logistic model**.

Study Questions (Q13.4) continued   Suppose we want to use mathematical modeling to assess the relationship between personality type (**E**) and CHD status (**D**) controlling for age, gender, ethnicity, diastolic blood pressure (DBP), smoking (SMK), and high-density lipoprotein (HDL).

6. True or False. The only possible choices for the independent variables in this model are E and the above 6 control variables.
7. True or False. In a mathematical model, continuous variables must be categorized.
8. True or False. In a case-control study, the dependent variable is exposure status.

Suppose $f(X_1, X_2, X_3, X_4, X_5, X_6, X_7)$ represents a mathematical formula that provides good prediction of CHD status, where X_1 through X_7 denote E and the 6 control variables described above.

9. True or False. If we substitute a person's specific values for X_1 through X_7 into the formula, we will determine that person's correct CHD status.

Summary
At the analysis stage, there are two options for control:
*   **Stratified analysis** - categorize the control variables and form combinations of categories or strata.
*   **Mathematical modeling** – use a mathematical expression for predicting the outcome from the exposure and the variables being controlled.
*   Stratified analysis has the drawback of running out of numbers when the number of strata is large.
*   Mathematical modeling has its drawbacks, including the choice of model and the variables to be included in the initial and final model.

Quiz (Q13.5) The three primary reasons for controlling in an epidemiological study, listed in the order that they should be assessed, are:

1. **???**
2. **???**
3. **???**

Choices: **Confounding** **Effect Modification** **Matching** **Stratification** **Mathematical Modeling**   **Precision Randomization**   **Restriction**

There are three options for control that can be implemented at the design stage.

4. **???** is a technique for balancing how unmeasured variables are distributed among exposure groups.
5. **???** limits the subjects in the study to a narrow range or values for one or more of the control variables.
6. In a case-control study, **???** ensures that the some or possibly all control variables have the same or similar distribution among case and control groups.

Choices **Matching** **Mathematical Modeling** **Optimization** **Randomization** **Restriction** **Stratification**

7. Stratification is an analysis technique that starts by dividing the subjects into different **???** based on categories of the **???** variables.
8. A major problem with stratified analyses is having too many **???** variables, which can result in **???** data in some strata.

Choices **control**   **diseaseexposure**   **large numbers**   **random samples** **sparse** **strata** **treatment**

9. In mathematical modeling we use a formula to predict a **???** variable from one or more **???** variables.
10. The problems with using a mathematical model include the choice of the **???** of the model, deciding what 111 to include in the model, and the **???** required for making statistical inferences from the model.

Choices **assumptions cases**   **complexity**   **control dependent**   **form** **independent subjects** **treatments** **variables**

Randomization

Randomization allocates subjects to exposure groups at random.   In epidemiologic research, randomization is used only in **experimental studies** such as **clinical** or **community trials**, and is never used in observational studies.

What does randomization have to do with the control of extraneous variables? The goal of randomization is **comparability**. Randomization tends to make the comparison groups similar on demographic, behavioral, genetic, and other characteristics **except** for exposure status. The investigator hopes, therefore, that if the study finds any difference in health outcome between the comparison groups, that difference can only be attributable to their difference in exposure status.

Randomization
- Allocates subjects to exposure groups at random
- Only in experimental studies
- Never in observational studies
- Comparison groups have similar characteristics except for exposure status
- Unmeasured variables are likely to be similarly distributed among exposure groups

For example, if subjects are randomly allocated to either a new drug or a standard drug for the treatment of hypertension, then it is hoped that other factors, such as age and sex, might have approximately the same distribution for subjects receiving the new drug as for subjects receiving the standard drug. Actually, there is no guarantee even with randomization that the distribution of age, for example, will be the same for the two treatment groups. The investigator can always check the data to see what has happened regarding any such characteristic, providing the characteristic is measured or observed in the study. If, for example, the age distribution is found to be different between the two treatment groups, the investigator can take this into account in the analysis by stratifying on age.

An important advantage of randomization is what it offers for those variables **not** measured in the study. Variables that are not measured obviously cannot be taken into account in the analysis. Randomization offers insurance, though no guarantee, that such unmeasured variables are similarly distributed among the different exposure groups. In observational studies, on the other hand, the investigator can account for only those variables that are measured, allowing more possibility for spurious conclusions because of unknown effects of important unmeasured variables.

Study Questions (Q13.6) Suppose you plan to do a case-control study to assess whether personality type is a risk factor for colon cancer.
1. Can you randomly assign your study subjects to different exposure groups?

Suppose you plan a clinical trial to compare two anti-hypertensive drugs. You wish to control for age, race, and gender, but you also wish to account for possible genetic factors that you cannot measure.

2. Can you control for specific genetic factors in your analysis?
3. Will the two drug groups have the same distributions of age, race, and gender?
4. What do you hope randomization will accomplish regarding the genetic factors you have not measured?

Summary
- ❖ **Experimental studies** use **randomization** whereas observational studies do **not** use randomization.
- ❖ The goal or randomization is comparability.
- ❖ Randomization tends to make comparison groups similar on other factors to be controlled.
- ❖ An important advantage of randomization is that it tends to make variable not measured similarly distributed among comparison groups.

❖ There is not guarantee that randomization will automatically make comparison groups similar on other factors.

Restriction

Restriction is another design option for control in which the eligibility of potential study subjects is narrowed by restricting the categories of one or more control variables. Restriction can be applied to both continuous and categorical variables. For a categorical variable, like gender, restriction simply means that the study is limited to one or more of the categories. For a continuous variable, restriction requires limiting the range of values, such as using a narrow age range, say from 40 to 50 years of age.

Restriction typically provides complete control of a variable. It is convenient, inexpensive, and it requires a simple analysis to achieve control. For example, if a study is restricted to females only, the analysis does not require obtaining an adjusted effect that averages over both genders. The main disadvantage of restriction is that we cannot generalize our findings beyond the restricted category. For continuous variables, another disadvantage is that the range of values being restricted may not be sufficiently narrow, so there may still be confounding to be controlled within the chosen range.

Restriction (Design Option)
  eligibility narrowed
Continuous Limiting the range of values

Categorical Limited to one or more of the categories

Advantages	**Disadvantages**
Complete control	Cannot generalize
Convenient	Not sufficiently narrow
Inexpensive	(continuous variables)
Simple analysis	

Given a list of several control variables to measure, we typically use restriction on a small number of variables. This allows hypotheses to be assessed over several categories of most control variables, thereby allowing for more generalizability of the findings.

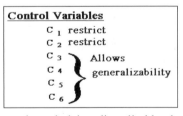

Control Variables
C_1 restrict
C_2 restrict
C_3
C_4 Allows generalizability
C_5
C_6

For example, if we want to control for age, gender, ethnicity, diastolic blood pressure, smoking, and HDL level, we would likely use restriction for no more than two or three of these variables, say age and gender.

Restriction may be used at the analysis stage even if not used at the design stage. For example, even though the study sample may include several ethnic groups, we may decide to only analyze the data for one of these groups, particularly if other ethnic groups have relatively few subjects. However, it's more advantageous to choose restriction at the design stage to gain precision in the estimated effect or to reduce study costs. For example, for a fixed study size or fixed study cost, restricting ethnicity to African-Americans at the design stage will provide more African-American subjects, and therefore more precision in effect measures for African-Americans, than would be obtained if the design allowed several ethnic groups to be eligible.

Summary
- ❖ Restriction is a design option that narrows the eligibility of potential study subjects by restricting the categories of one or more control variables.
- ❖ Restriction can be applied to both categorical and continuous variables.
- ❖ Restriction typically provides complete control, is convenient, inexpensive, and requires a simple analysis to achieve control.
- ❖ The main disadvantage of restriction is not being able to generalize findings beyond the restricted category.
- ❖ For continuous variables, another disadvantage is the possibility of residual confounding within the range of restricted values.
- ❖ Restriction may be used in the analysis stage, but if used at the design stage, precision may be gained and/or study costs may be reduced.

Quiz (Q13.7) Label each of the following statements as **True** or **False**.

1. Restriction can only be used with categorical variables.   **???**
2. An advantage of restriction is that it requires only a simple analysis to achieve control.   **???**
3. One disadvantage of restriction is that it can be expensive to administer. **???**
4. Restriction can be used at both the design and analysis stage.   **???**

Matching

Matching is a design option that can be used in **experimental studies** and in **observational cohort studies**, but is most widely used in **case-control studies**. A general definition of matching that allows other designs is given in Chaptersson 15.

There are generally two types of matching: **individual matching** and **frequency matching**. When individual matching is used in a case-control study, one or more controls are chosen for each case so that the controls have the same or similar characteristics on each of the variables involved in the matching. For example, if we match on age, race, and sex, and a given case is, say, 40 years old, black, and male, then the one or more controls matched to this case must also be close to or exactly 40 years old, black, and male. For continuous variables, like age, the categories used for matching must be specified prior to the matching process. For age, say, if the matching categories are specified as 10-year age bands that include the age range 35-45, then the control match for a 40-year-old case must come from the 35-45 year old age range.

Here, we are restricting the distribution of age, race, and gender in the control group to be the same as in the case group. But we are **not** restricting either the values or the distribution of age, race, and sex for the **cases**. That's why we say that matching imposes a **partial restriction** on the control variables being matched.

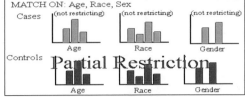

MATCH ON: Age, Race, Sex

Cases   (not restricting)   (not restricting)   (not restricting)

          Age   Race   Gender

Controls   Partial Restriction

          Age   Race   Gender

If **frequency matching** is used in a case-control study, then the matching is done on a group rather than individual basis. For example, suppose we wish to frequency match on race and gender in a case-control study, where the cases have the race-by-gender breakdown shown here:

	White Male	White Female	Black Male	Black Female
Cases	100 (33%)	100 (33%)	40 (13%)	60 (20%)

The controls then must be chosen as a group to have the same distribution as the cases over the four races by gender strata. If we want to have twice as many controls as cases, then the race by gender breakdown for controls will follow the same distribution pattern as the cases.

Several issues need to be considered when matching.

✓ First, what are the **advantages** and **disadvantages** of matching? A major reason for matching is to gain efficiency or precision in the estimate of effects, say, the odds ratio.

✓ **Should we match** at all, or should we choose the cases and controls without matching? There is no simple answer to this question, but a rough guideline is to only match on variables that you think will be strong confounders in your data.

✓ **How many controls** should we choose for each case? A rough guideline here is that usually no more than four controls per case will be necessary in order to gain precision.

✓ How do we **analyze matched data**? The answer here depends in part on whether or not there are other variables to be controlled in the analysis besides the matching variables. In particular, if the only variables being controlled are involved in the matching, than the appropriate analysis is a special kind of **stratified analysis**. But if in addition to the matching variables, there are other variables to be controlled, then the appropriate analysis involves **mathematical modeling**, usually using **logistic regression** methods.

> **Matching** - Issues
>
> **What are the Advantages/Disavantages?**
> Gain precision (efficiency)
> **Should we match at all?**
> Match on variables that are strong confounders
> **How many controls for each case?**
> 4 controls per case
> **How do we analyze matched data?**
> No other variables: Stratified analysis
> Other variables: Mathematical modeling

Summary

❖ Matching can be used in both experimental and observational studies, and is most often used in case-control studies.

❖ There are two types of matching: **individual matching** and **frequency matching**.

❖ A major reason for matching is to gain efficiency or precision in the estimate of effect.

❖ Usually no more than four controls per case will be necessary in order to gain precision.

❖ If the only variables being controlled are involved in the matching, then use stratified analysis.

❖ If there are other variables to be controlled, then use mathematical modeling.

Quiz (Q13.8) Label each of the following statements as **True** or **False**.

1. Matching is used mostly with observational cohort studies. **???**
2. For continuous variables, the ranges used for creating matching categories must be specified prior to the matching process. **???**
3. For frequency matching, there can be more controls than cases. **???**
4. Stratified Analysis is typically used for matched data to control for variables other than those involved in the matching. **???**

Stratified Analysis

Stratified analysis is an analysis option for control that involves categorizing all study variables, and forming combinations of categories called **strata**. If both the exposure and the disease variables are dichotomous, then the strata are in the form of several two by two tables. The number of strata will depend on how many variables are to be controlled and how many categories are defined for each variable.

Study Questions (Q13.9)

1. If three variables are to be controlled and each variable is dichotomized, how many strata are obtained?

2. If the control variables are age, race, and gender, give an example of one of the strata.

Once the strata are defined, a stratified analysis is carried out by making **stratum-specific** simple analyses and, if appropriate, by making an overall summary assessment of the **E→D** relationship that accounts for all control variables simultaneously. Both the stratum-specific analyses and the overall summary analyses will typically involve computing and interpreting a point estimate of the effect, say a risk ratio, a confidence interval for the point estimate, and a test of hypothesis for the significance of the point estimate.

For an overall **summary assessment**, the point estimate is an adjusted estimate that is some form of weighted average of stratum-specific estimates. The confidence interval is an interval estimate around this weighted average, and the test of hypothesis is a generalization of the Mantel-Haenszel chi-square that now considers several strata.

Summary
Stratified analysis involves the following steps:
- ❖ Categorize all variables
- ❖ Form combinations of categories (i.e., strata)
- ❖ Carry out stratum-specific analyses
- ❖ Carry out an overall E→D assessment, if appropriate
- ❖ Both stratum-specific analyses and overall assessment require point and interval estimates, and a test of hypothesis.

For overall assessment:
- ❖ The point estimate is an adjusted estimate that is a weighted average of stratum-specific estimates.
- ❖ The confidence interval is an interval estimate around the adjusted (weighted) estimate.
- ❖ The test of hypothesis is a generalization of the Mantel-Haenszel chi square test.

Quiz (Q13.10) Label each of the following statements as **True** or **False**.

1. Stratified analysis is an analysis option for control that involves categorizing all study variables, and forming combinations of categories called strata.   **???**
2. Tests of hypothesis are not appropriate for stratified analyses.   **???**
3. When carrying out stratum-specific analyses, the point estimate is typically computed as a weighted average.   **???**
4. When carrying out stratum-specific analyses, an appropriate test statistic for large samples is a Mantel-Haenszel chi square statistic.   **???**
5. If it is appropriate to carry out overall assessment over all strata, a recommended test statistic for large samples is a Mantel-Haenszel chi square statistic.   . . .   **???**
6. When carrying out overall assessment over all strata, a Mantel-Haenszel chi square statistic is always appropriate for large samples.   **???**

Mathematical Modeling

See lesson page 13-3 in the ActivEpi CD ROM for an introduction to mathematical modeling, including the terms independent and dependent variables, and expected value of a model. Also, a brief introduction to the logistic model is also provided.

References

Feinstein AR. Clinical Biostatistics. Mosby Publishers, St. Louis, 1977.

Hoes AW, Grobbee DE, Valkenburg HA, Lubsen J, Hofman A. Cardiovascular risk and all-cause mortality: a 12 year follow-up study in the Netherlands. Eur J Epidemiol 1993;9(3):285-92.

Kleinbaum DG, Kupper LL, Morgenstern H. Epidemiologic Research: Principles and Quantitative Methods. John Wiley and Sons Publishers, New York, 1982.

Kleinbaum DG, Klein M. Logistic Regression: A Self-Learning Text, 2nd Ed. Springer Verlag Publishers, 2002.

Miettinen OS. Matching and design efficiency in retrospective studies. Am J Epidemiol 1970;91(2):111-8.

Answers to Study Questions and Quizzes

Q13.1
1. 3 x 2 = 6 combinations
2. Approach 2 controls for age and smoking, since it considers what happens when variables are controlled. Approach 1 ignores control of age and smoking.

Q13.2
1. False. The statement addresses the question of interaction/ effect modification, not confounding.
2. False. The precision obtained will depend on the data; there is no guarantee that precision is always gained by controlling for extraneous variables.
3. Confounding, since the statement concerns what happens when we compare a crude estimate of effect with an adjusted estimate of effect.
4. If age and smoking are risk factors for lung cancer (they are), then the OR of 3.5 is more appropriate because it controls for confounding, even though it is less precise than the crude estimate; i.e., validity is more important than precision.
5. No, estimated OR's of 5.7 for smokers and 1.4 for non-smokers indicate strong interaction due to smoking (provided the observed interaction is statistically significant). An assessment of confounding would require comparing a crude estimate to an adjusted estimate, but use of the latter would not be appropriate because it would mask the presence of strong interaction.

Q13.3
1. You cannot generalize your results to men; that is, generalizing to men is an "external validity" problem.

2. The age group of persons over 50 is not necessarily narrow enough to completely control for age. In particular, there may still be "residual" confounding due to age within the age group over 50.
3. The control will have the same smoking status and gender as the case, i.e., the control will be a non-smoking male.
4. 220, since there will be 110 cases and 110 matched controls.
5. No, cases can be either male or female and either smokers or non-smokers, and they can have any distribution possible of each of these variables.
6. Yes, the controls are restricted to have the same distribution of both smoking status and gender as the cases.

Q13.4
1. It would not be appropriate to compute an overall adjusted estimate of there is strong evidence of interaction, e.g., if the estimated risk ratios in two or more strata are both statistically and meaningfully different.
2. Carry out a simple analysis for the given stratum by computing a point estimate of effect (e.g., a risk ratio), a confidence interval around the point estimate, and a test of hypothesis about the significance of this estimate.
3. There are 96 strata in all, so that it is highly likely that the entire dataset will be greatly thinned out upon stratification, including many strata containing one or more zero cells.
4. Do a stratified analysis one variable or two variables at a time, rather than all the variables being controlled simultaneously.

5. An advantage is that you can make some preliminary insights about confounding and interaction for every control variable. A disadvantage is that you will not be controlling for all variables simultaneously.
6. False. If age is continuous, then age^2 might also be used. Similarly for other continuous variables. Also, product terms like E x age, age x gender might be used.
7. False. Continuous variables can be treated as either continuous or categorical, depending on the investigator's judgment. However, for a stratified analysis, continuous variables must be categorical.
8. False. Even though cases and controls are selected first and previous exposure then determined, case-control status is the dependent variable in a mathematical model because it represents the health outcome variable being predicted.
9. False. Mathematical models rarely, if ever, perfectly predict the outcome variable. There is always some amount of error that represents the difference between a predicted value and the observed value.

Q13.5
1. Effect modification
2. Confounding
3. Precision
4. Randomization
5. Restriction
6. Matching
7. Strata, Control
8. Control, Sparse
9. Dependent, Independent
10. Form, Variables, Assumptions

Q13.6
1. No. In a case-control study, exposure status is determined only after cases and controls are selected. Therefore, randomization to exposure groups (i.e., personality types) is not possible in case-control studies.
2. No. You cannot control for factors in your analysis that you have not measured.
3. Not necessarily. Randomization would tend to make the distribution of age, race, and gender similar in the two drug groups, but there is no guarantee that they will be the same.
4. You hope that the distribution of genetic factors is similarly distributed within the two drug groups, even though these factors have not been measured. Moreover, you hope that, for any other unmeasured factors, randomization will distribute such factors similarly over the groups being considered.

Q13.7
1. False – Restriction can also be used to limit the range of values of a continuous variable.

2. True – An advantage of restriction is that it is inexpensive to administer.
3. False
4. True

Q13.8
1. False – Matching is used mostly with case-control studies.
2. True
3. True
4. False – If in addition to the matching variables, there are other variables to be controlled, then the appropriate analysis involves mathematical modeling using logistic regression methods.

Q13.9
1. 2 x 2 x 2 = 8 strata
2. One stratum would contain all study subjects who are in a categorized age group and have the same race and gender (e.g., white females 30-40 years old).

Q13.10
1. True
2. False – both the stratum-specific and the overall summary statistics will typically involve computing a point estimate, a confidence interval, and a test of hypothesis.
3. False – when carrying out stratum-specific analyses, the point estimate is a simple point estimate calculated for a specific stratum.
4. True
5. True
6. False – a Mantel-Haenszel test is not appropriate if there is significant and meaningful interaction over the strata.

CHAPTER 14

HOW TO DEAL WITH LOTS OF TABLES? STRATIFIED ANALYSIS

This is an analysis option for the control of extraneous variables that involves the following steps:
1. *Categorize all variables.*
2. *Form combinations of categories (i.e., strata).*
3. *Perform stratum-specific analyses.*
4. *Perform overall E-D assessment if appropriate.*

Both stratum-specific analyses and overall assessment require a **point estimate**, an **interval estimate**, and a **test of hypothesis**. In this chapter we focus on **overall assessment**, which is the most conceptually and mathematically complicated of the four steps. For overall assessment, the point estimate is an **adjusted estimate** that is typically in the form of a **weighted average** of stratum-specific estimates. The **confidence interval** is typically a large-sample interval estimate around the adjusted (weighted) estimate. The test of hypothesis is a generalization of the **Mantel-Haenszel chi square test**.

An Example – 1 Control Variable

We illustrate the four steps of a **stratified analysis** with an example:

STRATIFIED ANALYSIS
1. Categorize all variables
2. Form combinations of categories (strata)
3. Perform stratum-specific analyses
4. Perform overall E → D assessment

The tables below show data from a hypothetical retrospective cohort study to determine the effect of exposure to a suspected toxic chemical called TCX on the development of lung cancer. Suppose here that the only control variable of interest is smoking. First, we categorize this variable into two groups, smokers and non-smokers. Second, we form two-way tables for each stratum. Third, we perform **stratum specific analyses** as shown here. These data illustrate confounding. The crude data that ignores the control of smoking yields a moderately strong risk ratio estimate of 2.1. This is meaningfully different from the two estimates obtained when smoking is controlled, both of which indicate no association.

```
┌─────────────────────────────────────────────────────────────────────┐
│  Retrospective Cohort Study    TCX ──▶ Lung Cancer                    │
│                                                                        │
│      Crude Data │ TCX  no TCX │ Total     Control variable:           │
│       LC          27    14       41           Smoking                  │
│      No LC        48    67      115        ^                           │
│      Total        75    81      156      c RR = 2.1                    │
│   1. Categorize all variables                                          │
│   2. Form combinations of categories (strata)                         │
│   3. Perform stratum-specific analyses                                │
│  Non-                                                                  │
│  smokers │TCX no TCX│ Total    Smokers │TCX no TCX│ Total             │
│    LC      1    2      3         LC       26   12     38               │
│   No LC   24   48     72        No LC     24   19     43               │
│   Total   25   50     75        Total     50   31     81               │
│          ^                               ^                             │
│          RR = 1.0                        RR = 1.3                      │
└─────────────────────────────────────────────────────────────────────┘
```

Step 3 also involves computing **interval estimates** and a **P-value** for each stratum and then interpreting the results separately for each stratum as well as for the crude data. Each **stratum-specific** analysis is essentially a simple analysis for a two-way table. Here are the computed results:

```
┌─────────────────────────────────────────────────────────────┐
│            TCX ──▶ Lung Cancer                                │
│                     ^                                         │
│          Crude Data cRR = 2.1                                 │
│                                                               │
│                    95% CI: (1.2,3.7)                          │
│   Non-                  P = 0.02                              │
│                  ^                       ^                    │
│   smokers      RR = 1.0     Smokers    RR = 1.3              │
│          95% CI: (0.1, 10.6)      95% CI: (0.8, 2.3)         │
│             P = 1.00                 P = 0.25                 │
└─────────────────────────────────────────────────────────────┘
```

Study Questions (Q14.1)
1. What is your interpretation of the stratum-specific results?
2. Does there appear to be interaction due to smoking?
3. Does there appear to be an overall effect of TCX exposure after controlling for smoking status?

Step 4, the overall **E→D** assessment, should only be performed when appropriate. When evidence of **confounding** is present, this assessment should be conducted. However, when there is sufficient evidence of **interaction** or **effect modification**, this step is considered inappropriate. In our example, the risk ratio estimates for both smoking groups are essentially the same, which indicates that it is reasonable to go ahead with a summary or overall assessment.

To perform this step, we must do three things: compute an **overall adjusted estimate** of the exposure-disease effect over all the strata, carry out a **test of hypothesis** of whether or not there is an overall effect controlling for the stratification, and compute and interpret an **interval estimate** around the adjusted point estimate.

---

4. Perform overall E-D assessment

a. Adjusted estimate : weighted average

b. Test procedure : Mantel-Haenszel test for
                    stratified analysis

c. Interval estimate : large sample confidence interval

The adjusted estimate typically is some form of **weighted average** of stratum-specific estimates. The test procedure is the **Mantel-Haenszel** test for stratified analysis. The interval estimate is typically computed as a large sample confidence interval based on percentage points of the normal distribution. These three components of overall assessment will be described further in the activities to follow.

Study Questions (Q14.1) continued   A precision-based adjusted risk ratio estimate of the TCX to lung cancer relationship is computer to be 1.25. A 95% confidence interval around this estimate turns out to be (.78, 2.00). The Mantel-Haenszel test statistic has a P-value of .28.

4. What do you conclude from these results about the overall assessment of the E-D relationship in this study?

Summary
❖ The simplest form of stratification occurs when there is a single dichotomous variable to be controlled.
❖ In this case, only one variable is categorized (step 1) and two strata are obtained (step 2).
❖ Step 3 typically involves computing a point estimate, an interval estimate, and a P-value for each stratum.
❖ Overall assessment (step 4) may not be appropriate if there is interaction/effect modification.
❖ Step 4 involves computing an overall adjusted estimate of effect, a large-sample confidence interval for the adjusted effect, and a test of significance (the Mantel-Haenszel test).

Overall Assessment?

Because the risk ratio estimates for both smoking groups are essentially the same, we have concluded that it is reasonable to go ahead with an overall assessment using an **adjusted estimate**, a **confidence interval** around this adjusted estimate, and a **Mantel-Haenszel** test for the stratified data. The results are presented below. They clearly indicate that there is no meaningful or significant effect of TCX on the development of lung cancer when controlling for smoking.

TCX ✗→ Lung Cancer when controlling for smoking

Non-smokers	Smokers	Crude
☑ $\hat{RR}=1.0$	$\hat{RR}=1.3$	$c\hat{RR}=2.1$

$a\hat{RR}=1.25,$
95% CI {.78,2.00},
$\chi^2=1.18$ (P=.28)

But, what if we obtained a different set of stratum specific estimates, for example, the results shown below (examples 2 and 3)? Would we still want to compute an adjusted estimate, obtain a confidence interval around it and compute a Mantel-Haenszel test?

Non-smokers	Smokers	Crude
☑ $\hat{RR}=1.0$	$\hat{RR}=1.3$	$c\hat{RR}=2.1$
☐ $\hat{RR}=.52$	$\hat{RR}=3.5$	$c\hat{RR}=1.2$
☐ $\hat{RR}=1.1$	$\hat{RR}=4.2$	$c\hat{RR}=2.7$

Note: The rows of risk ratio results are, from top to bottom, examples 1, 2, and 3, respectively.

These two examples show a very strong interaction due to smoking. And, the type of interaction in example 2 is quite different from the interaction in example 3. The stratum-specific risk ratio estimates of 0.52 and 3.5 in example 2 are on the opposite side of the null value of 1. In contrast, the stratum-specific risk ratio estimates of 1.1 and 4.2 from example 3 are on the same side of the null value, although they are also quite different.

When stratum specific effects are on opposite sides of 1, as in example 2, it is possible that they can cancel each other in the computing of an adjusted effect. Consequently, in this situation, the use of such an adjusted estimate, corresponding confidence interval, and Mantel-Haenszel test is **not** recommended. The important results in this case are given by the contrasting stratum-specific effects, and these are likely to be masked by carrying out overall assessment.

When stratum specific effects are all in the same direction, as in example 3, a spurious appearance of no association cannot arise from cancellation of opposite effects. It may therefore be worthwhile, despite the interaction, to perform overall assessment, depending on the investigator's judgment of how large the difference between stratum-specific effects is or how stable these estimates are.

Summary

❖ Overall assessment (step 4) may not be appropriate if there is interaction/effect modification.
❖ The most compelling case for not carrying out an overall assessment is when significant stratum-specific effects are on opposite sides of the null value.
❖ When all stratum-specific effects are on the same side of the null value, overall assessment may be appropriate even if there is interaction.
❖ The most appropriate situation for performing overall assessment is when stratum-specific effects are all approximately equal, indicating no interaction over the strata.

An Example – Several Explanatory Variables

In recent years, antibiotic resistance has become a major problem in the treatment of bacterial infections. Many antibiotics that used to provide effective treatment against certain bacteria, particularly Staphylococcus aureus, or Staph, no longer work because newer strains of Staph aureus are resistant to antimicrobial drugs. When someone is diagnosed with infection due to Staph aureus, the first line of treatment typically involves methicillin-based antimicrobial drugs. However, strains of Staph aureus resistant to those drugs are now are considered a major problem for patients seen in emergency rooms. Resistant bacteria of this type are called methicillin-resistant Staph infections or MRSA.

We may wonder what are the characteristics or risk factors associated with having an MRSA infection? To study this question, a cross-sectional study was carried out at Grady Hospital in Atlanta, Georgia involving 297 adult patients seen in an emergency department whose blood cultures taken within 24 hours

Analysis on Several Variables
• MRSA status: (1=yes, 0=No)
• Previous Hospitalization: (1=yes, 0=No)
• Age: (continuous) ⟶ 1=age>55, 0=age ≤55
• Gender: (1=male, 0=female)
• Antimicrobial Drugs: (1=yes, 0=no)

of admission were found to have Staph aureus infection. Information was obtained on several variables, some of which were previously described risk factors for methicillin resistance:

We use this information to illustrate a stratified analysis to assess whether previous hospitalization is associated with methicillin resistance, controlling for age, gender, and prior use of antimicrobial drugs. Age is continuous so we will categorize age into two groups (1=age greater than 55 years; 0=age less than or equal to 55 years).

We first consider the crude data relating previous hospitalization to MRSA status:

Crude Data	Prev Hosp Yes	No	Total
MRSA Yes	103	12	115
MRSA No	75	102	177
Total	178	114	292

CRUDE DATA

Prev Hosp ⟶ MRSA Status

$cOR = 11.67\ (5.99,\ 22.77)$

$\chi^2_{MH} = 65.01\ (p < 0.001)$

Study Questions (Q14.2)

1. Looking at the crude data only, is previous hospitalization associated with methicillin resistance?
2. What reservations should you have about your answer to question 1?
3. Should you automatically stratify on age, sex, and prior antimicrobial use since they were measured in the study?
4. Since there were 297 persons in the study, why does the overall total equal 292?

Now let's see what happens when we stratify separately on age, sex, and prior antimicrobial drug use? Each stratified table is depicted separately in the following.

Relation between MRSA and Previous Hospitalization Stratified on Age

		age ≤ 55					age > 55		
	Crude Data	Prev Hosp				Crude Data	Prev Hosp		
		Yes	No	Total			Yes	No	Total
MRSA	Yes	51	6	57	MRSA	Yes	52	6	58
	No	52	72	124		No	23	30	53
	Total	103	78	181		Total	75	36	111

$\hat{OR}=11.77$ $\chi^2_{MHS}= 62.49 \ (P < .0001)$ $\hat{OR}=11.30$

$a\hat{OR}= 11.56 \ (5.87, \ 22.76)$

B-D Test for Interaction (P=.95)

5. Focusing on stratifying age only, does there appear to be interaction/effect modification due to age based on the stratum-specific results?
6. The Breslow Day (BD) Test for Interaction provides a P-value for testing the null hypothesis that there is no interaction over the strata. Based on this test with stratifying on age, is there evidence of interaction?
7. Based on your answers to the above questions, is an overall assessment of the E-D relationship appropriate when stratifying on age?
8. Is there confounding due to age? (Hint: $c\hat{OR} = 11.67$.)
9. Does there appear to be a significant effect of previous hospitalization on MRSA when controlling for age?
10. What does the confidence interval for the adjusted estimate say about this estimate?

Relation between MRSA and Previous Hospitalization Stratified on Sex

		Gender = 1 (Male)					Gender = 0 (Female)		
	Crude Data	Prev Hosp				Crude Data	Prev Hosp		
		Yes	No	Total			Yes	No	Total
MRSA	Yes	69	9	78	MRSA	Yes	34	3	37
	No	44	70	114		No	31	32	63
	Total	113	79	192		Total	65	35	100

$\hat{OR}=12.20$ $\chi^2_{MHS}= 65.66 \ (P < .0001)$ $\hat{OR}=11.70$

$a\hat{OR}= 12.06 \ (6.15, \ 23.62)$

B-D Test for Interaction (P=.96)

11. Is an overall assessment of the E-D relationship appropriate when stratifying only on gender?
12. Is there confounding due to gender? (Hint: $c\hat{OR} = 11.67$.)
13. Does there appear to be a significant effect of previous hospitalization on MRSA status when controlling for gender?

Relation between MRSA and Previous Hospitalization Stratified on Prior Antimicrobial Drug use ("PAMDU")

Crude Data	PAMDU = 1 Prev Hosp				Crude Data	PAMDU = 0 Prev Hosp		
	Yes	No	Total			Yes	No	Total
MRSA Yes	92	3	95		MRSA Yes	10	9	19
MRSA No	47	13	60		MRSA No	27	89	116
Total	139	16	155		Total	37	98	135

$$\hat{OR} = 8.48 \qquad \chi^2_{MHS} = 20.08 \ (P < .0001) \quad \hat{OR} = 3.66$$

$$a\hat{OR} = 5.00 \ (2.26, 11.04)$$

B-D Test for Interaction (P=.31)

14. Is an overall assessment of the E-D relationship appropriate when stratifying only on PAMDU?
15. Is there confounding due to PAMDU? (Hint: $c\hat{OR} = 11.67$.)
16. Does there appear to be a significant effect of previous hospitalization on MRSA status when controlling for PAMDU?

Summary
❖ When several variables are being controlled using stratified analysis, the typical first step in the analysis is to analyze and interpret the crude data.
❖ The next step typically is to stratify separately on each control variable including carrying out an overall assessment of the E-D relationship, if appropriate.
❖ One approach to determine whether overall assessment is appropriate is to assess whether stratum-specific effects are more or less the same.
❖ Another approach is to carry out a Breslow Day test of the null hypothesis that there is no interaction/effect modification due to the variable(s) being stratified.

An Example – Several Explanatory Variables (Continued)

Here is a summary table that results from stratifying on each control variable separately.

STRATIFIED ANALYSIS FOR ASSOCIATION OF PREV. HOSP. WITH MRSA STATUS

Control Variable	aOR (95% CI)	MH P-Value	B-D P-Value
None	11.67 (5.99, 22.77)	P<.0001	–
Age	11.56 (5.87, 22.76)	P<.0001	.95
Gender	12.06 (6.15, 23.62)	P<.0001	.96
PAMDU	5.00 (2.26, 11.04)	P<.0001	.31
Crude Odds Ratio = 11.67 (5.99, 22.77)			

Study Questions (Q14.3)

1. Based on the information in the above table, which, if any, of the variables age, gender, and previous antimicrobial drug use needs to be controlled?
2. Is there a gain in precision from the control of any of the variables age, gender, and previous antimicrobial drug use?

We now add to the summary table the results from controlling for two and three variables at a time.

```
STRATIFIED ANALYSIS FOR ASSOCIATION
OF PREV. HOSP. WITH MRSA STATUS

Control Variable  aOR (95% CI)          MH P-Value   B-D P-Value
       None       11.67 (5.99, 22.77)   P<.0001         -
        Age       11.56 (5.87, 22.76)   P<.0001        .95
     Gender       12.06 (6.15, 23.62)   P<.0001        .96
      PAMDU        5.00 (2.26, 11.04)   P<.0001        .31
  Age, Gender     11.59 (5.91, 22.76)*  P<.0001        .90
  Age, PAMDU       4.63 (2.08, 10.29)   P<.0001        .59
 Gender, PAMDU     5.04 (2.31, 11.03)*  P<.0001        .60
Age, Gender, PAMDU 4.66 (2.14, 10.14)*  P<.0001        .74
Crude Odds Ratio = 11.67 (5.99, 22.77)
* These estimates use a correction of .5 in every cell
of those strata that contain a zero frequency
```

3. Does controlling for age, gender, or both have an affect on the results after already controlling for previous antimicrobial drug use (PAMDU
4. Using the BD P-value, is there any evidence that there is interaction when stratifying on any or all of these three variables being controlled?
5. Why do you think it is necessary to use a correction factor such as .5 in strata that contain a zero frequency?
6. Based on all the information in the table, what is the most appropriate estimate of the odds ratio of interest? (You may choose two alternatives here.)
7. Is there evidence that previous hospitalization has an effect on whether or not a person is methicillin resistant to Staph aureus?

The stratum-specific results when simultaneously controlling for age, gender, and previous antimicrobial drug use are shown in the box at the end of this chapter. There are 8 strata, because three variables are being controlled and each variable has two categories.

Study Questions (Q14.3) continued (Note: there is no question 8)
9. What is the most obvious characteristic that describes the stratified results just shown?
10. What does your answer to the previous question indicate about stratum-specific analyses with these strata?
11. Based on comparing stratum-specific odds ratio estimates, does there appear to be interaction within the stratified data?
12. Give three reasons that justify doing an overall Mantel-Haenszel test using these data?

Summary

- ❖ When several variables are being controlled simultaneously using stratified analysis, not all of these variables may need to be controlled depending on whether a variable contributes to confounding or precision.
- ❖ The simultaneous control of several variables typically leads to strata with small numbers and often zero cell frequencies.
- ❖ When there are small numbers in some strata, stratum-specific conclusions may be unreliable.
- ❖ There are three things to consider when assessing interaction in stratified data:
  - o Are stratum-specific estimates essentially the same?
  - o Is the Breslow-Day test for interaction significant?
  - o Are stratum-specific estimates unreliable because of small numbers?

Stratum Specific Results

Here are the stratum specific results when simultaneously controlling for age, gender, and previous antimicrobial drug use.

1. Age ≤ 55, Male, PAMDU=Yes

Prev. Hosp.

		Yes	No	
MRSA	Yes	37	2	39
	No	22	7	29
		59	9	68

$\hat{OR}$ =5.89

2. Age ≤ 55, Male, PAMDU = No

Prev. Hosp.

		Yes	No	
MRSA	Yes	5	4	9
	No	13	49	62
		18	53	71

$\hat{OR}$ =4.71

3. Age ≤ 55, Female, PAMDU=Yes

Prev. Hosp.

		Yes	No	
MRSA	Yes	9	0	9
	No	14	3	17
		23	3	26

$\hat{OR}$ =4.59*

4. Age ≤ 55, Female, PAMDU = No

Prev. Hosp.

		Yes	No	
MRSA	Yes	0	0	0
	No	2	13	15
		2	13	15

$\hat{OR}$ =5.4*

5. Age > 55, Male, PAMDU=Yes

Prev. Hosp.

		Yes	No	
MRSA	Yes	24	1	25
	No	2	2	4
		26	3	29

$\hat{OR}$ =24.00

6. Age > 55, Male, PAMDU = No

Prev. Hosp.

		Yes	No	
MRSA	Yes	2	2	4
	No	7	12	19
		9	14	23

$\hat{OR}$ =1.71

7. Age > 55, Female, PAMDU=Yes

Prev. Hosp.

		Yes	No	
MRSA	Yes	22	0	22
	No	9	1	10
		31	1	68

$\hat{OR}$ =7.11*

*with .5 adjustment

8. Age > 55, Female, PAMDU = No

Prev. Hosp.

		Yes	No	
MRSA	Yes	3	3	6
	No	5	15	20
		8	18	26

$\hat{OR}$ =3.00

Quiz (Q14.4) Label each of the following statements as **True** or **False**.

1. Stratification only involves categorizing variables into two groups and conducting separate analysis for each group.   **???**
2. One of the four steps of a stratified analysis is to compute an overall summary E-D assessment when appropriate.   **???**
3. The calculation of an overall summary estimate may be considered inappropriate if there is considerable evidence of statistical interaction.   **???**
4. The calculation of an overall summary estimate may be considered inappropriate if there is considerable evidence of confounding.   **???**
5. When considering the appropriateness of computing overall summary results, the investigator must exercise some judgment regarding the clinical importance of the observed differences among stratum-specific estimates as well as to the stability of these estimates.   **???**

6. Compare the stratum specific RR estimates for each of the three situations below. Fill in the blank with **yes**, **no** or **maybe** regarding the appropriate use of a summary estimate.

Situation:	RR: Stratum 1	RR: Stratum 2	Overall Est.
Opposite direction	0.7	3.5	**???**
Same direction	1.5	4.8	**???**
Uniform effect	2.3	2.9	**???**

See Lesson pages 14-2 through 14.6 in the ActivEpi CD ROM for a detailed discussion of the following topics:
- *The Mantel-Haenszel (MH)Chi Square Test for Stratified Analysis*
- *When Not to Use the MH Test*
- *The MH Test for Person-time Cohort Studies*
- *Overall Assessment Using Adjusted Estimates*
- *Mantel-Haenszel Adjusted Estimates (e.g., mOR)*
- *Interval Estimation of Adjusted Estimates*

References

Clayton DG. Some odds ratio statistics for the analysis of ordered categorical data. Biometrika 1974;61:525-31.

Kleinbaum DG, Kupper LL, Morgenstern H. Epidemiologic Research: Principles and Quantitative Methods. John Wiley and Sons Publishers, New York, 1982.

Mantel N. Chi-square tests with one degree of freedom: Extensions of the Mantel-Haenszel procedure. J Am Stat Assoc 1963;58:690-700.

Mantel N, Haenszel W. Statistical aspects of the analysis of data from retrospective studies of disease. J Natl Cancer Inst 1959;22(4):719-48.

Rezende NA, Blumberg HM, Metzger BS, Larsen NM, Ray SM, and McGowan JE, Jr. Risk factors for methicillin-resistance among patients with Staphylococcus aureus bacteremia at the time of hospital admission. Am J Med Sci 2002; 323(3):117-23.

Answers Study Questions and Quizzes

Q14.1

1. For both smokers and non-smokers separately, there appears to be no association between exposure to TXC and the development of lung cancer. Never the less, it may be argued that the RR of 1.3 for smokers indicates a moderate association; however, this estimate is highly non-significant.

2. No, the two stratum-specific risk ratio estimates are essentially equal. Again, the RR of 1.3 for smokers indicates a small effect, but is highly non-significant.

3. No, even though the crude estimate of effects is 2.1, the correct analysis requires that smoking be controlled, from which the data show no effect of TCX exposure. An adjusted estimate over the two strata would provide an appropriate summary statistic that controls for smoking.

4. Since the adjusted point estimate is close to the null value of 1 and the Mantel-Haenszel test statistic is very non-significant, you should conclude that there is no evidence of and E-D relationship from these data

Q14.2

1. Yes, the odds ratio of 11.67 is very high and the MH test is highly significant and, even though the confidence interval is wide, the interval does not include the null value.

2. The association may change when one or more variables are controlled. If this happens and the control variables are risk factors, then an adjusted estimate or estimates would be more appropriate.

3. Not necessarily. If one or more of these variables are not previously known risk factors for MRSA status, then such variables may not be controlled.

4. Some (n=5) study subjects had to having missing information on either MSRA status or on previous hospitalization information. In fact, it was on the latter variable that 5 observations were missing.

5. No, the stratum-specific odds ratios

within different age groups are very close (around 11).

6. No, the P-value of .95 is very high, indicating no evidence of interaction due to age.

7. Yes, overall assessment is appropriate because there is no evidence of interaction due to age.

8. No, the crude and adjusted odds ratios are essentially equal.

9. Yes, the Mantel-Haenszel test for stratified data is highly significant (P<.0001).

10. The confidence interval is quite wide, indicating that even though the adjusted estimate is both statistically and meaningfully significant, there is little precision in this estimate.

11. Yes, overall assessment is appropriate because there is no evidence of interaction due to gender.

12. No confounding since the crude and adjusted odds ratios are essentially equal when controlling for gender.

13. Yes, the Mantel-Haenszel test for stratified data is highly significant (P<.0001).

14. The answer to this question is "maybe." There appears to be interaction because the odds ratio is 8.48 with previous drug use but only 3.66 with no previous drug use. However, both odds ratio estimates are on the same side of 1, so an adjusted estimate will not be the result of opposite effects canceling each other. Moreover, the BD test for interaction is non-significant, which supports doing overall assessment.

15. Yes, when controlling for previous drug use, the crude odds ratio of 11.67 is quite different than the much smaller odds ratio of 5.00.

16. Yes, the Mantel-Haenszel test for stratified data is highly significant (P<.0001), and although the confidence interval is wide, it still does not contain the null value.

Q14.3

1. Previous antimicrobial drug use needs to be controlled because it is a confounder.

2. Yes, precision is gained from controlling for previous antimicrobial drug use, since the width of the confidence interval for the adjusted estimate is much narrower than the width of the corresponding confidence for the crude data.

3. No, neither the adjusted odds ratio nor the confidence interval nor the MH P-value changes either significantly or meaningfully when comparing the results that control for PADMU alone with results that control for additional variables.

4. No, all P-values are quite large, indicating that the null hypothesis of no interaction should not be rejected. However, perhaps a comparison of stratum-specific estimates may suggest interaction when more than one variable is controlled.

5. Because the estimated odds ratio is undefined in a stratum with a zero cell frequency.

6. OR=4.66 is an appropriate choice because it controls for all three variables. being considered for control. Alternatively, OR=5.00 is also appropriate because it results from controlling only for previous antimicrobial drug use, which is the only variable that affects confounding and precision.

7. Yes, the adjusted odds ratio (close to 5.00) indicates a strong effect that is also statistically significant. The 95% confidence interval indicates a lack of precision, but the results are overall indicative of a strong effect.

8. (Note: there is no question 8)

9. There are small numbers, including a number of zeros in almost all tables.

10. Stratum-specific analyses, even when there are no zero cells, are on the whole unreliable because of small numbers.

11. Yes, the odds ratio estimate in table 5 is 24.00 whereas the odds ratio in table 6 is 1.71 and the odds ratio in table 1 is 5.89, all quite different estimates.

12. The BD test is not significant, all odds ratio estimates, though different, are all on the same side of the null value, and the strata involve very small numbers.

Q14.4

1. F – Stratification also involves performing an overall assessment when appropriate.

2. T

3. T

4. F – An overall summary estimate may be considered inappropriate if there is considerable evidence of interaction.

5. T

6. No, Maybe, Yes

CHAPTER 15

MATCHING - SEEMS EASY, BUT NOT THAT EASY

*Matching is an option for control that is available at the study design stage. We previously introduced matching in Chapter 13. We suggest that you review that chapter before proceeding further with this chapter. The primary goal of matching is to gain **precision** in estimating the measure of effect of interest. There are other advantages to matching as well, and there are disadvantages. In this chapter, we define matching in general terms, describe different types of matching, discuss the issue of whether to match or not match, and describe how to analyze matched data.*

Definition and Example of Matching

Reye's syndrome is a rare disease affecting the brain and liver that can result in delirium, coma, and death. It usually affects children and typically occurs following a viral illness.

To investigate whether aspirin is a determinant of Reye's syndrome, investigators in a 1982 study carried out a matched case-control study that used a statewide surveillance system to identify all incident cases with Reye's syndrome in Ohio. Population-based matched controls were selected as the comparison group. Potential controls were first identified by statewide sampling of children who had experienced viral illnesses but who had not developed Reye's syndrome. Study controls were then chosen by individually matching to each case one or more children of the same age and with the same viral illness as the case. Parents of both cases and controls were asked about their child's use of medication, including aspirin, during the illness.

Study Questions (Q15.1)
1. Why do you think that **type of viral illness** was considered as one of the matching variables in this study?
2. Why do you think **age** was selected as a matching variable?

This study is a classic example of the use of individual matching in a case-control study. Although the simplest form of such matching is **one-to-one** or **pair matching**, this study allowed for more than one control per case.

Matching typically involves two groups being compared, the index group and the comparison group. In a case-control study, the index group is the collection of cases, for example, children with Reye's syndrome, and the comparison group is the collection of controls.

If the study design was a cohort study or clinical trial, the index group would instead be the collection of exposed persons and the comparison group would be the collection of unexposed persons. Because matching is rarely used in either cohort or clinical trial studies, our focus here will be on case-control studies.

Matching	Case-Control	Cohort / Clin. Trial
INDEX GROUP	Cases	Exposed
versus		
COMPARISON GROUP	Controls	Unexposed

No matter what type of matched design is used, the **key feature** is that the **comparison group is restricted to be similar to the index group** on the matching factors. Thus, in the Reye's Syndrome study, the controls were restricted to have the same distribution as the cases with regard to the variables age and type of viral illness. But we are not restricting the distribution of age or viral illness for the cases. That's why we say that matching imposes a **partial** restriction on the control group in a case-control study.

Summary
- ❖ A 1982 study of the relationship of aspirin to Reye's syndrome in children is a classic example of individually matching in a case-control study.
- ❖ The simplest form of individual matching is one-to-one or pair matching, but can also involve more than one control per case.
- ❖ Typically, matching compares an *index group* with a *comparison group*.
- ❖ In a case-control study, the index group and the comparison group are the cases and controls, respectively.
- ❖ In a cohort study or clinical trial, the index group and the comparison are the exposed and unexposed, respectively.
- ❖ The key feature of matching is that the comparison group is restricted to be similar to the index group with regards to the distribution of the matching factors.

Types of Matching

There are two types of matching, **individual matching** and **frequency matching**. **Individual matching**, say in a case-control study, is carried out one case-at-a-time by sequentially selecting one or more controls for each case so that the controls have the same or similar characteristics as the case on each matching variable. For example, if we match on age, race, and sex, then the controls for a given case are chosen to have the same or similar age, race and sex as the case.

When matching on continuous variables, like age, we need to specify a rule for deciding when the value of the matching variable is "close-enough." The most popular approach for continuous variables is **category matching**. (Note: category matching is one of several ways to carry out individual matching involving a continuous variable. See the box at the end of this section for a description of other ways to match on a continuous variable.) The categories chosen for this type of matching must be specified prior to the matching process. For example, if the matching categories for age are specified as 10-year age bands then the control match for a 40-year-old case must come from the 36-45 year old age range.

The first step is to categorize each of the matching variables, whether continuous or discrete. Then for each index subject match by choosing one or more comparison subjects who are in the same category as the index subject for every one of the matching variables.

Study Questions (Q15.2) Consider a case-control study that involves individual category matching on the variables age, gender, smoking status, blood pressure, and body size.

1. What do you need to do first before you can carry out the matching?
2. How do you carry out the matching for a given case?
3. If the case is a 40-year-old male smoker who is obese and has high blood pressure, can its matched control be a 40-year-old male smoker of normal body size with low blood pressure? Explain.

In frequency matching the matching is done on a group rather than individual basis. The controls are chosen as a group to have the same distribution as the cases on the matching variables. For example, we might frequency match on blood pressure and age in a case-control study where the cases have the blood pressure-by-age category breakdown shown below, by insuring that the controls have the same breakdown:

	HiBP, Age>55	HiBP, Age<55	NormBP, Age>55	NormBP, Age<55	Total
Cases	40	60	50	50	200

Study Questions (Q15.2) continued Suppose you wish to have three times as many total controls as cases. Answer the following questions.

4. What is the BP group by age group breakdown for the number of controls?
5. What is the percentage breakdown by combined BP group and age group for the controls?

How do you decide between individual matching and frequency matching? The choice depends primarily, on which type of matching is more convenient in terms of time, cost, and the type of information available on the matching variables. The choice also depends on how many variables are involved in the matching. The more matching variables there are, the more difficult it is to form matching groups without finding matches individual by individual.

Study Questions (Q15.2) continued Suppose cases are women with ovarian cancer over 55 years of age in several different hospitals and you wanted to choose controls to be women hospitalized with accidental bone fractures matched on age and hospital.

6. Which would be more convenient, frequency matching or individual matching?

Suppose cases are women with ovarian cancer over 55 years of age in one hospital and controls were women hospitalized with accidental bone fractures and matched on age, race, number of children, age at first sexual intercourse, and age at first menstrual period.

7. Which would be more convenient, frequency matching or individual matching?

Summary
- There are two general types of matching, **individual** versus **frequency matching**.
- **Individual matching** in a case-control study is carried out one case at a time.
- With individual matching, we sequentially select one or more controls for each case so that the controls have the same or similar characteristics as the given case on each matching variable.
- For continuous variables, matching can be carried out using caliper matching, nearest neighbor matching, or category (the most popular) matching.
- **Frequency matching** involves category matching on a group basis, rather than using individual matching.

Matching Ratios

An important design issue for a matched study is the ratio of the number of comparison subjects to the number of index subjects in each matched stratum. We call this ratio the **matching ratio** for the matched study. Here is a list of different matching ratios that are possible:

Matching ratio =	# Comparison Subjects			
		# Index subjects		
Name	# Cases	# Controls	Type	Why?
1 to 1 (pair-matching)	1	1	Individual	Gain precision (vs. no matching)
R to 1	1	R	Individual	Gain precision (increase n)
R_i to 1	1	R_i	Individual	Try for R, but find < R
R_i to S_i	S_i	R_i	Frequency or Individual	Convenience or 'Pooling'

The smallest and simplest ratio is **1 to 1**, also referred to as **pair matching**. In a case-control study, pair matching matches 1 control to each case and requires individual matching. Why use pair matching? Pair matching can lead to a gain in precision in the estimated effect measure when compared to not matching at all for a study of the same total size. Also, it is easier to find one match than to find several matches per index subject.

R to 1 matching in a case-control study involves choosing **R** controls for each case using individual matching. For example, 3 to 1 matching in a case-control study would require three controls for each case. R to 1 matching is preferable to pair matching because even more precision can be gained from the larger total sample size would be increased. However, from a practical standpoint, it may be difficult to find more than several matched controls for each case.

R_i to 1 matching allows for a varying number of matched subjects for different cases using individual matching. For example, 3 controls may be found for one case, but only 2 for another and perhaps only one control for a third. R_i to

1 matching is often not initially planned but instead results from trying to carry out R to 1 matching and then finding fewer than **R** matches for some cases.

R_i by S_i matching allows for one or more controls to be matched as a group to several cases also considered as a group The letter **i** here denotes the **i-th** matched group or stratum containing R_i controls and S_i cases. This matching ratio typically results from frequency matching but can also occur from individual matching when **pooling exchangeable matched strata.**

Study Questions (Q15.3)   A detailed discussion of **pooling** is given in a later section. Consider an individually matched case-control study involving 2 to 1 matching, where the only matched variable is smoking status (i.e., SMK = 0 for non-smokers and SMK = 1 for smokers). Suppose there are 100 matched sets in which 30 sets involve all smokers and 70 sets involve all non-smokers. Suppose further that we *pool* the 30 ("exchangeable") sets involving smokers into one combined stratum and the 70 ("exchangeable") sets involving non-smokers into another combined stratum.

1. How many cases and controls are in the first matched stratum (that combine 30 matched sets)?
2. How many cases and controls are in the second matched stratum (that combines 70 matched sets)?
3. What type of matching ratio scheme is being used involving pooled data, R to 1 or R_i to S_i?

Consider the following table determined by **frequency matching** on race and gender in a case-control study.

Frequency Matching on Race and Gender
Case-Control Study

	White Male	White Female	Black Male	Black Female
Cases	100 (33%)	100 (33%)	40 (13%)	60 (20%)
Controls	200 (33%)	200 (33%)	80 (13%)	120 (20%)

4. How many matched strata are there in this frequency-matched study?
5. What type of matching ratio describes this design: R to 1 or R_i to S_i?
6. What are the numbers of controls and cases in each stratum?

Summary
❖ The **matching ratio** for a matched design is the ratio of the number of comparison subjects to the number of index subjects in each matching stratum.
❖ Matching ratios may be **1 to 1, R to 1, R_i to 1**, or **R_i to S_i**.
❖ The simplest matching ratio is 1 to 1, also called pair matching.
❖ **R to 1 matching** gives more precision than 1 to 1 matching because of increased sample size, but finding R matches per index subject may be difficult.
❖ **R_i to 1 matching** typically occurs when trying for R to 1 matching but finding less than R comparison subjects for some index subjects.

❖ R_i **to** S_i **matching** typically results from frequency matching but may also result from pooling artificially matched strata from individual matching.

How Many Matched Should You Select?

If **R to 1 matching** is used, how large should R be? The widely accepted answer to this question is that there is little to gain in terms of precision by using an R larger than four. The usual justification is based on the **Pitman Efficiency criterion**, which is approximately the ratio of the variance of an adjusted odds ratio computed from pair matching to the corresponding variance computed from R to 1 matching. Here is the Pittman efficiency formula:

Pitman Efficiency Criterion
approximately
$$\frac{\mathrm{Var}\,(\mathrm{a\hat{O}R}_{1\ to\ 1})}{\mathrm{Var}\,(\mathrm{a\hat{O}R}_{R\ to\ 1})} = \frac{2R}{(R+1)}$$

Computing this criterion for several values of **R** yields the following table:

R	1	2	3	4	5	6	...	∞
2R/(R+1)	1.000	1.333	1.500	1.600	1.667	1.714	...	2
% increase	-	33.3	12.5	6.7	4.2	2.8		-

This table shows diminishing returns once **R** exceeds 4. The Pittman efficiency increases 33.3 percent as **R** goes from 1 to 2, but only 4.2 percent as **R** goes from 4 to 5. The percent increase in efficiency clearly is quite small as **R** gets beyond 4. Moreover, the maximum possible efficiency is 2 and at R = 4 the efficiency is 1.6.

Study Questions (15.4)
1. Why does the Pittman efficiency increase as **R** increases?
2. What does the previous table say about the efficiency of 2 to 1 matching relative to pair-matching?

Summary
❖ For **R to 1 matching**, there is little to gain in precision from choosing R to be greater than 4.
❖ A criterion used to assess how large R needs to be is the **Pittman Efficiency criterion**, which compares the precision of R to 1 matching relative to pair matching.
❖ A table of **Pittman Efficiency** values computed for different values of **R** indicates a diminishing return regarding efficiency once R exceeds 4.

1. If we match in a case-control study, the index group is composed of exposed subjects.   **???**
2. If we match in a cohort study, the comparison group is composed of non-cases.
                                                                                ???
3. If we individually category match on age and gender in a case-control study, then the control for a given case must be either in the same age category or have the same gender as the case.   **???**
4. When frequency matching on age and race in a case-control study, the age distribution of the controls is restricted to be the same as the age distribution of the cases.   **???**
5. Five-to-one matching will result in a more precise estimate of effect than obtained from 4-to-one-matching for the same number of cases.   **???**
6. Ri-to-1 matching may result when trying to carry out R-to-1 matching.   **???**
7. Pair matching is a special case of R_i-to-S_i matching.   **???**
8. Not much precision can be gained from choosing more than one control per case.   **???**

Reasons for Matching

Why should we use matching to control for extraneous variables when designing an epidemiologic study? The primary advantage of matching is that it can be used to gain **precision** in estimating the effect measure of interest. Matching can allow you to get a **narrower confidence interval** around the effect measure than you could obtain without matching.

Why use matching ?
- Gain precision
- Control for variables difficult to measure
- Practical aspects - convenience, time-saving, cost-saving
- Control for confounding (?)

Another reason for matching is to control for variables that are difficult to measure. For example, matching on neighborhood of residence would provide a way to control for social class, which is difficult to measure as a control variable. Matching on persons from the same family, say brothers or sisters, might be a convenient way of controlling for genetic, social, and environmental factors that would be otherwise difficult to measure.

A third reason for matching is to take advantage of practical aspects of collecting the data, including convenience, timesaving, and cost-saving features.

For example, if cases come from different hospitals, it may be practical to choose controls matched on the case's hospital at the same time as you are identifying cases from the hospital's records. In an occupational study involving different companies in the same industry, controls can be conveniently matched to cases from the same company. Such controls will likely have social and environmental characteristics similar to the cases.

Another reason often given for matching is to control for **confounding**. We have placed a question mark after this reason because, even if matching is not

264 Chapter 15. Matching – Seems Easy, but not That Easy

used, confounding may be controlled using stratified analysis or mathematical modeling. Also, if you match in a case-control study, you must make sure to do what we later describe as a **matched analysis** in order to properly control for confounding.

Matching is usually limited to a restricted set of control variables. There are typically other variables not involved in the matching that we might want to control. Matching does not preclude controlling for confounding from those risk factors that are measured but not matched.

<u>Summary</u> The reasons for matching include:
- ❖ Gain precision
- ❖ Control for variables difficult to measure
- ❖ Practical aspects: convenience, time-saving, cost-savings
- ❖ Can control confounding for both matched and unmatched variables.

Reasons Against Matching

Why might we decide not to use matching when designing an epidemiologic study? One reason is that matching on a weak or non-risk factor is unlikely to gain precision and might even lose precision relative to not matching. If all potential control variables are at best weak risk factors, the use of matching will not achieve a gain in precision.

Study Questions (Q15.6) Suppose you match on hair color in a case-control study of occupational exposure for bladder cancer.

1. Do you think hair color is a risk factor for bladder cancer?
2. Based on your answer in the previous question, would you expect to gain precision in your estimate by matching on hair color? Explain.

Another reason not to use matching is the cost of time and labor required to find the appropriate matches, particularly when individual matching is used. To actually carry out the matching, a file that lists potential controls and their values on all matching variables must be prepared and a selection procedure for matching controls to cases must be specified and performed. This takes time and money that would not be required if controls were chosen by random sampling from a source population.

A third reason for not matching is to avoid the possibility of what is called **overmatching**. Overmatching can occur if one or more matching variables are highly correlated with the exposure variable of interest. For example, in an occupational study, if we match on job title, and job title is a surrogate for the exposure being studied, then we will 'match out' the exposure variable. That is, when we overmatch, we are effectively matching on exposure, which would result in finding no exposure-disease effect even if such an effect were present.

Study Questions (Q15.6) continued
3. If the exposure variable is cholesterol level, how might **overmatching** occur from matching on a wide variety of dietary characteristics, including average amount of fast-food products reported in one's diet?

Another drawback of matching is that your study size might be reduced if you were **not** able to find matches for some index subjects. The precision that you hoped to gain from matching could be compromised by such a reduction in the planned study size.

Study Questions (Q15.6) continued
4. What study size problem might occur if you category-match on several variables using very narrow category ranges?

Summary
Reasons for **not** matching:
❖ Matching on weak risk factors is unlikely to gain (and may lose) precision.
❖ Matching may be costly in terms of time and money required to carry out the matching process.
❖ You may inappropriately overmatch and therefore effectively match on exposure.
❖ You may have difficulty finding matches and consequently lose sample size and correspondingly the precision you were hoping to gain from matching.

To Match or Not to Match?

How do we decide whether or not we should use matching when planning an epidemiologic study? And if we decide to match, how do we decide which variables to match on? The answer to both of these questions is "**it depends**". Let's consider the list of reasons for and against matching that we described in the previous activities:

Your decision whether to match or not to match should be based on a careful review of the items in both columns of this list and on how you weigh these different reasons in the context of the study you are planning.

Reasons For Matching	Reasons Against Matching
Gain precision	Matching on weak risk factors may lose precision
Control for variables difficult to measure	Matching may be costly in terms of time and money
Practical aspects	You may have difficulty finding matches
Control for confounding of both matched and unmatched variables	You may overmatch
	Can control for confounding even without matching

Study Questions (Q15.7)   Suppose the practical aspects for matching are outweighed by the cost in time and money for carrying out the matching. Also suppose that previously identified risk factors for the health outcome are not known to be very strong predictors of this outcome.

1. Should you match?

Suppose age and smoking are considered very strong risk factors for the health outcome:

2. Should you match or not match on age and smoking?

Suppose you want to control for social and environmental factors.

3. Should you match or not match on such factors?

   Although all items listed for or against matching are important, the primary statistical reason for matching is to gain precision. The first items on both lists concern precision and they suggest that whether or not matching will result in a gain in precision depends on the investigator's prior knowledge about the important relationships among the disease, exposure, and potentially confounding variables. If such prior knowledge, is available, for example from the literature, and is used properly, a reasonable decision about matching can be made.

   It is widely recommended that, with regards to precision, the safest strategy is to match only on strong risk factors expected to show up as confounders in a study. This recommendation clearly requires subjective judgment about what is likely to happen in one's study regarding the distribution of potential confounders. In practice, a decision to use matching for precision gain applies to only those factors identified in the literature as strong predictors of the health outcome.

Summary

❖ The answer to the question "to match or not to match?" is "**it depends**".

❖ Your decision depends on a careful review of the reasons for and against matching and how you weigh these different reasons.

❖ Whether or not you will gain precision depends on the investigators' prior knowledge about the relationships of the variables being measured.

❖ Recommendation regarding precision: match only on strong risk factors expected to show up as confounders in one's study.

Quiz (15.8)   <u>**True**</u> or <u>**False**</u>:

1. One reason for deciding to match in a case-control study is to obtain a valid estimate of the odds ratio of interest.   <u>???</u>
2. An advantage of matching over non-matching is that your sample size may be smaller from not matching.   <u>???</u>
3. Matching on a weak risk factor may result in a loss of precision when compared to non-matching.   <u>???</u>
4.

Fill in the Blanks

5. Which of the following choices are reasons against using matching.   <u>???</u>
    a. You match on a non-risk factor.
    b. You want to control for a variable difficult to measure.
    c. You want to control for both matched and unmatched variables.
    d. Your matching variable is highly correlated with the exposure variable.
    e. It is costly to carry out the matching.

Choices   <u>a only</u>   <u>a, b and c</u>   <u>a, b and d</u>   <u>a, d and e</u>   <u>b only</u>   <u>b, c and d</u>   <u>c only</u>   <u>d only</u>   <u>e only</u>

6. If matching is convenient and inexpensive to carry out, it should always be preferred to non-matching. **???**

7. If your primary reason for considering matching is to gain precision in your estimated odds ratio, should you match or not match in a case-control study? **???**

Choices   **False**   **It depends**   **True**   **Don't match if costly**   **Match always**
Match if convenient **Never match**

Analysis of Matched Data – Options and General Principles

There are two options for analyzing matched data with dichotomous outcomes: **stratified analysis** using **Mantel-Haenszel** methods and **mathematical modeling** using **logistic regression**. Mantel-Haenszel methods are appropriate whenever all the variables being controlled are involved in the matching. Logistic regression methods are appropriate if some variables being controlled have not

> **Two options for analyzing matched data:**
>
> **Stratified Analysis**
> (using Mantel-Haenszel methods)
> • All variables being controlled
>   are involved in matching
>
> **Mathematical modeling**
> (using logistic regression)
> • Some variables being controlled
>   have not been matched-on

been matched-on and some variables have been matched-on.

For example, if we match in case-control study on age, race and sex and these three variables are the only ones being considered for control, then the Mantel-Haenszel methods, for stratified analysis, are appropriate. In contrast, if we match on age, race and sex and we also want to control for other non-matched variables, such as physical activity level, body size, and blood pressure, then it is necessary to use logistic regression methods.

When carrying out a matched analysis, we must consider **four** important principles. **First**, a matched analysis requires that you actually "control" for the matching variables. In particular, if you fail to control for the matching variables in a case-control study, you will not have addressed confounding due to these variables and your estimated odds ratio will be biased towards the null. And, if you don't control for the matching variables in a follow-up study, you are likely not to gain the precision in your estimated risk ratio that you had intended to achieve through matching.

Second, a **matched analysis** is a **stratified analysis**. The strata are the matched sets or pooled matched sets. For example, if you pair match in a case-control study and you have 100 cases, then there are 100 matched sets or strata to analyze. Each matched set would contain two persons, the case and the control:

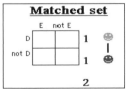

Third, when using logistic regression to do a matched analysis, the strata are defined using dummy or indicator variables. The number of dummy variables will be one less than the number of matching strata.

For example, if we pair-match in a case-control study and we have l00 cases, a logistic model for such data will require 99 dummy variables to incorporate the l00 matching strata.

Study Questions (Q15.9)
1. State the logit form of a logistic model that allows for the analysis of 100 case-control matched-pairs to describe the relationship of a dichotomous exposure variable E to a dichotomous outcome D.

Fourth, a key advantage to using logistic modeling with matched data is that you can control for variables involved in the matching as well as variables not involved in the matching. If you use a stratified analysis instead, you will typically have to drop some matching strata from the analysis, and consequently will lose precision in your estimate.

Study Questions (Q15.9) continued
Suppose you match on age, race, and sex in a case-control study involving 100 matched pairs. For your analysis, you wish to control for systolic blood pressure (SBP) and cholesterol level (CHL), neither of which is involved in the matching, as well as controlling for the matching variables.

2. State the logit form of a logistic model for carrying out the analysis described above.
3. What information will be lost if a stratified analysis is carried out to control for the matching as well as for SBP and CHL?

Summary
* Two options for analyzing matched data are stratified analysis using Mantel-Haenszel methods and mathematical modeling using logistic regression.
* A matched analysis requires that you control for the matching variables.
* A matched analysis is a stratified analysis.
* When using logistic regression to do a matched analysis, the strata are defined using dummy (i.e., indicator) variables.
* When using logistic modeling with matched data, you can control for variables involved in the matching as well as variables not involved in the matching.

Does Matching Control for Confounding?

The answer to this question is clearly **no** if we wish to control for variables not matched on in addition to the variables involved in the matching. If, however, we **assume that the only variables being controlled are involved in the matching**, then the answer requires us to consider cohort and case-control studies separately.

In a **cohort study, matching automatically controls for confounding** without the need to control for the matching variables. Nevertheless, you still need to control for the matching in order to gain the precision that you expected to gain by matching (assuming you made a good decision on which variables to match).

In a **case-control study, matching does not automatically control for confounding**, so that it is necessary to control for the matching variables in order to control for confounding.

Moreover, it can be shown (details omitted here) that the **crude odds ratio for matched case-control data is always biased towards the null value of 1**. Thus, it is necessary to control for the matching variable **F** (using stratified analysis or logistic regression) since ignoring the control of **F** (by using a crude odds ratio estimate) will give a biased answer tending towards concluding an absence of an effect.

What are the Consequences from Not Doing a Matched Analysis (Case-Control Data)?

There are two ways to not carry out a matched analysis:

1. **Ignore the matching**
2. **Break the matching**

1. If we match on one or more variables, but we analyze the resulting study data without controlling for any of the matched variables, then we are **ignoring the matching**. As an example, suppose we have dichotomous **E** and **D** variables, 100 cases, and we pair-match on age and sex. If we ignore the matching and ignore controlling for any other risk factors not matched on, then we are effectively doing a "crude analysis" of the data, i.e., our estimate is a crude odds ratio, **cOR** 'hat'. There are two fundamental criticisms of ignoring the matching:

   a. The estimated **cOR** is always biased towards the null value of 1 in matched (case-control and cohort) studies. Thus, the estimated **cOR** is expected to give a different (biased) odds ratio from the odds ratio (i.e., **mOR**) expected from a matched analysis.

   b. If the matching does its job (i.e., helps precision), the **mOR** estimate is expected to give better precision than the corresponding **cOR** estimate.

2. If we match, but control for the matched variables without doing a matched analysis, then we are **breaking the matching**. As an example, suppose, as above, we have dichotomous **E** and **D** variables, 100 cases, and we pair-match on age and sex. If we break the matching, then we control for age and sex by forming strata from combinations of these 2 variables, and then do a stratified analysis. The number of resulting strata is likely to be considerably less than 100, e.g., if age has 3 categories and sex has 2 categories, then the number of strata is six. If we do not break the matching, we control for age and sex by treating each matched set as a single stratum. Since there are 100 case-control pairs, a matched analysis would then be a stratified analysis involving 100 strata with 2 persons per strata.

   What is a good reason to break the matching? In the above example, where age has 3 categories and sex has 2 categories, breaking the matching is equivalent to pooling exchangeable matched sets, which is more appropriate than assuming that there are 100 distinct matching strata. [See the activity on "Pooling" on Lesson Page 15-4 of the ActivEpi CD]. **What are some of the problems with breaking the matching?**

   a. If you break the matching, then it is possible that the precision of the estimated odds ratio might be less than the precision obtained by doing a matched analysis (with or without pooling).

   b. The strata resulting from breaking the matching may not be equivalent to the strata that would result from pooling exchangeable matched sets (the correct analysis).

   c. As a consequence of b, the estimated odds ratio obtained from a stratified analysis resulting from breaking the matching may be meaningfully different from the estimated odds ratio obtained from a pooled analysis.

   d. If you wish to control for variables that have not been matched in addition to the matching variables, then breaking the matching will require you to break up matched sets for those pairs that are in different categories of the unmatched variable(s).

Analysis of Pair-Matched Case-Control Data

*We now illustrate a matched analysis using **pair-matched case-control** data. The data can be analyzed using a stratified analysis to obtain a **mOR**, a **MH test** of hypothesis, and a **confidence interval** around the mOR.*

In the 1970s, several studies were carried out to evaluate whether the use of estrogen as a hormone replacement for menopausal women leads to endometrial cancer. One such study used **individual matching** to carry out a **pair-matched case-control study** involving women living in a Los Angeles retirement community between 1971 and 1975. There were 63 cases. Controls were chosen by individual matching to cases on age, marital status, and date of entry into the retirement community. Each of the 63 matched-pairs represents 63 strata containing 2 persons per stratum. For each stratum, we form the 2 by 2 table that relates exposure, here estrogen use, to disease outcome, here, endometrial cancer status. Each of these strata can take on one of the four forms shown below, depending on the exposure status determined for the case and control persons in a given stratum.

Stratum Type 1 holds any matched pair where **both** the case and the controls are exposed, that is, both used estrogen. A matched pair of this type is called a **concordant** matched pair. We denote the number of concordant matched pairs of this type **W**. The study actually found 27 matched pairs of this type.

Stratum Type 4 holds those matched pairs where **neither** the case nor the control used estrogen. This type of stratum also holds concordant matched pairs since both cases and controls have the same exposure status, this time unexposed. We denote the number of **concordant** matched pairs of this type **Z**. The study actually found 4 matched pairs of this type.

The other two stratum types hold what are called **discordant pairs**. In stratum type 2, the case uses estrogen but the control does not. In stratum type 3, the case did not use estrogen, and the control did. In both these types of strata, the case has a different exposure than its matched control. The numbers of discordant pairs of each type are called **X** and **Y**, respectively. The study found **X** equal to 29 and **Y** equal to 3. Notice that the sum of **W**, **X**, **Y**, and **Z** is 63, the number of matched pairs in the study.

How do we analyze these data? A simple answer to this question is that we use a computer to carry out a stratified analyses of these 63 strata to obtain a **Mantel-Haenszel odds ratio**, a **Mantel-Haenszel test of hypothesis**, and a **95% confidence interval** around the estimated odds ratio. We will carry out this analysis in the next section.

Study Question (Q15.10)

1. Why is it necessary to compute an mOR instead of a precision-based adjusted odds ratio (i.e., aOR)?

Summary

❖ We illustrate a matched analysis using pair-matched case-control data.

❖ The study involved 63 matched-pairs or strata with 2 persons per stratum.

❖ There were 4 types of strata, 2 of which involved **concordant** matched pairs and 2 of which involved **discordant** matched pairs.

❖ **W** = the number of concordant pairs where both the case and control are exposed.

❖ **X** = the number of discordant pairs where the case is exposed and control unexposed.

❖ **Y** = the number of discordant pairs where the case is unexposed and the control exposed.

❖ **Z** = the number of concordant pairs where both the case and control are unexposed.

❖ The data can be analyzed using a stratified analysis to obtain a mOR, a MH test of hypothesis, and a confidence interval around the mOR.

Analysis of Pair-Matched Case-Control Data (continued)

A stratified analysis of the 63 strata can be carried out using a computer to obtain a **Mantel-Haenszel odds ratio**, a **Mantel-Haenszel test of hypothesis**, and a **95% confidence interval** for the mOR. Each of the 63 strata is of one of the four types shown in

McNemar's Table (pair-matched case-control)		Control	
		E	not E
Case	E	W	X
	not E	Y	Z

the table in the previous section. A convenient way to carry out this analysis without using a computer is to form the following table using the numbers of **concordant** and **discordant** pairs **W**, **X**, **Y**, and **Z**.

This table is called **McNemar's table for pair-matched case-control data**. The numbers in this table represent pairs of observations rather than individual observations. Using this table, simple formulas can be written for the mOR,

$$m\hat{OR} = \frac{X}{Y}$$

$$\chi^2_{MHS} = \frac{(X-Y)^2}{X+Y}$$

$$m\hat{OR} \exp\left[\pm 1.96\sqrt{\frac{1}{X}+\frac{1}{Y}}\right]$$

Mantel-Haenszel test statistic, and for a 95 percent confidence interval for the mOR (see table following this paragraph). Notice that all these formulas involve information only on the numbers of **discordant** pairs, **X** and **Y**; the **concordant** pair information is not used.

Substituting the values for **X** and **Y** into each of these formulas, we obtain the results shown here:

$$m\hat{OR} = \frac{29}{3} = 9.67$$

$$\chi^2_{MHS} = \frac{(29-3)^2}{29+3} = 21.13$$

$$95\% \text{ CI: } (2.94, 31.73)$$

Study Question (Q15.11)

1. How do you interpret the above results in terms of the relationship between estrogen use (E) and endometrial cancer (D) that was addressed by the pair-matched case-control study?

Summary
❖ A convenient way to carry out a matched-pairs analysis for case-control data is to use **McNemar's** table containing concordant and discordant matched pairs.
❖ Using only the discordant pairs **X** and **Y**, simple formulae can be used to compute the mOR, the MH test of hypothesis, and a 95% CI around the mOR.

The Case-Crossover Design

The **case-crossover design** is a variant of the **matched case-control study** that is intended to be less prone to bias than the standard case-control design because of the way controls are selected. The design incorporates elements of both a matched case-control study and a **nonexperimental retrospective crossover experiment**. (Note: In, a **crossover design**, each subject receives at least two different exposures/treatments at different occasions.) The fundamental aspect of the case-crossover design is that each case serves as its own control. Time-varying exposures are compared between intervals when the outcome occurred (case intervals) and intervals when the outcome did not occur within the same individual.

The case-crossover design was designed to evaluate the effect of brief exposures with transient effects on acute health outcomes when a traditional control group is not readily available. The primary advantage of the case-crossover design lies in its ability to help control confounding. Self-matching subjects against themselves automatically eliminates confounding between subjects and from both measured and unmeasured fixed covariates.

As an example of a case-cross over design, Redlemeier and Tibshirani studied whether the use of a cellular telephone while driving increases the risk of a motor vehicle collision. Their data considered 699 drivers who had cellular telephones and who were involved in motor vehicle collisions resulting in substantial property damage but no personal injury. Each person's cellular-telephone calls on the day of the collision and during the previous week were analyzed through the use of detailed billing records.

Overall, 170 of the 699 subjects had used a cellular telephone during the 10-minute period immediately before collision, 37 subjects had used the telephone during the same period on the day before the collision, and 13 subjects had used the telephone during both periods. This information provided the following McNemar table for analysis:

	Day Before		
Crash Day	**Use**	**Not Use**	
Use	13	157	170
Not Use	24	505	529
	37	662	699

The above results indicates a very strong and significant effect that indicates that cell phone use while driving increases the risk for motor vehicle collision. Furthermore, the primary analysis, which adjusted for intermittent driving, yielded an estimated **mOR** of 6.5 with a 95% confidence interval of 4.5 to 9.9.

See Lesson pages 15-3 through 15.5 in the ActivEpi CD ROM for a detailed discussion of the following topics:

- *Analysis of R-to-1 Matched Case-Control Data*
- *Pooling Matched Data*
- *Analysis of Frequency Matched Data*
- *Analysis of Matched Cohort Data*
- *Logistic Regression – Matched and Unmatched Covariates for Matched Case-Control Studies*

アA Pocket Guide to Epidemiology **273**

References

References on Matching
Breslow NE, Day NE. Statistical Methods in Cancer Research. Volume 1. The Analysis of Case-Control Studies. International Agency for Research in Cancer, Lyon, 1980.

Brock KE, Berry G, Mock PA, MacLennan R, Truswell AS, Brinton LA. Nutrients in diet and plasma and risk of in situ cervical cancer. J Natl Cancer Inst 1988 Jun 15;80(8):580-5.

Diaz T, Nunez JC, Rullan JW, Markowitz LE, Barker ND, Horan J. Risk factors associated with severe measles in Puerto Rico. Pediatr Infect Dis J 1992;11(10):836-40. (Example of frequency matching)

Donovan JW, MacLennan R, Adena M. Vietnam service and the risk of congenital anomalies. A case-control study. Med J Aust 1984;140(7):394-7.

Halpin TJ, Holtzhauer FJ, Campbell RJ, Hall LJ, Correa-Villasenor A, Lanese R, Rice J, Hurwitz ES. Reye's syndrome and medication use. JAMA 1982;248(6):687-91.

Kleinbaum DG, Klein M. Logistic Regression: A Self-Learning Text, 2nd Ed. Springer Verlag Publishers, 2002.

Kleinbaum DG, Kupper LL, Morgenstern H. Epidemiologic Research: Principles and Quantitative Methods. John Wiley and Sons Publishers, New York, 1982.

Kupper LL, Karon JM, Kleinbaum DG, Morgenstern H, Lewis DK, Matching in epidemiologic studies: validity and efficiency considerations. Biometrics 1981;37(2):271-291.

McNeil D. Epidemiologic Research Methods. John Wiley and Sons Publishers, 1996. (Example of pair matching in a cohort study)

Miettinen OS. Individual matching with multiple controls in the case of all-or-none responses. Biometrics 1969;25(2):339-55.

Miettinen OS. Estimation of relative risk from individually matched series. Biometrics 1970;26(1):75-86.

Ury HK. Efficiency of case-control studies with multiple controls per case: continuous or dichotomous data. Biometrics 1975;31(3):643-9.

Case-Crossover Design
Maclure M, Mittleman MA. Should we use a case-crossover design? Annu Rev Public Health 2000;21:193-221.

Maclure M. The case-crossover design: a method for studying transient effects on the risk of acute events. Am J Epidemiol 1991;133(2):144-53.

Redelmeier DA, Tibshirani RJ. Association between cellular-telephone calls and motor vehicle collisions. N Engl J Med 1997;336(7):453-8.

Answers to Study Questions and Quizzes

Q15.1
1. Reye's syndrome was associated with only certain types of viruses, so "virus type" was an important risk factor for the outcome.
2. Older children were less likely to develop Reye's syndrome, i.e., age was an important risk factor.

Q15.2
1. You need to categorize the continuous variables age, blood pressure, and body size.
2. Choose one or more controls to be in the same category of age, gender, smoking status, blood pressure, and body size as the case.
3. No. The case and controls have to be in the same category for each of the matching variable. The control choice in the question is not appropriate because both body size and blood pressure categories of the control are different categories than observed on the case.
4. {High BP, age ≥ 55} = 120; {High BP, age < 55} = 180; {Normal BP, age ≥

55} = 150; {Normal BP, age < 55} = 150

5. {High BP, age $\geq$ 55} = 20%; {High BP, age < 55} = 30%; {Normal BP, age $\geq$ 55} = 25%; {Normal BP, age < 55} = 25%

6. Frequency matching because it should be logistically easier and less costly to find groups of control subjects, particularly by hospital than to find controls one case at a time.

7. Individual matching because there are many variables to match on, many of which are quite individualized.

Q15.3

1. 30 cases and 60 controls
2. 70 cases and 140 controls
3. R_i to S_i, since R_1 = 60, S_1 = 30, and R_2 = 140, S_2 = 70
4. Four
5. R_i to S_i matching ratio. Even though there are twice as many controls overall as there are cases, the numbers of cases and controls vary within each stratum.
6. White Male: R = 200, S = 100; White Female: R = 200, S = 100; Black Male: R = 80, S = 40; Black Female: R = 120, S = 60.

Q15.4

1. For a fixed number of index subjects, total sample size for the study increases as R increases
2. There is a 33% increase in going from R = 1 to R = 2. This indicates that there is considerable precision to be gained by using 2 to 1 matching instead of 1 to 1 matching.

Q15.5

1. False – in a case-control study, the index group is composed of cases.
2. False – in a cohort group, the comparison group is composed of unexposed individuals.
3. False – The control of a given case in this situation would need to be the same regarding both matching factors.
4. True
5. True – Five to one matching will result in an increase in precision of 4.2% compared to four to one matching.
6. True
7. True
8. False – Choosing 2 controls per case

versus 1 per case will increase precision by 33%. This increase in precision will continue with each added control per case. However, the table of Pittman Efficiency, values computed for different values of R (number of controls per case) indicates a diminishing return regarding efficiency once R exceeds 4.

Q15.6

1. No, hair color has no known relationship to bladder cancer.
2. Because hair color has no known relationship to bladder cancer, and is not a risk factor needing to be controlled, matching on hair color is unlikely to have any effect on the precision of the estimated exposure-disease effect, i.e., even though matching on hair color will make cases and controls "balanced" with respect to hair color, the estimated effect is unlikely to be more precise than would result from "unbalanced" data obtained from not matching.
3. Fast-food products tend to be high in saturated fats, so if you match on amount of fast-food products in one's diet, you may effectively be matching on cholesterol level.
4. You will have difficulty finding matches for some index subjects and are likely to obtain a smaller sample size than originally planned.

Q15.7

1. There is no strong reason for matching, and the reasons against outweigh the reasons for.
2. You might expect to gain precision from matching, but you also need to weigh the other reasons listed, particularly the cost in time and money to carry out the matching.
3. Again, your decision depends on how you weight all the reasons for and against matching. Matching on neighborhood of residence may be a convenient way to control for social and environmental factors that are difficult to measure. However, if the exposure variable has a behavioral component, you must be careful that you won't overmatch in this situation.

Q15.8

1. False – one reason for deciding to match in a case-control study is to obtain a more precise estimate of the odds ratio of interest.
2. False – a reduction in the sample size due to not finding an appropriate match would be a disadvantage of matching.
3. True
4. a, d, and e
5. False – you still need to be concerning about matching on weak risk factors and overmatching.
6. It depends – it depends on at what cost you gain the precision. It is important to consider other things such as cost, money, time, how strong or weak are the risk factors, overmatching, etc.

Q15.9

1. Logit $P(X) = b_0 + b_1(D1) + b_2(D2) + \ldots + b_{99}(D99) + b_{100}(E)$ where D1 through D99 are 99 dummy variables that distinguish the 100 matched pairs. In particular, the Di may be defined as follows: Di=1 for a subject in the i-th matched pair and Di = 0 for a subject not in the i-th matched pair. Thus, for each of the two subjects in the first matched pair, D1 = 1, D2 = D3 =…= D99 = 0 and for each subject in the 100-th matched pair, D1 = D2 =…D99 = 0.
2. Logit $P(X) = b_0 + b_1(D1) + b_2(D2) + \ldots + b_{99}(D99) + b_{100}(SBP) + b_{101}(CHL) + b_{102}(E)$ where D1 through D99 are 99 dummy variables that distinguish the 100 matched pairs.
3. Any matched pair in which the case is in a different SBP or CHL category than is the corresponding control will have to be dropped from such a stratified analysis. The only matched pairs to be kept for analysis will be those in which both the case and control are in the same SBP and CHL categories.

Q15.10

1. All strata have zero cells, so it is not possible to compute stratum-specific odds ratios.

Q15.11

1. The mOR estimate of 9.67 indicates a very strong relationship between estrogen usage and endometrial cancer, controlling for the matching variables. The MH test has a P-value equal to zero to four decimal places. Therefore, the point estimate is highly significant. The 95% CI is quite wide, so there is considerable imprecision in the point estimate. Overall, however, the results suggest a strong effect of estrogen use on the development of endometrial cancer.

Index

Printed in the United States of America